Cardiovascular Nuclear Medicine and MRI

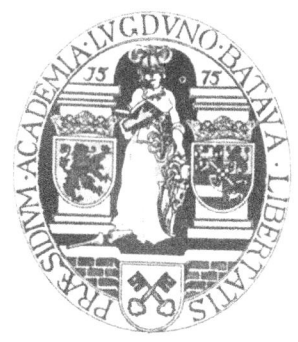

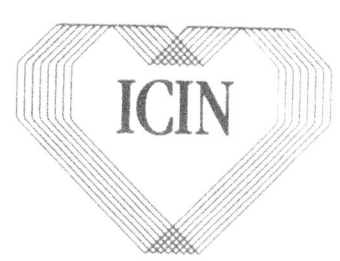

Developments in
Cardiovascular Medicine

VOLUME 128

The titles published in this series are listed at the end of this volume.

Cardiovascular Nuclear Medicine and MRI

Quantitation and Clinical Applications

edited by

JOHAN H.C. REIBER
Department of Diagnostic Radiology and Nuclear Medicine,
University Hospital Leiden, Leiden, The Netherlands

and

ERNST E. VAN DER WALL
Department of Cardiology,
University Hospital Leiden, Leiden, The Netherlands

SPRINGER SCIENCE+BUSINESS MEDIA, B.V.

Library of Congress Cataloging-in-Publication Data

Cardiovascular nuclear medicine and MRI : quantitation and clinical
  applications / edited by Johan H.C. Reiber and Ernst E. van der
  Wall.
        p.   cm. -- (Developments in cardiovascular medicine ; v. 128)
  Based on a meeting of the Working Group on Nuclear Cardiology,
which was held Mar. 22-23, 1991 under the auspices of the European
Society of Cardiology and the Interuniversity Cardiology Institute
of the Netherlands, and on the Second International Symposium on
Computer Applications in Nuclear Medicine and Cardiac Magnetic
Resonance Imaging, which was held Mar. 20-22, 1991 in Rotterdam, the
Netherlands.
    Includes index.
    ISBN 978-0-7923-1467-7   ISBN 978-94-011-2666-3 (eBook)
    DOI 10.1007/978-94-011-2666-3
    1. Heart--Radionuclide imaging--Congresses. 2. Heart--Magnetic
resonance imaging--Congresses. 3. Heart--Tomography--Congresses.
I. Reiber, J. H. C. (Johan H. C.) II. Wall, E. van der.
III. Working Group on Nuclear Cardiology. IV. European Society of
Cardiology. V. Interuniversitair Cardiologisch Instituut (Utrecht,
Netherlands) VI. International Symposium on Computer Applications
in Nuclear Medicine and Cardiac Magnetic Resonance Imaging (2nd :
1991 : Rotterdam, Netherlands) VII. Series.
    [DNLM: 1. Cardiovascular Diseases--diagnosis--congresses.
2. Cardiovascular Diseases--radionuclide imaging--congresses.
3. Magnetic Resonance Imaging--congresses. 4. Tomography, Emission
-Computed, Single-Photon--congresses.   W1 DE997VME v.128 / WG 141
C2697 1991]
RC683.5.I42C38 1992
DNLM/DLC
for Library of Congress   91-35321

ISBN 978-0-7923-1467-7

This publication has also been made possible by support of Hoechst Pharma Cardiovasculars and Du Pont Pharmaceuticals.

Contents

Foreword

In recent years there have been major advances in the fields of cardiovascular nuclear medicine and cardiac magnetic resonance imaging. In Nuclear cardiology more adequate tomographic systems have been designed for routine cardiac use, as well as new or improved quantitative analytic software packages both for planar and tomographic studies implemented on modern state-of-the-art workstations. In addition, artificial intelligence techniques are being applied to these images in attempts to interpret the nuclear studies in more objective and reproducible manners. Various new radiotracers have been developed such as antimyosin, labeled isonitriles, metabolic compounds, etc. Furthermore, alternative stress testing with dipyridamole and dobutamine has received much attention in clinical cardiac practice. Magnetic resonance imaging is a relative newcomer in cardiology and has already shown its merits, not only for anatomic information but more and more for the functional aspects of cardiac performance.

Previous to the annual meetings of the European Society of Cardiology (ESC), which started in Vienna 1988, separate meetings had been organized by the Working Group on Nuclear Cardiology, the first meeting being in Tours 1978, followed by several other successful symposia (Vienna 1982, Rotterdam 1983, Edinburgh 1987). These meetings were quite intimate and reunited a number of experts in a given field, enhancing the flow and exchange of information. At the ESC meeting in Nice 1989, it was decided by the Working Group on Nuclear Cardiology to continue the organization of its own meetings of the Working Group on a biennial basis. As a result, the first biennial meeting of the Working Group on Nuclear Cardiology was organized in 1991, March 22–23.

The meeting was held under the auspices of the ESC and the Interuniversity Cardiology Institute of the Netherlands (ICIN).

This first biennial meeting has highlighted the substantial progress in the cardiac nuclear techniques with major emphasis on clinical applications. The clinical aspect was underscored, particularly since the meeting was directly preceded by the Second International Symposium on Computer Applications in Nuclear Medicine and Cardiac Magnetic Resonance Imaging which was held on March 20–22, 1991. In the preceding meeting the computer aspects were discussed with specific emphasis on three-dimensional (3–D)-reconstruction and filtering methods, quantitation, quality control, artificial intelligence applications, 3D-displays, workstations, multi-modality imaging and image compression techniques in nuclear medicine in general and cardiovascular imaging in particular. This joint venture of both meetings proved very advantageous as it also attracted many physicists, programmers, image processing specialists, and technicians active in these fields. Therefore, this 'coincidence' provided a larger forum for the advance of cardiovascular nuclear medicine and cardiac magnetic resonance imaging.

During both meetings, excellent tutorials have been presented by invited experts from Europe and the United States. This book consists of a compilation of manuscripts based on the presentations of all tutorial speakers. It is a perfect representation of both symposia, covering almost every aspect of cardiovascular nuclear medicine and cardiac magnetic resonance imaging. The book is intended to assist the nuclear medicine physician, the radiologist, the physicist/image processing specialist, and the clinical cardiologist in understanding the nuclear medicine techniques, particularly those used in cardiovascular medicine, and in increasing the knowledge of cardiac magnetic resonance imaging.

We thank the contributors for making every effort in providing superb state-of-the-art chapters, and we hope that this book will be a valuable contribution to the progress in noninvasive imaging of human heart disease.

August 1991   JOHAN H.C. REIBER
                                                  ERNST E. VAN DER WALL

List of contributors

JOSEPH AREEDA, M.D.
Cedars Sinai Medical Center, Department of Nuclear Medicine, Box 48750,
Los Angeles, CA 90048–0750, USA

FRANK-MICHAEL BAER, M.D.
III Clinic Internal Medicine, University of Cologne, Joseph-Stelzl-Mannstr.
9, D-5000 Köln, Germany

GEORGE A. BELLER, M.D.
Division of Cardiology, Department of Medicine, University of Virginia
Health Sciences Center, Box 158, Charlottesville, VA 22908, USA

DANIEL S. BERMAN, M.D.
Department of Nuclear Medicine, Cedars Sinai Medical Center, Box 48750,
Los Angeles, CA 90048–0750, USA

JAKOBUS A.K. BLOKLAND, Ph.D.
Department of Nuclear Medicine, University Hospital Leiden, Building 1,
C4–Q, Rijnsburgerweg 10, 2333 AA Leiden, The Netherlands

SIMON H. BRAAT, M.D.
Department of Cardiology, Academic Hospital Maastricht, P.O. Box 5800,
6202 AZ Maastricht, The Netherlands

EMMA C.M.L. BRACEY
Division of Radiological Sciences, Guy's Hospital, London Bridge, London
SE1 9RT, United Kingdom

ALBERT V.G. BRUSCHKE, M.D.
Department of Cardiology, University Hospital Leiden, Building 1, C5–P31,
Rijnsburgerweg 10, 2333 AA Leiden, The Netherlands

C. DAVID COOKE, M.S.E.E.
Department of Radiology, Emory University School of Medicine, 1364 Clifton Road NE, Atlanta, GA 30322, USA

JAMES R. CORBETT, M.D.
Department of Radiology, University of Texas, Southwestern Medical Center at Dallas, 5323 Harry Hines Blvd, Dallas, TX 75235–9058, USA

E. GORDON DEPUEY, M.D.
Department of Radiology, Emory University School of Medicine, 1364 Clifton Road NE, Atlanta, GA 30322, USA

JOOST DOORNBOS, Ph.D.
Department of Radiology, University Hospital Leiden, Building 1, C2–S, Rijnsburgerweg 10, 2333 AA Leiden, The Netherlands

PAUL R.M. VAN DIJKMAN, M.D.
Department of Cardiology, University Hospital Leiden, Building 1, C5–P25, Rijnsburgerweg 10, 2333 AA Leiden, The Netherlands

DUNCAN S. DYMOND, M.D.
Department of Cardiology, St. Bartholomew's Hospital, London EC1A 7BE, United Kingdom

HERMANN EICHSTAEDT, M.D., Ph.D.
Department of Cardiology, University Clinic Rudolf Virchow, Free University of Berlin, Spandauer Damm 130, 1000 Berlin 19, Germany

NORBERTO F. EZQUERRA, Ph.D.
Department of Radiology, Emory University School of Medicine, 1364 Clifton Road NE, Atlanta, GA 30322, USA

TRACY L. FABER, Ph.D.
Department of Radiology, University of Texas, Southwestern Medical Center at Dallas, 5323 Harry Hines Blvd., Dallas, TX 75235–9058, USA

RUSSELL D. FOLKS, B.Sc.
Department of Radiology, Emory University School of Medicine, 1364 Clifton Road NE, Atlanta, GA 30322, USA

JOHN FRIEDMAN, M.D.
Department of Nuclear Medicine, Cedars Sinai Medical Center, Box 48750, Los Angeles, CA 90048–0750, USA

ERNEST V. GARCIA, Ph.D.
Department of Radiology, Emory University School of Medicine, 1364 Clifton Road NE, Atlanta, GA 30322, USA

L. STEPHEN GRAHAM, Ph.D.
Department of Nuclear Medicine, VA Medical Center, 16111 Plummer Street, Sepulveda, CA 91343, USA

DAVID J. HAWKES, M.D.
Division of Radiological Sciences, Guy's Hospital, London Bridge, London SE1 9RT, United Kingdom

JAEKYEONG HEO, M.D.
Noninvasive Cardiac Imaging, Philadelphia Heart Institute, Presbyterian Medical Center of Philadelphia, 39th & Market Streets, Philadelphia, PA 19104, USA

KITHSIRI B. HERATH
Department of Nuclear Medicine, VA Medical Center, 16111 Plummer Street, Sepulveda, CA 91343, USA

MARK D. HERBST, M.D., Ph.D.
Department of Radiology, Emory University School of Medicine, 1364 Clifton Road NE, Atlanta, GA 30322, USA

DEREK L.G. HILL
Division of Radiological Sciences, Guy's Hospital, London Bridge, London SE1 9RT, United Kingdom

ABDULMASSIH S. ISKANDRIAN, M.D.
Noninvasive Cardiac Imaging, Philadelphia Heart Institute, Presbyterian Medical Center of Philadelphia, 39th & Market Streets, Philadelphia, PA 19104, USA

HOSEN KIAT, M.D.
Department of Nuclear Medicine, Cedars Sinai Medical Center, Box 48750, Los Angeles, CA 90048–0750, USA

MICHAEL A. KING, Ph.D.
Department of Nuclear Medicine, University of Massachusetts Medical Center, 55 Lake Avenue North, Worcester, MA 01655, USA

RICHARD LIM
Department of Cardiology, St. Bartholomew's Hospital, London EC1A 7BE, United Kingdom

DAVID T. LONG, B.S.E.E.
Department of Nuclear Medicine, University of Massachusetts Medical Center, 55 Lake Avenue North, Worcester, MA 01655, USA

JAMSHID MADDAHI, M.D.
Division of Nuclear Medicine and Biophysics, Department of Radiological Sciences, UCLA School of Medicine, CHS 17215, Los Angeles, CA 90024, USA

PIOTR MANIAWSKI, M.Sc.
Department of Cardiology, Nuclear Medicine, Yale University School of Medicine, 333 Cedar Street, New Haven, CT 06520, USA

NIELS A.A. MATHEIJSSEN, M.A.
Department of Radiology, University Hospital Leiden, Building 1, C2–S, Rijnsburgerweg 10, 2333 AA Leiden, The Netherlands

JUDY NEGRETE
Department of Nuclear Medicine, VA Medical Center, 16111 Plummer Street, Sepulveda, CA 91343, USA

MENCO G. NIEMEYER, M.D.
Department of Nuclear Medicine, University Hospital Leiden, Building 1, C4–Q, Rijnsburgerweg 10, 2333 AA Leiden, The Netherlands

RODERIC I. PETTIGREW, Ph.D.
Department of Radiology, Emory University School of Medicine, 1364 Clifton Road NE, Atlanta, GA 30322, USA

ERNEST K.J. PAUWELS, Ph.D.
Department of Nuclear Medicine, University Hospital Leiden, Building 1, C4–Q, Rijnsburgerweg 10, 2333 AA Leiden, The Netherlands

PIERRE RIGO, M.D.
Department of Cardiology, Academic Hospital Maastricht, P.O. Box 5800, 6202 AZ Maastricht, The Netherlands

PAUL ROOS
Department of Applied Mathematics, Delft University of Technology, P.O. Box 5031, 2600 GA Delft, The Netherlands

ALBERT DE ROOS, M.D.
Department of Radiology, University Hospital Leiden, Building 1, C2–S, Rijnsburgerweg 10, 2333 AA Leiden, The Netherlands

F. PAUL VAN RUGGE, M.D.
Department of Radiology, University Hospital Leiden, Building 1, C2–S, Rijnsburgerweg 10, 2333 AA Leiden, The Netherlands

HARALD SCHICHA, M.D.
Department of Nuclear Medicine, University of Cologne, Joseph-Stelzl-Mannstr. 9, D-5000 Köln, Germany

UDO SECHTEM, M.D.
III Clinic Internal Medicine, University of Cologne, Joseph-Stelzl-Mannstr. 9, D-5000 Köln, Germany

PETER THEISSEN, M.D.
Department of Nuclear Medicine, University of Cologne, Joseph-Stelzl-Mannstr. 9, D-5000 Köln, Germany

KENNETH VAN TRAIN, M.Sc.
Department of Nuclear Medicine, Cedars Sinai Medical Center, Box 48750, Los Angeles, CA 90048–0750, USA

BENJAMIN M.W. TSUI, Ph.D.
Department of Radiology and Department of Biomedical Engineering, The University of North Carolina at Chapel Hill, Campus Box 7575, 152 MacNider Hall, Chapel Hill, NC 27599–7575, USA

RICHARD M.A. UNDERWOOD, M.D.
Royal Brompton National Heart and Lung Hospitals, Dovehouse Street, London SW3 6LY, United Kingdom

MAX A. VIERGEVER, Ph.D.
Department of Radiology and Nuclear Medicine, University Hospital Utrecht, E02.222, Heidelberglaan 100, 3584 CX Utrecht, The Netherlands

FRANS J.Th. WACKERS
Department of Cardiology, Nuclear Medicine, Yale University School of Medicine, 333 Cedar Street, New Haven, CT 06520, USA

ERNST E. VAN DER WALL, M.D.
Department of Cardiology, University Hospital Leiden, Building 1, C5–P25, Rijnsburgerweg 10, 2333 AA Leiden, The Netherlands

JEROLD W. WALLIS, M.D.
Mallinckrodt Institute of Radiology, Washington University School of Medicine, St. Louis, MO 63110, USA

HEIN J.J. WELLENS, M.D.
Department of Cardiology, Academic Hospital Maastricht, P.O. Box 5800, 6202 AZ Maastricht, The Netherlands

1. Cardiovascular imaging in the nineties

HERMANN EICHSTAEDT

Summary

The boundaries for the future of cardiac imaging and image processing have been enumerated with great ambitions, but the attainment of those goals will require a unique approach to further investigations. To reach these goals, the future approach should focus on the biological and technical problems that remain to be solved before complete characterization of cardiac structure, function, perfusion, and metabolism by imaging techniques will become a reality. These goals can only be met by interdisciplinary teams of investigators, representing expertise in the divergent areas of physics, electrical and computer engineering, physiology, biochemistry, computer science and the clinicians in cardiology, radiology, and nuclear medicine. The successful attainment of our shared objectives depends on a close interaction among the several academic disciplines cited, including collaboration with industrial research and development laboratories.

The achievements of coordinate cardiac imaging research to date are extraordinary and suggest that the application of quantitative analytical techniques to cardiovascular images will continue to yield impressive and meaningful results which should increase our knowledge of the cardiovascular system and the subjective utility for our patients.

1. Introduction

Prodigious breakthrough in cardiovascular imaging has occurred in the past two decades. As evidenced by the other chapters in this volume, the cardiovascular researcher and the clinician caring for patients with cardiac disease dispose of a widely divergent set of tools to evaluate many aspects of cardiac structure and function. To facilitate a broad overview of the several currently available imaging modalities, their current contribution to cardiovascular science and various aspects of the future of cardiac imaging and image processing, several important goals of cardiac imaging have to be defined. By examining these goals and by determining how near we are to their

Johan H.C. Reiber & Ernst E. van der Wall (eds.), Cardiovascular Nuclear Medicine and MRI, 1–26.
© 1992 *Kluwer Academic Publishers.*

Table 1. Objectives of cardiovascular imaging

Anatomy of chambers, walls, valves, great vessels
Size
Shape
Relationships (congenital disease)
Function
Systolic
Diastolic
Valvular
Myocardial metabolism
Macro- and microperfusion
Tissue characterization
Injury
Scar
Neoplasm
Thrombus
Infiltration
Cardiomyopathy

attainment, we may conjecture about likely directions for future cardiac imaging.

The ideal ambitions of clinical cardiac imaging include the complete structural, functional, and metabolic characterization of the heart, great vessels, and the pulmonary vasculature in a noninvasive manner (Table 1). To achieve these goals the following requirements are needed: 1) the depiction of cardiac morphology (chambers, walls, great vessels, valves, and the anatomy of the coronary arteries); 2) the delineation of systolic and diastolic chamber and valvular function; 3) the assessment of myocardial metabolism and perfusion; and 4) the characterization of myocardial structure, so-called tissue characterization.

At present, cardiac morphology and function can quite well be assessed using a variety of conventional techniques (Table 2). Twenty-five years ago, the only clinically useful approach to examining cardiac chamber morphology and function involved angiographic procedures that required direct injection of contrast media into the heart during cardiac catheterization. Currently, diagnostic information of this type can often be obtained with less invasive procedures such as echocardiography and conventional radionuclide imaging. Recent research and clinical practice have shown that digital angiography with an intravenous contrast injection, cine-computed tomography, and magnetic resonance imaging are able to provide quantitative information on cardiac morphology on a routine basis. These procedures may gradually replace conventional angiography for the purpose of assessing left ventricular ejection fraction, right ventricular ejection fraction, quantification and local-

Table 2. Established methods and methods under development of cardiac imaging

	Anatomy	Function	Metabolism	Perfusion	Tissue-characterization
Established methods					
X-ray	+	+	–	–	–
ultrasound	+ +	+ + +	–	(contrast)	+
isotopes	+	+ + +	+ +	+ + +	+
angiography	+ +	+ + +	–	+	–
Methods under development					
Color-Doppler	+ + +	+ + +	–	(contrast)	+
PET	+	+	+ + +	+ + +	–
SPECT	+	+	+ +	+ + +	+
DA	+ +	+ +	–	+ + +	+ +
CT (Cine)	+ + +	+ + +	–	+ + +	+ +
MR (I + S)	+ + +	+ + +	+ +	+	+ + +

PET: Positron Emission Tomography; SPECT: Single-Photon Emission Computed Tomography; DA: Digital Angiography; CT: transmission Computed Tomography; MR: Magnetic Resonance, I: Imaging; S: Spectroscopy.

ization of intracardiac shunts, and assessment of right and left ventricular mass.

As indicated in Table 2, we are still far from attaining the goals of measuring metabolism and of characterizing myocardial tissue. Using selective angiography, we can delineate coronary anatomy. To date, noninvasive approaches to the depiction of coronary anatomy have not been successful. Furthermore, the standard approach to assessing the severity of coronary stenoses – estimation of percent diameter narrowing of the stenotic segment compared to a presumably normal segment – does not correlate with the physiological significance of the obstruction [1]. Therefore, estimation of percent diameter stenosis from standard coronary cine-angiograms is not the optimal independent standard against which to judge newer modalities.

Based on these considerations, investigative efforts in cardiac imaging and image processing will focus to an increasing degree upon three major purposes: 1) anatomic and metabolic characterization of myocardium, 2) assessment of regional myocardial perfusion, and 3) the noninvasive definition of coronary arterial anatomy. I would like to discuss each of these major objectives, along with the imaging modalities likely to result in attainment of these intentions.

2. Characterization of myocardial tissue

The majority of conventional cardiac imaging procedures visualize either the silhouette of the cavities (angiography, radionuclide techniques) or the anatomical position of the subendocardium and subepicardium (echocardiography). Definition of the characteristics of the tissues comprising the walls of the cardiac chambers is either achieved with these methods in a limited fashion or not at all. Magnetic resonance imaging has filled up this space in the last ten years.

Coronary artery disease, the most common heart disease in the civilized world, has major effects on the tissue of the left ventricular wall. Coronary artery disease can result in regional infarction, left ventricular aneurysm, and multifocal cardiac necrosis [2]. Other important cardiac diseases, such as cardiomyopathies and congenital defects, also alter the composition of tissue in the ventricular walls. The effects of these important clinical entities on the composition of the ventricular wall cannot be defined quantitatively with echocardiography and radionuclide methods, but tissue characterization is becoming a realistic measure with magnetic resonance imaging and spectroscopy.

Most likely, one specific and particularly critical need with respect to tissue characterization is to quantitate the size of myocardial infarction.

2.1. *Extent of myocardial infarction*

Of decisive importance to the individual is the size of a region of necrotic myocardium. The mass of necrotic myocardium, expressed as a percentage of the entire left ventricle, has a major impact on the patient's prognosis, since cardiac functional impairment [3–6] and electrical instability [7,8] correlate closely with infarct size. The major clinical need and use for measurements of infarct size in living humans is to estimate the impact of interventions on the mass of infarcted myocardium. The ideal method would enable us to obtain an early predicted infarct size and then to compare it 2 to 4 weeks later with a final observed infarct size. If these measurements are made in a control group of patients to show a good prediction of final infarct size by a measurement obtained early, this group of patients can be compared with a second group treated by interventional therapy applied between measurements to learn whether final observed infarct size was indeed less than the infarct size that would have been predicted from the early measurement. This type of methodology is sorely needed to evaluate drugs, thrombolytic therapy, coronary angioplasty and coronary bypass graft surgery, and other potential means used for reducing infarct size in humans. For human studies during acute myocardial infarction, such a measurement has to be safe and rapid in order to avoid interference with the care of these mostly ill patients.

The most factual way to measure infarct size experimentally is by postmortem studies with or without dyes such as nitrophenyltetrazolium to stain intact mitochondria in the myocardium [8,9]. In regions with no functioning mitochondria, there will be an absence of stain, while in regions with functioning myocardium, there will be a clear uptake of the stain to distinguish the two regions. This is confirmed by histologic study of tissue under the microscope to confirm that stained regions are normal and that unstained regions are necrotic. Using this technique, it has been possible to perform experiments in animals to assess the effects of different interventions on infarct size.

An auxiliary way to assess infarct size in animals has been to measure the content of the creatine kinase enzyme in the tissue [10,11]. This enzyme is normally present in tissue to catalyze the transfer of high-energy phosphate bonds. Since the large enzyme molecule leaks out when the cell membrane is irreversibly injured, the concentration of creatine kinase in the myocardial sample is a good indicator of its viability [9–11].

In humans the methods available to estimate infarct size are limited. The electrocardiogram is the oldest and most widely used method. The electrocardiographic pattern of acute myocardial infarction (ST-elevation, T-wave inversion, and Q-waves) allows the qualitative detection of transmural infarcts fairly reliably [12]. The problem occurs when trying to quantitate the amount of myocardium infarcted. This has been estimated by maps of ST-elevation at multiple sites over the precordium or Q-waves over the precordium for anterior infarcts, but the methods do not work at all for inferior infarcts [13]. Furthermore, there have been several challenges to the validity of electrocardiographic mapping to quantitate the mass of infarcted myocardium [14]. In general, it appears that electrocardiographic methods do not offer enough to be useful for quantitative clinical investigation.

A more indirect approach is required clinically, which involves measuring the amount of creatine kinase released into the venous blood from the necrotic myocardium. Based on this measurement, one is able to reconstruct the total amount of creatine kinase washed out by performing frequent sampling at different times [11]. Another method to identify infarcted myocardium includes the pyrophosphate staining of calcium around the border of an infarct [15]. Yet another approach, devised by Khaw et al. [16], is to use an antibody to the myocardial contractile protein myosin. Normally, myosin is covered by its intact cell membrane and would not be available for binding by an antibody. If the cell membrane is irreversibly damaged and is leaking, the antibody molecule can enter the cell and be detected if the antibody is labeled [16–19]. These techniques have been used clinically in the last ten years to allow the detection of regions of the heart that appear to be necrotic.

Impaired tissue perfusion represented by a thallium-201 perfusion defect of a certain degree of severity offers one approach that is at least measurable in vivo. Silverman et al. [20] showed that a semiquantitatively estimated defect on the thallium-201 scintigram performed during the early phase of acute myocardial infarction predicts the patient's ultimate prognosis with a fair degree of reliability. In the seventies, technetium-99m pyrophosphate hot-spot imaging has been more difficult to quantitate, but the tomographic methods nowadays may make this approach more useful. Technetium-99m SestaMIBI studies have also been obtained after myocardial infarction [21].

Magnetic resonance tomography has been shown a useful method for imaging acute myocardial infarction, when the relaxation substance or contrast agent gadolinium-DTPA was used. Although this might be a promising scientific method, the clinical use has yet to be settled [22–26].

The more unfailing way to estimate infarct size is to appraise its impact on left ventricular function. It has been known that simply the presence of acute shortness of breath with a myocardial infarction is a bad prognostic sign; this was taken advantage of in a clinical classification of infarct severity based on symptoms and signs [27]. In addition, the presence of rales and gallops on physical exam and of interstitial pulmonary edema on chest radiography are other markers of a fairly large infarct causing congestive heart failure. More sophisticated measurements also confirm the same trends more reliably. Measurement of pulmonary capillary wedge pressure by the Swan-Ganz catheter and cardiac output by the thermodilution technique has been performed extensively in the coronary care unit and shown to characterize patients with different severities of myocardial infarction and different prognoses [3,4]. Indeed, there is a correlation between the elevation of pulmonary capillary wedge pressure and the amount of creatine kinase enzyme released to the blood [4]. In addition, both indexes appear to correlate with other estimates of impaired global or regional left ventricular function 1 month after acute myocardial infarction [28]. For example, left ventricular ejection fraction in radionuclide ventriculography shows a rough correlation with infarct size experimentally and with prognosis in humans. However, the ejection fraction that correlates with infarct size must be measured 2 weeks to 2 months after an infarct at a time when the infarcted tissue is clearly separate from ischemic or stunned myocardium [5,29]. This stunned myocardium can produce more severe initial reduction of left ventricular function than will result from the final infarct.

The estimation of regional function in a quantitative way is even more unequivocal to assess infarct size. This can be expressed either as a perimeter of the left ventricular outline on contrast angiography that does not contract well [28] or as the area of poorly contracting left ventricle on a radionuclide ventriculography [30]. Several measurements of this type have been shown to correlate roughly with infarct size in animals and with the cruder measurements available in humans.

Electrophysiologic variables such as the ease of producing arrhythmias by programmed electrical stimulation have also been shown to correlate with the mass of myocardium that is infarcted experimentally. In studies in dogs, a close linear correlation ($r = 0.92$) has been found between infarct size measured by tetrazolium and histology versus a quantitative index of electrical instability measured during programmed electrical stimulation 4 days after acute myocardial infarction in the dog [8]. Califf et al. [31] found that the frequency and type of ventricular premature beats measured on Holter electrocardiographic monitoring correlated roughly with the regional abnormalities of contraction measured on contrast angiograms a few weeks after infarction. Finally, the presence and quantitative importance of infarction can approximately be assessed by imaging with indium-111 antimyosin [16–18]. After acute myocardial infarction, it is necessary to apply several of these physiologic principles of the patient for follow-up evaluation of the patient [32]. In general, the patient's prognosis is determined by the amount of irreversible myocardial damage and by the amount of myocardium that becomes reversibly ischemic during stress.

2.2. *Area at risk*

Complementary to the importance of infarct size in determining clinical outcome after infarction, the so-called "risk area" (the volume of myocardium supplied by the stenotic or occluded artery) is another critical determinant of the consequences of coronary occlusion [33]. Many studies aimed at limiting infarct size have not taken into account the risk area of individual coronary arteries. Since risk area is a potent predictor of infarct size after coronary occlusion, and since risk areas of the same coronary artery differ widely from subject to subject, the definition of risk area is an important additional goal.

A number of new techniques hold promise in providing important information concerning the anatomic and metabolic characteristics of myocardial tissue. Quantitative echocardiography including transesophageal technique and echocontrast has been shown capable of identifying acute ischemia [34,35], infarction [36,37], and myocardial contusion [38], and may achieve similar results in other disorders. However, because of the nonstandard instrumentation used in most of the previous research, and due to a host of biological and technical problems, ultrasound tissue characterization is still an investigative technique.

Magnetic resonance imaging has contributed with interesting data to characterize infarcted tissue [39,40]. It is safe to predict that magnetic resonance contrast agents like gadolinium-DTPA provide further tissue characterization utilizing gated imaging techniques. To maximize myocardial localization of such contrast agents and to reduce toxic systemic side effects, magnetic resonance contrast agents that localize in the myocardium could be injected directly into the heart during coronary angiography for later magnetic resonance imaging. Tissue characteristics that appear to be definable by magnetic resonance imaging techniques include acute ischemia, infarction, and fibrosis. Magnetic resonance contrast agents linked to monoclonal antibodies specific for ventricular myosin are in the experimental stage. This might also be of use in transplant rejection [41].

With radionuclide techniques infarct sizing is likely to be considerably improved by the application of methods utilizing single photon emission computed tomography (SPECT). Results of SPECT imaging techniques utilizing intravenously injected thallium-201 and technetium-99m pyrophosphate indicate considerable progress in accurately defining infarct size [42,43]. Furthermore, SPECT imaging has been applied to quantify infarct size with considerable success using iodine-131 or indium-111 labeled monoclonal antibodies to ventricular myosin heavy chain [44].

Comparable progress in infarct sizing has been reported with the use of positron emission tomography, utilizing new tracers as rubidium-82 [45]. The success of the strontium-82/rubidium-82 generator is likely to spark the commercial development of other specialized generators that produce positron emitters as well as the development of minicyclotrons that produce short-lived tracers such as carbon-11, nitrogen-15, and oxygen-15. The final result might be the design and manufacture of less expensive imaging systems that would allow broader utilization of positron techniques and would markedly expand the role of radionuclide methods in cardiac imaging [46,47]. Myocardial metabolic activities can also be measured with positron imaging techniques, including myocardial oxygen utilization, fatty acid metabolism, glucose utilization, and other aspects of myocardial metabolism.

Cine-computed tomography with contrast enhancement also appears capable of defining regional deficits in myocardial perfusion, which likely are predictive of infarct size [48].

The evaluation of coronary risk area has been accomplished using a variety of techniques that will be clinically applicable to a variable degree. These methods of analysis of risk area include the assessment of regional wall motion [49], the use of radioactive microspheres injected into the coronary arteries [50], contrast echocardiography [51], and contrast enhanced cine-computed tomography.

3. Regional myocardial perfusion

Calculation of myocardial perfusion in humans continues to be remarkably crude. Although it is now possible to measure total flow to most or all of the left ventricle, using techniques such as thermodilution and gas clearance methods, available techniques for assessing regional perfusion have been limited to qualitative or semiquantitative determinations of thallium-201 distribution or xenon-133 clearance in the myocardium. Efforts to assess the transmural distribution of myocardial perfusion in humans have thus far been uniformly unsuccessful.

The assessment of regional and transmural myocardial perfusion in a quantitative pattern is greatly needed to characterize the regulation of the coronary circulation in humans. The dominant heart disease of our time, coronary artery disease, frequently manifests itself by regional perfusion abnormalities that primarily involve the subendocardial layers of the left ventricle. The inability to measure differentially the perfusion in the inner and outer layers of the left ventricular wall will continue to limit the diagnostic value and applicability of various imaging approaches for diagnosing and determining the severity of abnormalities in coronary perfusion due to coronary atherosclerosis. In addition, the inability to measure regional myocardial perfusion accurately makes it virtually impossible to determine the relative importance of the coronary collateral circulation in patients with obstructive coronary disease.

Presently obtainable approaches to assess regional myocardial perfusion in humans are limited to radionuclide techniques. Although exercise planar thallium-201 imaging has had moderate success in the diagnosis of coronary artery disease, it is far too imprecise to define blood flow changes reliably in the territories of the individual coronary vessels for the purposes of studying the regulation of myocardial blood flow [52,53]. The recent development of quantitative computer techniques, especially when combined with the use of SPECT systems, promises significant improvement in the determination of regional myocardial blood flow by thallium-201 scintigraphy [54–57]. The rapid improvement of the emission tomography techniques and the high probability for the development of better myocardial perfusion tracers (e.g. technetium-99m labeled agents) are likely to result in much more accurate assessment of regional myocardial perfusion during stress, rest, and pharmacologic intervention [58–60].

The bulging improvements and increasing utilization of positron emission tomography should also result in a more accurate technique for defining regional myocardial perfusion, which could be favourably combined with parallel determinations of myocardial metabolism. It is unlikely, however, that either positron or SPECT techniques will ever achieve the spatial resolution necessary to define perfusion differentially for inner and outer layers of the myocardial wall.

The potential to study contrast clearance curves from the myocardial wall has been demonstrated by cine-computed tomography [48]. Whether computed tomography is capable of achieving the resolution necessary for defining perfusion by analysis of clearance curves from the various layers of the myocardium is uncertain. The initial encouraging results and the intense current investigation using cine-computed tomographic techniques in a few institutions will likely lead to progress toward the goal of perfusion measurements.

Magnetic resonance imaging is another technique that promises to achieve the goal of myocardial perfusion determination. The nowadays available magnetic resonance imaging systems have excellent spatial and contrast resolution and the dependence of signal intensity on blood flow is well documented [61]. Measurement of regional magnetic resonance signal intensities or relaxation times after infusion of a paramagnetic contrast agent may prove to be a robust method of assessment of myocardial perfusion. One significant problem in the cardiac applications of magnetic resonance is the relatively long data acquisition time in most of the sequences and, thus, the need for electrocardiographic gating during data acquisition. Rapid acquisition in magnetic resonance imaging has been used for a few years now [62] and may prove to be a solution to this problem [63,64].

Besides measurement of myocardial perfusion under basal conditions, it is important to be able to assess maximal coronary dilator capacity. This is essential because abnormalities in coronary reserve (differences between basal and maximal coronary flow) are the hallmarks necessary to assess the physiological significance of individual coronary obstruction. Unfortunately, several techniques that can accurately measure resting myocardial blood flow (gas clearance, xenon-133 clearance, etc.) underestimate maximal coronary flow. Promising approaches to measuring coronary reserve with imaging techniques include positron emission tomography, fast-computed tomography, and digital angiography [65].

3.1. *Differentiation between ischemic and scar tissue*

Whether a region of myocardium is irreversibly infarcted, reversibly ischemic, or normal is absolutely crucial in deciding to perform interventions such as thrombolytic therapy, angioplasty, or coronary bypass graft surgery on patients early and late in the course of infarction. A very common reason that patients are sent for stress radionuclide studies is to distinguish irreversibly infarcted from reversibly ischemic myocardium. Although changes in the severity of a defect on thallium from early to delayed rest images have some value in this regard, they are not perfect arbiters of viability. Thirty to 40 percent of fixed defects that show no redistribution from exercise to delayed rest thallium imaging can disappear entirely after a successful coronary angioplasty [66] or coronary bypass graft surgery [67]. Therefore, late imaging with or without a second injection after 24 hr has been performed [68–69]. Some redistribution can certainly occur in the myocardium overlying an infarct and may cause overestimation of the amount of reversible tissue. Assessment of regional contraction at rest and exercise or with nitroglycerin, postextrasystolic potentiation [70], or catecholamines [71] may also be useful but these interventions are not sufficiently specific to solve this diagnostic dilemma.

Occlusion of a coronary artery induces experimental infarction in the endocardial third to half of the left ventricular wall thickness supplied by that artery [72]. There will still be surviving normal tissue in the outer two-thirds to one-half. Yet, because the artery is still totally occluded and collaterals may not be adequate, some ischemia may develop with stress in the middle third of the ventricular wall thickness between the infarct in the endocardium and normal tissue in the epicardium [72]. When performing which low-level exercise thallium-201 imaging studies 10 days after an acute myocardial infarction, reversible thallium-201 defects identify patients who are at high risk of future development of unstable angina, infarction, or sudden death. These results are encouraging because they suggest that thallium-201 imaging can, in this setting, distinguish infarct from ischemia or stunned myocardium. It is difficult to detect these fine gradations by the available techniques and the mixture of infarcted, ischemic, and normal tissue may not be differentiated accurately by current radionuclide methods [73].

3.2. *Ischemic myocardium*

The situation where blood flow cannot meet myocardial oxygen demands is defined as myocardial ischemia,, and this situation leads to the following abnormalities.

3.2.1. *Wall motion abnormalities*

In the region supplied by an occluded coronary artery abnormal contraction has first been demonstrated in the dog by Tennant and Wiggers in 1933 [74]. This developed within a minute of the occlusion. The finding was confirmed by contrast left ventriculography in humans with coronary artery disease in 1967 by Herman and Gorlin [75]. In addition, they pointed out that the larger and more severe regional contractile deficits led to impaired overall function of the left ventricle [76]. The cause of the early contractile failure of ischemic myocardium has not been determined with certainty but may be related to an accumulation of hydrogen ions which displace calcium from its binding sites on contractile proteins [77,78]. The earliest contractile defect does not depend on a depletion of tissue ATP, when the total concentration of ATP in heart muscle is considered [79].

The myocardium that is dependent on the stenotic coronary artery is affected primarily by this impairment of contraction. The ischemic zone shows impaired systolic wall inward motion on gated equilibrium or first-pass bloodpool scans [80], echocardiography, digital and analogue contrast ventriculography [81], dynamic cine-computed tomography, and dynamic magnetic resonance imaging. Corresponding changes in left ventricular regional systolic wall thickening can be seen on echocardiography, computed tomography or magnetic resonance imaging. The greater the abnormality of left ventricular regional function, the greater the impairment of left ventricular global function [76]. Global function can be assessed by any of the above methods as the left ventricular ejection fraction. Left ventricular ejection fraction is a major predictor of patient prognosis in coronary artery disease [14]. Global cardiac function can also be assessed by cardiac output and left ventricular filling pressures after insertion of appropriate intravascular catheters, such as Swan-Ganz balloon-tipped thermodilution catheter in the pulmonary artery [3,4]. Left ventricular global function can remain nearly normal despite impaired contraction of the ischemic zone because of a compensatory increase in contraction of nonischemic myocardium. Thus, measurement of regional contraction is more sensitive than measurement of global function to assess the effects of coronary artery disease on the heart [6]. In patients with coronary artery disease, regional contraction is often normal at rest but becomes abnormal during stress imposed by exercise or drugs that increase the work of the heart [71,82].

Particularly coronary artery disease also affects the diastolic function of the left ventricle, making it functionally stiffer. It appears that the diastolic function of the heart is influenced by native, ATP-dependent, and passive elastic properties of the myocardium [83]. Acute ischemia can impair ATP availability for active relaxation during early diastole, and prior infarction can destroy elastic tissue that is needed for passive relaxation [84,85]. These abnormalities can be measured as decreased peak filling rate and delayed time from endsystole until peak filling rate. In addition, one of the major abnormalities of ischemic myocardium is delayed contraction [86]. The ischemic zone may contract after the remainder of the left ventricle has begun its early diastolic filling phase. This competition between different left ventricular regions during early diastole impairs the normal increase in left ventricular diastolic filling volume but increases left ventricular diastolic pressure. This may cause further inhibition of left ventricular filling from the left atrium by making the pressure gradient between left atrium and left ventricle less favorable for left ventricular filling.

Impaired left ventricular diastolic and/or systolic function during acute ischemia or infarction will cause dyspnea [4]. As the left ventricle becomes functionally stiffer, a higher filling pressure is required to achieve the same diastolic left ventricular volume. This higher filling pressure is transmitted from the left ventricle to the left atrium to the pulmonary veins, and to the pulmonary capillaries. The higher pressure causes fluid to leak out into the interstitial spaces of the lung where it impinges upon alveolar air spaces and increases the work of breathing [87]. In addition, exercise-induced left ventricular dysfunction is associated with an abnormal increase in thallium-201 lung uptake during exercise [88], or with increased pulmonary blood volume by gated blood pool scanning [89]. The latter two markers during exercise are often associated with three-vessel disease.

The influence of acute myocardial ischemia on contractile function appears to precede measurable metabolic effects [78,90]. The effects of ischemia on contractile function, however, can persist even after coronary blood flow is restored [91]. The cause of this prolonged inhibition of contraction by transient ischemia is uncertain, but it may be depletion of the precursors of ATP during ischemia [92]. This phenomenon has been referred to as stunned myocardium because the contractile function will improve gradually over time after restoration of coronary blood flow [29]. An important clinical consequence of this prolonged effect of ischemia on contractile behavior is that it complicates interpretation of regional left ventricular contraction as an index of myocardial viability shortly after a prolonged ischemic event. For example, regional left ventricular wall motion may remain quite abnormal for a few days after a myocardial infarction interrupted by acute reperfusion and then recover substantially a few weeks later [5,6]. Practically, this fact limits the clinical value of regional wall motion measurements a few hours or days after thrombolytic therapy in deciding whether the patient has viable but jeopardized myocardium that might benefit from angioplasty or bypass surgery. There have been suggestions that inotropic stimulation can overcome the prolonged effect of ischemia on regional myocardial contraction [70,93].

3.2.2. *Changes in cellular metabolism*

Decrease of coronary blood flow causes two types of problems for myocardial metabolism: 1) inadequate delivery of oxygen and other nutrients, and 2) inadequate washout of carbon dioxide, lactic acid, and other metabolic breakdown products.

In ischemic myocardium metabolic abnormalities occur rapidly, but measurable abnormalities do lag somewhat behind contractile defects [79]. There is a depletion of high energy phosphates such as ATP and creatine phosphate [9,94]. This presumably results because of the lack of oxygen to serve as the final electron acceptor for mitochondrial oxidative phosphorylation. When oxidative phosphorylation is impaired, high-energy phosphate bonds cannot be produced, leading to depletion of ATP and creatine phosphate. Ischemic metabolic abnormalities are often characterized by abnormal lactate metabolism. Normally some lactate is present in arterial blood, and is taken up by the heart muscle and used as an energy substrate. This is because lactate can be converted in the presence of oxygen to pyruvate and metabolized. In contrast, in ischemic myocardium, where little oxygen is available, the lactate cannot be taken up for production of pyruvate, but pyruvate is degraded to lactate. When pyruvate is degraded to lactate, it cannot be metabolized and pyruvate is released into coronary venous blood. Thus, under ischemic circumstances, more lactate is released from the heart than is taken up. The accumulation of lactate leads to tissue acidosis, which may contribute to further contractile dysfunction and to inhibition of anaerobic glycolysis. The accumulation of lactic acid impairs the further production of energy in the absence of oxygen in the heart muscle.

The main energy substrates of heart muscle are fatty acids, which supply about 70 % of the energy requirements under normal circumstances [94]. However, during ischemia, when oxygen is not available, fatty acids cannot be metabolized to produce ATP. Thus, ischemic myocardium cannot use fatty acids because of the absence of oxygen as a final electronic receptor for mitochondrial oxidative phosphorylation. For this reason, fatty acids accumulate in the heart and are not taken up when labeled exogenous fatty acids are injected into the circulation. Knowledge of this fact can be used for nuclear imaging of cardiac fatty acid metabolism [95].

4. Reactions on coronary stenoses

Lumen obstruction of coronary arteries by any mechanism leads to several consequences: 1) limitation of coronary blood flow, 2) development of coronary collaterals, and 3) the potential for coronary steal. Myocardial ischemia (with abnormalities of contraction, metabolism and electrophysiology), and finally, myocardial infarction are the consequences of these obstructions.

4.1. *Reduction of flow*

Coronary artery disease manifests itself as a reduction in the maximum coronary blood flow that can be carried by an artery when the lumen obstruction is moderate [96]. The ability of coronary blood flow to increase from its baseline to its maximum value is called coronary blood flow reserve capacity. About half the lumen diameter can be obstructed before there is any reduction in coronary blood flow reserve of the maximum blood flow under exercise conditions. The artery must be obstructed by 80 to 90 % before there is any reduction in the flow available at rest. These findings have emerged from studies in animals in which coronary blood flow can be measured precisely by an electromagnetic flow probe and coronary lumen diameter can be measured mechanically. Such precise measurements are not available in humans.

A major indication for radionuclide studies during stress is to determine the functional significance of coronary arterial narrowing observed on angiography. The angiographer calls a lesion significant when it reduces lumen diameter by 50 to 70 % [97]. However, it is well known that the angiographic appearance of coronary arterial narrowing, especially when interpreted subjectively, is not a precise predictor of reduction in coronary blood flow. Studies comparing coronary arteriography with postmortem analysis of the coronary arteries showed a very poor correlation between experienced angiographers' readings of the coronary arteriogram and the postmortem appearance of the coronary artery [98]. More importantly, White et al. [1] correlated coronary arteriographic findings with the peak coronary blood flow velocity during stress measured in the coronary artery at the time of open heart surgery by a minimally invasive ultrasonic Doppler flowmeter. They found a very poor correlation between peak flow velocity and angiographic estimates, such as a computer program to characterize the coronary arterial lumen size and shape more accurately [99], as well as videodensitometric methods to estimate coronary blood flow from dye injections during coronary angiography [100].

Estimating the functional significance of a coronary lesion in clinical practice, however, often falls to nuclear studies. The angiographer most often seeks help in assessing the significance of borderline lesions that reduce lumen diameter by 30 to 70 %. The idea is to impose a stress on the circulation so that coronary blood flow is increased to near maximal values. This can be done by exercise in most circumstances but may occasionally be better performed by intravenous administration of dipyridamole, a coronary vaso-dilator drug [101]. When coronary blood flow is increased to a maximum value in normal arteries, it is easier to detect a difference in flow between a normal artery and an artery that is blocked by atherosclerotic plaque. In this way, it is easier to appreciate the contrast between the blood flow rates in normal versus partially occluded coronary arteries. The common interpreta-tion is that if a patient shows a defect on exercise thallium-201 imaging or a wall motion abnormality or decrease in ejection fraction on exercise measure-ment of left ventricular function, the anatomic lesion observed by angiogra-phy is functionally significant.

Qualitative planar thallium-201 imaging [101,102] and studies with qualita-tive SPECT imaging by Shonkoff et al. [103] showed a significant increase in the number of positive tests as the severity of coronary narrowing mea-sured by calipers on arteriograms increased. In another preliminary study of SPECT thallium-201 imaging, in animals, Cedarholm et al. [104] found that quantitative analysis by the bull's-eye ischemic score correlated well with the severity of reduction in maximum coronary blood flow during isoproterenol infusion and could distinguish between coronary stenoses that did or did not impair regional myocardial contraction as measured by ultrasonic crystals. These data suggest that a defect on SPECT thallium-201 images during catecholamine stress in an animal with a coronary stenosis implies ischemia, and not merely a difference in perfusion. Also clinical studies show the high value of quantitative programs in thallium-201 scintigraphy [105,106].

Radionuclide imaging procedures for defining a functionally significant coronary stenosis in humans assume that the nuclear test may be the gold standard and that the coronary arteriogram has become the variable to be assessed. This approach is the opposite of the standard approach, whereby nuclear cardiology procedures are validated against the coronary arterio-graphic gold standard. For example, there have been several indications during the past years that patients with mild 20 to 60 % narrowing of lumen diameter will often be those who exhibit positive exercise thallium scans, consistent with the idea that thallium-201 scintigraphy may provide a better 'gold standard' than does the coronary arteriogram, under some circum-stances. The issue of whether coronary angiography or stress radionuclide imaging provides the better reference method is not yet settled [107]. Clinical practice in many centers, however, allows for the referral of patients for angioplasty or coronary bypass surgery on the basis of abnormalities demon-strated on stress radionuclide imaging when coronary arteriography shows a borderline significant lesion.

4.2. *Inception of coronary collaterals*

When antegrade coronary flow is reduced by an atherosclerotic plaque, the opening of coronary arterial collateral vessels is starting in consequence of and compensation for coronary arterial lumen obstruction [108]. The collateral coronary arteries are present in rudimentary form from birth onward and are called upon to enlarge and carry larger volumes of flow when there is an obstruction developing in the normal channels. The collaterals can then take flow from a normal coronary artery around an obstruction in another coronary branch to perfuse the distal vascular bed. Thus, the collaterals are relatively large channels that supply blood to a major coronary arterial branch and distribute the blood within the same vascular distribution as that major arterial branch with the occlusion. Coronary collaterals are not small arteries but their size is larger than the size of capillaries [109].

There is a high degree of variability in the development of collaterals in members of any one species as well as differences among species (e.g., dogs, pigs, sheep, primates, and humans). The variability among different individuals of the same species may outweigh the variability among different species. Any comparison of different species with humans must first take note of the major methodologic problem of measuring collateral blood flow in humans [108]. Thus, the most obvious species difference between humans and animals is the ability to measure collateral coronary blood flow accurately in animals by radioactive plastic microspheres and other techniques, used in controlled conditions, in contrast to the very limited methods and conditions available for estimating collateral perfusion in humans [108].

In animals it has clearly been demonstrated that when the collateral circulation is well developed, it can restore resting coronary blood flow to normal after a gradual total occlusion of a coronary artery [108–110]. Thus, if an artery is gradually occluded by controlled coronary constriction, the myocardium supplied by that vessel will not undergo infarction, and collaterals will be well developed. Under stress conditions many of these animals that show adequate protection of the myocardium at rest, show that blood flow does not increase as much through collaterals as it does through native vessels supplying normal myocardium [109,110]. This has been most clearly demonstrated by exercise tests in dogs measuring collateral coronary blood flow by the radioactive plastic microsphere method with in vitro postmortem counting, which measures flow per gram of tissue supplied by normal arteries compared with flow per gram of tissue supplied by collaterals [109,111].

Problems with techniques to estimate collateral function limit such studies in humans. Any human study that attempts to assess the functional significance of large collaterals seen on angiography in patients with partial or total occlusion of a coronary artery is subject to serious misinterpretation [108,112]. First, partial occlusion permits a variable amount of antegrade flow, which is not measured. As a result, the contractile function of the myocardium distal to the stenosis will depend not only on collaterals but on a variable amount of antegrade flow as well. Second, the criteria to identify functionally adequate collaterals on angiography are poor. Several such criteria of the adequacy of collateral filling include the size of the vessel beyond the point of stenosis, subjective grading of the intensity of visualization of contrast material in the artery beyond the occlusion [97,112,113], and the time required for a dye to pass from the normal artery to the obstructed artery (which appears to be inversely related to collateral perfusion measured by intracoronary xenon) [112,113]. Finally, one way to determine whether the myocardium supplied by collaterals functions adequately is to assess its regional contraction from a contrast angiogram [97].

Coronary collaterals in general are not adequate to supply the demands of the myocardium in humans [97]. The relevant studies have generally been flawed by trying to assess collaterals in the presence of some antegrade flow, by the difficulty in assessing the degree of collateral development, and by the difficulty in determining whether the myocardium supplied by the collaterals is necrotic (and therefore does not need collateral flow) or viable (and therefore does need collateral flow) [108,112]. For example, one study found that in a group of 22 patients with totally occluded coronary arteries, 6 patients showed normal planar thallium-201 scintigrams in the distribution of the occluded coronary artery during exercise [112]. This normal exercise thallium-201 image correlated with shorter dye appearance times on coronary arteriography as another index of the adequacy of their collateral development. An interesting finding in that study was that people with totally occluded left anterior descending coronary arteries rarely had adequate collaterals defined by exercise thallium-201 scintigraphy, whereas patients with totally occluded right or circumflex coronary arteries usually had adequate protection by collaterals measured by exercise thallium-201 scintigrams [112]. There was no differential sensitivity of the planar thallium-201 imaging technique for the anterior versus inferior walls of the heart in a group of patients with myocardial infarctions represented by Q-waves and akinetic segments of the contrast ventriculogram. In those patients, there was an equal sensitivity of planar thallium-201 imaging to detect the infarct in the anterior wall (92 %) versus the inferior or posterolateral walls (88 %). It appears that the left anterior descending coronary artery cannot be protected as well by collaterals as can the right or circumflex coronary arteries [112]. The most likely explanation for this difference is that the mass of myocardium supplied by the left anterior descending coronary artery in normal cases is larger than the mass supplied by the right or circumflex coronary artery in humans. This is supported by animal studies that have shown that the collateral flow per gram of tissue is lower when the mass of the left ventricle supplied by the occluded coronary artery is larger [9].

4.3. *The phenomenon of coronary steal*

The experiment defining coronary steal was first performed by Fam and MacGregor [114], who showed that when one artery was totally occluded and dependent for its blood flow on collaterals from an adjacent artery, they could demonstrate a reduction in collateral flow, under certain circumstances.

In their experiments, they produced a severe partial occlusion in the artery that was supplying collaterals to an artery with total occlusion. During administration of the vasodilator dipyridamole, these investigators were able to show a reduction in collateral flow measured directly as retrograde flow from the cut end of the occluded artery distal to the site of ligation, which was proposed to be as follows: Dipyridamole increased flow velocity through the partially occluded coronary artery, and this increase in flow velocity would be expected to cause a decrease in pressure in that partially occluded artery. If one recalls from physics that total energy in such a system must remain constant and is the sum of kinetic energy (roughly equivalent to flow velocity) and potential energy (roughly equivalent to the pressure gradient), this is easy to understand. As dipyridamole dilates the small arterioles in the myocardium supplied by the partially occluded artery, it can have no further effect on the arterioles in the ischemic region, which are already maximally dilated by the process of ischemia itself. With the dilation of these arterioles, more blood rushes through the artery; therefore, flow velocity must increase as flow crosses the partial coronary stenosis. In that partially occluded artery, there is a further drop in pressure distal to the stenosis. This drop in pressure distal to the partial stenosis means that the pressure at the origin of the collateral vessels will now be decreased. Collateral vessels are quite dependent on the pressure gradient across these vessels to drive blood flow into the ischemic myocardium; thus, collateral flow will drop when pressure in the artery from which the collaterals originate decreases.

Becker indicated in following studies [115] that coronary steal would not occur when only one artery was occluded and other arteries were normal. His experiments were based on microsphere studies designed to identify the ischemic zone and to measure collateral blood flow during administration of dipyridamole plus methoxamine to hold aortic pressure constant. Patterson and Kirk [116] performed studies using adenosine as a vasodilator while holding left main coronary artery pressure constant with a special cannula and perfusion pump. When one artery was occluded and the left main coronary artery pressure was maintained constant, adenosine was able to induce a small coronary steal, indicating that there is some pressure gradient across the coronary circulation proximal to the origins of the coronary collaterals. This pressure drop would predict that about 10 % of the resistance of the coronary circulation is present in the large coronary arteries proximal to the origin of the collaterals.

When one artery is totally occluded and other arteries are normal, the magnitude of coronary steal is small or not existing. The magnitude of coronary steal is amplified greatly when there is a partial stenosis in the coronary circulation in another artery proximal to the origin of collateral vessels. There is a roughly linear relationship between the magnitude of coronary steal and the severity of stenosis of the left main coronary artery proximal to the origin of the collaterals. This phenomenon helps explain why multivessel coronary disease, and especially left main coronary disease, has such a serious impact on the coronary circulation and the life expectancy of the patient. Multivessel disease jeopardizes the origin of collateral vessels and thus further decreases perfusion of the myocardium.

During thallium-201 imaging with dipyridamole, the myocardium does not need to be ischemic in order to produce a thallium-201 defect in contrast to exercise or catecholamine stress [101]. Dipyridamole dilates normal vessels, delivers more flow through normal arteries, and gives a brighter image at thallium-201 scintigraphy in those regions. In contrast, myocardium supplied by a stenotic coronary artery will not show as great an increase in blood flow or thallium-201 distribution so that it will appear as a defect [117]. Furthermore, in the occasional patient in whom evidence of ischemia such as chest pain and/or electrocardiographic changes do develop during dipyridamole imaging, one mechanism could be arterial hypotension and bradycardia [118]. When blood pressure is reduced below the level that sustains coronary blood flow across the stenotic coronary lesions, the patient may well experience ischemia. Coronary steal cannot be differentiated in these circumstances. When arterial pressure is reduced, the reduced arterial pressure is transmitted down the partially occluded coronary artery, further reducing collateral perfusion of the area supplied by the collateral vessels. Thus, one cannot distinguish coronary steal when arterial pressure has also decreased. This mechanism, however, of increased flow velocity reducing the pressure at the origin of collaterals probably contributes to ischemia under these conditions. In fact, recent studies have demonstrated development of transient abnormalities of left ventricular regional contraction during dipyridamole infusion to confirm ischemia in a few patients.

4.4. Noninvasive quantification of coronary anatomy

The anatomy of coronary arteries can at present be studied only by selective analogue or digital contrast angiography. This investigation remains mandatory and is there to stay in patients who are candidates for coronary bypass surgery or percutaneous transluminal coronary angioplasty.

Various techniques make it possible to visualize proximal segments of coronary vessels noninvasively. Such techniques include echocardiography [119], digital subtraction angiography with peripheral or central intravenous contrast administration [81,120], computed tomography [121], and magnetic resonance imaging. In addition, intravenous digital subtraction angiography [122] and computed tomography [123] can be utilized to visualize aortocoronary bypass grafts [81,124]. The only technique that may someday provide a noninvasive approach to image coronary anatomy directly is digital angiography with intravenous injection of contrast media. However, we are unaware of successful attempts to date of visualizing the smaller branches of the coronary arteries using any imaging technique other than selective coronary angiography.

5. Conclusion

The boundaries for the future of cardiac imaging and image processing have been enumerated with great ambitions, but the attainment of those goals will require a unique approach to further investigations. To succeed, this approach must focus on the biological and technical problems remaining to be solved before complete characterization of cardiac structure, function, perfusion, and metabolism by imaging techniques will become a reality. These goals can only be met by interdisciplinary teams of investigators, representing expertise in the divergent areas of physics, electrical and computer engineering, physiology, biochemistry, computer science and the clinicians in cardiology, radiology, and nuclear medicine. Although there is precedent for such wideranging collaboration, the problems inherent in interdisciplinary investigation can be formidable. Nonetheless, for the successful attainment of our shared objectives, a close interaction will be necessary among the several academic disciplines cited, including collaboration with industrial research and development laboratories.

Interdisciplinary investigative groups are now developed in our European Society of Cardiology, increasing attention will need to be addressed especially to methods of computerized quantitative image analysis. Traditional imaging research has focused on the hardware of image acquisition, with less emphasis on innovations in analytical procedures. Increased effort at developing interactive or fully automated computer-assisted quantitative image analysis techniques promises to yield substantial benefits to clinical imaging, such as improved reproducibility, standardization of methods, and an enhanced ability to compare data among institutions. Computer-based quantitative methods will also allow the clinician and investigator to evaluate certain types of information not readily appreciated by simple visual inspection. This will be particularly true for time-related data, for example, such as thallium-201 wash-out curves.

The achievements of imaging research to date are extraordinary and suggest that the application of quantitative analytical techniques to cardiovascular images will continue to yield impressive and meaningful results which should increase our knowledge of the cardiovascular system and the subjective utility for our patients.

References

1. White CW, Wright CB, Doty DB, et al. Does visual interpretation of the coronary arteriogram predict the physiologic importance of a coronary stenosis? N Engl J Med 1984;310:819–24.
2. Alpert JS, Braunwald E. Acute myocardial infarction: pathological, pathophysiological, and clinical manifestations. In: Braunwald E, editor. Heart disease: a textbook of cardiovascular medicine. 2nd ed. Philadelphia: Saunders, 1984:1262–1300.

3a. Forrester JS, Diamond G, Chatterjee K, Swan HJ. Medical therapy of acute myocardial infarction by application of hemodynamic subsets (first of two parts). N Engl J Med 1976;295:1356–62.

3b. Forrester JS, Diamond G, Chatterjee K, Swan HJ. Medical therapy of acute myocardial infarction by application of hemodynamic subsets (second of two parts). N Engl J Med 1976;295:1404–13.

4. Russel RO Jr, Mantle JA, Rogers WJ, Rackley CE. Current status of hemodynamic monitoring: indications, diagnosis, complications. In: Rackley CE, editor. Critical care cardiology. FA Davis 1981:1–13.

5. Stack RS, Phillips HR 3d, Grierson DS, et al. Functional improvement of jeopardized myocardium following intracoronary streptokinase infusion in acute myocardial infarction. J Clin Invest 1983;72:84–95

6. Sheehan FH, Bolson EL, Dodge HT, Mathey DG, Schofer J, Woo HW. Advantages and applications of the centerline method for characterizing regional ventricular function. Circulation 1986;74:293–305.

7. Williams DO, Scherlag BJ, Hope RR, El-Sheriff N, Lazzara R. The pathophysiology of malignant ventricular arrhythmias during acute myocardial ischemia. Circulation 1974;50:1163–72.

8. Jones-Collins BA, Patterson RE. Quantitative measurement of electrical instability as a function of myocardial infarct size in the dogs. Am J Cardiol 1981;48:858–63.

9. Kirk ES, Jennings RB. Pathophysiology of myocardial ischemia. In: Hurst JW, editor. The heart, arteries and veins. 5th ed. New York: McGraw-Hill 1982:979–95.

10. Hirzel HO, Sonnenblick EH, Kirk ES. Absence of a lateral border zone of intermediate creatine phosphokinase depletion surrounding a central infarct 24 hr after acute coronary occlusion in the dog. Circ Res 1977;41:673–83.

11. Roberts R, Sobel BE. Creatine kinase isoenzymes in the assessment of heart disease. Am Heart J 1978;95:521–8.

12. Savage RM, Wagner GS, Ideker RE, Podolsky SA, Hackel DB. Correlation of postmortem anatomic findings with electrocardiographic changes in patients with myocardial infarction: retrospective study of patients with typical anterior and posterior infarcts. Circulation 1977;55:279–85.

13. Holland RP, Brooks H. TQ-ST segment mapping: critical review and analysis of current concepts. Am J Cardiol 1977;40:110–29.

14. Risk stratification and survival after myocardial infarction. N Engl J Med 1983;309:331–6.

15. Willerson JT, Parkey RW, Lewis SE, Bonte FJ, Buja LM. Hot-spot imaging for patients with acute myocardial infarction. J Cardiovasc Med 1982;7:291.

16. Khaw BA, Beller GA, Haber E. Experimental myocardial infarct imaging following intravenous administration of iodine-131 labeled antibody (Fab')$_2$ fragments specific for cardiac myosin. Circulation 1978;57:743–50.

17. Van Vlies B, van Royen EA, Visser CA, et al. Frequency of myocardial Indium-111 antimyosin uptake after uncomplicated coronary artery bypass grafting. Am J Cardiol 1990;66:1191–5.

18. Jain D, Crawley JC, Lahiri A, Raftery EB. Indium-111–antimyosin images compared with triphenyl tetrazolium chloride staining in a patient six days after myocardial infarction. J Nucl Med 1990;31:231–3.

19. Johnson LL, Seldin DW, Keller AM. Dual isotope thallium and indium antimyosin SPECT imaging to identify acute infarct patients at further ischemic risk. Circulation 1990;81:37–45.

20. Silverman KJ, Becker LC, Bulkley BH, et al. Value of early thallium-201 scintigraphy for predicting mortality in patients with acute myocardial infarction. Circulation 1980;61:996–1003.

21. Pellikka PA, Behrenbeck T, Verani MS, Mahmarian JJ, Wackers FJ, Gibbons RJ. Serial changes in myocardial perfusion using tomographic technetium-99m hexakis-2-methoxy-

2-methylpropyl-isonitrile imaging following reperfusion therapy of myocardial infarction. J Nucl Med 1990;31:1269–75.

22. Eichstaedt H, Felix R, Steiner-Peleny G, Langer M. MR-Diagnostik des Myokardinfarktes mit Gadolinium-DTPA. Zentralbl Radiol 1985;129:960–6.

23. Eichstaedt H, Felix R, Langer M, Peleny G. Heart-imaging with magnetic resonance tomography using the paramagnetic contrast medium Gadolinium-DTPA. In: Lemke HU, Rhodes ML, Jaffee CC, Felix R, editors. Computer assisted radiology. Berlin: Springer, 1985:56–78.

24. Eichstaedt HW, Felix R, Dougherty FC, Langer M, Rutsch W, Schmutzler H. Magnetic resonance imaging (MRI) in different stages of myocardial infarction using the contrast agent gadolinium-DTPA. Clin Cardiol 1986;9:527–35.

25. de Roos A, Matheijssen NA, Doornbos J, van Dijkman PRM, van Voorthuisen AE, van der Wall EE. Myocardial infarct size after reperfusion therapy: Assessment with Gd-DTPA-enhanced MR Imaging. Radiology 1990;176:517–21.

26. Van der Wall EE, van Dijkman, PR, de Roos A, et al. Diagnostic significance of gadolinium-DTPA (diethylenetriamine penta-acetic acid) enhanced magnetic resonance imaging in thrombolytic treatment for acute myocardial infarction: its potential in assessing reperfusion. Br Heart J 1990;63:12–17.

27. Norris RM, Brandt PW, Caughey DE, Lee AJ, Scott PJ. A new coronary prognostic index. Lancet 1969;1:274–8.

28. Rackley CE. Quantitative evaluation of left ventricular function by radiographic techniques. Circulation 1976;54:862–79.

29. Braunwald E, Kloner RA. The stunned myocardium: prolonged, postischemic ventricular dysfunction. Circulation 1982;66:1146–9.

30. Green MV, Bacharach SL. Functional imaging of the heart: methods, limitations and examples from gated blood pool scintigraphy. Prog Cardiovasc Dis 1986;28:319–48.

31. Califf RM, Burks JM, Behar VS, Margolis JR, Wagner GS. Relationship among ventricular arrhythmias, coronary artery disease, and angiographic and electrocardiographic indicators of myocardial fibrosis. Circulation 1978;57:725–32.

32. Epstein SE, Palmeri ST, Patterson RE. Current concepts: evaluation of patients after acute myocardial infarction: indications for cardiac catheterization and surgical intervention. N Engl J Med 1982;307:1487–92.

33. Lee JT, Ideker RE, Reimer KA. Myocardial infarct size and location in relation to the coronary vascular bed at risk in man. Circulation 1981;64:526–34.

34. Mimbs JW, Bauwens D, Cohen RD, O'Donnell M, Miller JG, Sobel BE. Effects of myocardial ischemia on quantitative ultrasonic backscatter and identification of responsible determinants. Circ Res 1981;49:89–96.

35. McPherson DD, Aylward PE, Knosp BM, et al. Ultrasound characterization of acute myocardial ischemia by polar texture analysis (abstract). Circulation 1984;70 (suppl 2):II396.

36. Mimbs JW, Yuhas DE, Miller JG, Weiss AN, Sobel BE. Detection of myocardial infarction in vitro based on altered attenuation of ultrasound. Circ Res 1977;41:192–8.

37. Skorton DJ, Collins SM, Nichols J, Pandian NG, Bean JA, Kerber RE. Quantitative texture analysis in two-dimensional echocardiography: application to the diagnosis of experimental myocardial contusion. Circulation 1983;68:217–23.

38. Skorton DJ, Melton HE Jr, Pandian NG, et al. Detection of acute myocardial infarction in closed-chest dogs by analysis of regional two-dimensional echocardiographic gray-level distributions. Circ Res 1983;52:36–44.

39. Higgins CB, Herfkens R, Lipton MJ, et al. Nuclear magnetic resonance imaging of acute myocardial infarction in dogs: alterations in magnetic relaxation times. Am J Cardiol 1983;52:184–8.

40. Higgins CB, Lanzer P, Stark D, et al. Imaging by nuclear magnetic resonance in patients with chronic ischemic heart disease. Circulation 1984;69:523–31.

41. Doornbos J, Verwey H, Essed CE, Balk AH, de Roos A. MR imaging in assessment of cardiac transplant rejection in humans. J Comput Assist Tomogr 1990;14:77–81.

42. Prigent F, Maddahi J, Sato Y, et al. Quantification of myocardial infarct size in the dog using single photon emission computerized tomography: slice-by-slice comparison of T1–201 tomograms and pathology (abstract). Circulation 1984;70 (suppl 2):II450.

43. Corbett JR, Lewis SE, Wolfe CL, et al. Measurement of myocardial infarct size by technetium pyrophosphate single-photon tomography. Am J Cardiol 1984;54:1231–6.

44. Yazaki Y, Isobe M, Tsuchimochi H, Takaku F, Nishikawa J, Iio M. A new method of myocardial infarct sizing by single photon emission tomography using labeled monoclonal antibody specific for ventricular myosin heavy chain (abstract). Circulation 1984;70 (suppl 2):II9.

45. Goldstein RA, Hicks CH, Kuhn JL, et al. Myocardial infarct imaging with rubidium-82 and PET in man (abstract). Circulation 1984;70 (suppl 2):II9.

46. Muehllehner G, Colsher JG, Lewitt RM. A hexagonal bar positron camera: problems and solutions. IEEE Trans Nucl Sci 1983;30:652–60.

47. Berger HJ, Eisner R, DePuey EG, Patterson R. New vistas in cardiovascular nuclear medicine. J Nucl Med 1984;25:1254–8.

48. Rumberger JA, Feiring AJ, Lipton MJ, Higgins CB, Marcus ML. Measurement of myocardial perfusion by ultrafast CT (abstract). J Am Coll Cardiol 1985;5:500.

49. Pandian NG, Koyanagi S, Skorton DJ, et al. Relations between 2–dimensional echocardiographic wall thickening abnormalities, myocardial infarct size and coronary risk area in normal and hypertrophied myocardium in dogs. Am J Cardiol 1983;52:1318–25.

50. Johnson MR, Feiring AJ, Kioschos JM, Bruch PM, Kirchner PT, White CW. Risk area determination in patients with acute myocardial infarction (abstract). Circulation 1984;70 (suppl 2):II275.

51. Armstrong WF, Mueller TM, Kinney EL, Tickner EG, Dillon JC, Feigenbaum H. Assessment of myocardial perfusion abnormalities with contrast-enhanced two-dimensional echocardiography. Circulation 1982;66:166–73.

52. Eichstaedt H, Schumacher M, Feine U, Kochsiek K. Rechnerunterstützte 201Tl-Myokardszintigraphie in der Routinediagnostik der koronaren Herzerkrankung. Nuklearmedizin 1978;17:233–7.

53. Niemeyer MG, Laarman GJ, van der Wall EE, et al. Is quantitative analysis superior to visual analysis of planar thallium 201 myocardial exercise scintigraphy in the evaluation of coronary artery disease? Analysis of a prospective clinical study. Eur J Nucl Med 1990;16:697–704.

54. Fintel DJ, Frank TL, DiPaula AF, McGaughey MM, Becker LC. Quantitation of regional myocardial thallium uptake by single photon emission computed tomography (abstract). Circulation 1984;70 (suppl 2):II9.

55. Fintel DJ, Links JM, Frank TL, Becker LC. Comparison of planar and tomographic thallium imaging for the detection of coronary artery disease (abstract). Circulation 1984;70 (suppl 2):II450.

56. Maddahi J, Prigent F, Staniloff H, et al. A new probabilistic approach to the quantitative interpretation of T1–201 rotational myocardial tomograms for assessment of coronary artery disease (CAD) (abstract). Circulation 1984;70 (suppl 2):II450.

57. Klein JL, Garcia EV, DePuey G, et al. Reversibility bull's-eye: a new polar bull's-eye map to quantify reversibility of stress-induced SPECT thallium-201 myocardial perfusion defects. J Nucl Med 1990;31:1240–6.

58. Iskandrian AS, Heo J, Kong B, Lyons E. Effect of exercise level on the ability of thallium-201 tomographic imaging in detecting coronary artery disease: analysis of 461 patients. J Am Coll Cardiol 1989;14:1477–86.

59. Hendel RC, McSherry B, Karimeddini M, Leppo JA. Diagnostic value of a new myocardial perfusion agent, teboroxime (SQ 30,217), utilizing a rapid planar imaging protocol: preliminary results. J Am Coll Cardiol 1990;16:855–61.

60. Koster K, Wackers FJ, Mattera JA, Fetterman RC. Quantitative analysis of planar technetium-99m-sestamibi myocardial perfusion images using modified background subtraction. J Nucl Med 1990;31:1400–8.

61. Kaufman L, Crooks L, Sheldon P, Hricak H, Herfkens R, Bank W. The potential impact

of nuclear magnetic resonance imaging on cardiovascular diagnosis. Circulation 1983;67:251–7.

62. Ordidge RJ, Mansfield P, Doyle M, Coupland RE. Real time movie images by NMR. Br J Radiol 1982;55:729–33.

63. Underwood SR. Cine magnetic resonance imaging and flow measurements in the cardiovascular system. Br Med Bull 1989;45:948–67.

64. Pettigrew RI. Dynamic cardiac MR imaging. Radiol Clin North Am 1989;27:1183–203.

65. Vogel R, LeFree M, Bates E, et al. Application of digital techniques to selective coronary arteriography: use of myocardial contrast appearance time to measure coronary flow reserve. Am Heart J 1984;107:153–64.

66. Cloninger KG, DePuey EG, Garcia EV, et al. Redistribution abnormalities in exercise thallium images: unresolved ischemia vs infarction? (abstract) J Nucl Med 1986;27:997.

67. Tillisch J, Marshall R, Schelbert H, Huang SC, Phelps M. Reversibility of wall motion abnormalities: Preoperative determination using positron tomography, 18–fluorodeoxyglucose and 13–NH$_3$ (abstract). Circulation 1983;68 (suppl 3):III387.

68. Dilsizian V, Rocco TP, Freedman NM, Leon MB, Bonow RO. Enhanced detection of ischemic but viable myocardium by the reinjection of thallium after stress-redistribution imaging. N Engl J Med 1990;323:141–6.

69. Yang LD, Berman DS, Kiat H, et al. The frequency of late reversibility in SPECT thallium-201 stress-redistribution studies. J Am Coll Cardiol 1990;15:334–40.

70. Dyke SH, Cohn PF, Gorlin R, Sonnenblick EH. Detection of residual myocardial function in coronary artery disease using post-extra systolic potentiation. Circulation 1974;50:694–9.

71. Horn HR, Teichholz LE, Cohn PF, Herman MV, Gorlin R. Augmentation of left ventricular contraction pattern in coronary artery disease by an inotropic catecholamine. The epinephrine ventriculogram. Circulation 1974;49:1063–71.

72. Patterson RE, Jones-Collins BA, Aamodt R. Impaired collateral blood flow reserve early after nontransmural myocardial infarction in conscious dogs. Am J Cardiol 1982;50:1133–40.

73. Moore CA, Cannon J, Watson DD, Kaul S, Beller GA. Thallium 201 kinetics in stunned myocardium characterized by severe postischemic systolic dysfunction. Circulation 1990;81:1622–32.

74. Tennant R, Wiggers CJ. Effect of coronary occlusion on myocardial contraction. Am J Physiol 1935;112:351–61.

75. Herman MV, Heinle RA, Klein MD, Gorlin R. Localized disorders in myocardial contraction. Asynergy and its role in congestive heart failure. N Engl J Med 1967;227:222–32.

76. Herman MV, Gorlin R. Implications of left ventricular asynergy. Am J Cardiol 1969;23:538–47.

77. Katz AM. Effects of ischemia on the contractile processes of heart muscle. Am J Cardiol 1973;32:456–60.

78. Auffermann W, Watters T, Wu S, Parmley WW, Higgins CB, Wikman-Coffelt J. The descending limb of the Frank-Starling curve is due to energy depletion and excess Ca^{2+} entry (abstract). J Am Coll Cardiol 1988;11 (suppl A):72A.

79. Carmeliet E. Myocardial ischemia: reversible and irreversible changes. Circulation 1984;70:149–51.

80. Reiber JH. Review of methods for computer analysis of global and regional left ventricular function from equilibrium gated blood pool scintigrams. In: Simoons ML, Reiber JHC, editors. Nuclear imaging in clinical cardiology. Boston: Nijhoff, 1984:173–217.

81. Eichstaedt H, Langer M, Felix R. Die digitale Subtraktions-Ventrikulographie bei der Bestimmung globaler und regionaler linksventrikulärer Parameter im Vergleich zur Katheter-Laevokardiographie. Radiologie 1984;24:277–85.

82. Borer JS, Bacharach SL, Green MV. Real-time radionuclide cineangiography in the noninvasive evaluation of global and regional left ventricular function at rest and during exercise in patients with coronary artery disease. N Engl J Med 1977;296:839–44.

83. Bonow RO, Bacharach SL. Left ventricular diastolic function: evaluation by radionuclide ventriculography. In: Pohost GM, Higgins CB, Morganroth J, editors: New concepts in cardiac imaging. Chicago: Year Book Medical Publishers, 1987:107–37.

84. Gaasch WH, Blaustein AS, Andrias CW, Donahue RP, Avitall B. Myocardial relaxation. II. Hemodynamic determinants of rate of the left ventricular isovolumic pressure decline. Am J Physiol 1980;239:H1–6.

85. Mirsky I. Assessment of diastolic function: suggested methods and future consideration. Circulation 1984;69:836–41.

86. Green MV, Jones-Collins BA, Bacharach SL, Findley SL, Patterson RE, Larson SM. Scintigraphic quantitation of asynchronous myocardial motion during the left ventricular isovolumic relaxation period: A study in the dog during acute ischemia. J Am Coll Cardiol 1984;4:72–9.

87. Fishman AP. Pulmonary edema. The water-exchanging function of the lung. Circulation 1972;46:390–408.

88. Boucher CA, Zir LM, Beller GA, et al. Increased lung uptake of thallium-201 during exercise myocardial imaging: clinical hemodynamic and angiographic implications in patients with coronary artery disease. Am J Cardiol 1980;46:189–96.

89. Okada RD, Pohost GM, Kirshenbaum HD, et al. Radionuclide-determined change in pulmonary blood volume with exercise. Improved sensitivity of multigated blood-pool scanning in detecting coronary-artery disease. N Engl J Med 1979;301:569–76.

90. Auffermann W, Chew WM, Tavares NJ, et al. ^{31}P-magnetic resonance spectroscopy and cine ^{1}H magnetic resonance imaging of dilated cardiomyopathy in humans. J Am Coll Cardiol 1989;13 (suppl A):199A.

91. Weiner JM, Apstein CS, Arthur JH, Pirzada FA, Hood WB Jr. Persistence of myocardial injury following brief periods of coronary occlusion. Cardiovasc Res 1976;10:678–86.

92. Swain JL, Sabina RL, McHale PA, Greenfield JC Jr, Holmes EW. Prolonged myocardial nucleotide depletion after brief ischemia in the open-chest dog. Am J Physiol 1982;242:H818–26.

93. Theroux P, Ross J Jr, Franklin D, Kemper·WS, Sasyama S. Regional myocardial function in the conscious dog during acute coronary occlusion and responses to morphine, propranolol, nitroglycerin and lidocaine. Circulation 1976;53:302–14.

94. Neely JR, Morgan HE. Relationship between carbohydrate and lipid metabolism 2nd energy balance of heartmuscle. Annu Rev Physiol 1974;36:413–59.

95. Van der Wall EE. Dynamic myocardial scintigraphy with 123–I-labeled free fatty acids [dissertation]. Amsterdam: Rodopi, 1981.

96. Gould KL, Lipscomb K. Effects of coronary stenoses on coronary flow reserve and resistance. Am J Cardiol 1974;34:48–55.

97. Gorlin R. Coronary artery disease. Philadelphia: Saunders, 1976.

98. Schwartz JN, Kong Y, Hackell DB, Bartel AG. Comparison of angiographic and post mortem findings in patients with coronary artery disease. Am J Cardiol 1975;36:174–8.

99. Brown BG, Bolson E, Frimer M, Dodge HT. Quantitative coronary arteriography: estimation of dimensions, hemodynamic resistance, and atheroma mass of coronary artery lesions using the arteriogram and digital computation. Circulation 1977;55:329–37.

100. Rutishauser W, Bussmann WD, Noseda G, Meier W, Wellauer J. Blood flow measurement through single coronary arteries by roentgen densitometry. I. A comparison of flow measured by a radiologic technique applicable in the intact organism and by electromagnetic flowmeter. Am J Roentgenol Radium Ther Nucl Med 1970;109:12–20.

101. Gould KL, Schelbert HR, Phelps ME, Hoffman EJ. Noninvasive assessment of coronary stenosis by myocardial perfusion imaging during pharmacologic coronary vasodilation. V. Detection of 47 percent diameter coronary stenosis with intravenous nitrogen-13 ammonia and emission computed tomography in intact dogs. Am J Cardiol 1979;43:200–8.

102. Ritchie JL, Trobaugh GB, Hamilton GW, et al. Myocardial imaging with thallium-201 at rest and during exercise. Comparison with coronary arteriography and resting and stress electrocardiography. Circulation 1977;56:66–71.

103. Shonkoff D; Eisner RL, Gober A, et al. What quantitative criteria should be used to read defects on the SPECT Tl-201 bullseye display in men?: ROC analysis (abstract). J Nucl Med 1987;28:674–5.

104. Cedarholm JC, Martin SE, Greene R, et al. Can SPECT Tl-201 determine the 'physiological significance' of a coronary stenosis? (abstract). J Nucl Med 1987;28:666–7.

105. Maddahi J, van Train K, Prigent F, et al. Quantitative single photon emission computed thallium-201 tomography for detection and localization of coronary artery disease: optimization and prospective validation of a new technique. J Am Coll Cardiol 1989;14:1689–99.

106. Van Train KF, Maddahi J, Berman DS, et al. Quantitative analysis of tomographic stress thallium-201 myocardial scintigrams: A multicenter trial. J Nucl Med 1990;31:1168–79.

107. Gerson MC. Test accuracy, test selection, and test result interpretation in chronic coronary artery disease. In: Gerson MC, editor. Cardiac nuclear medicine. New York: McGraw-Hill, 1987;309–47.

108. Gregg DE, Patterson RE. Functional importance of the coronary collaterals. N Engl J Med 1980;303:1404–6.

109. Schaper W. The collateral circulation of the heart. Amsterdam: North-Holland, 1971.

110. Fedor JM, Rembert JC, McIntosh DM, Greenfield JC Jr. Effects of exercise- and pacing-induced tachycardia on coronary collateral flow in the awake dog. Circ Res 1980;46:214–20.

111. Eichstaedt H, Felix R. Survey of techniques for measuring myocardial microperfusion. In: Heuck HW, editor. Radiological functional analysis of the vascular system: contrast media, methods, results. Berlin: Springer, 1983;150–62.

112. Eng C, Patterson RE, Horrowitz SF, et al. Coronary collateral function during exercise. Circulation 1982;66:309–16.

113. Smith SC Jr, Gorlin R, Herman MV, Taylor WJ, Collins JJ Jr. Myocardial blood flow in man: effects of coronary collateral circulation and coronary artery bypass surgery. J Clin Invest 1972;51:2556–65.

114. Fam WM, McGregor M. Effect of coronary vasodilator drugs on retrograde flow in areas of chronic myocardial ischemia. Circ Res 1964;15:355–64.

115. Becker LC. Conditions for vasodilator-induced coronary steal in experimental myocardial ischemia. Circulation 1978;57:1103–10.

116. Patterson RE, Kirk ES. Coronary steal mechanisms in dogs with one-vessel occlusion and other arteries normal. Circulation 1983;67:1009–15.

117. Niemeyer MG, van der Wall EE, Leijtens JP, Wever J, van der Pol JM, Willekens FG. Myocardial imaging using thallium 201 scintigraphy after dipyridamole infusion: a case story. Angiology 1989;40:1065–71.

118. Pennell DJ, Underwood SR, Ell PJ. Symptomatic bradycardia complicating the use of intravenous dipyridamole for thallium-201 myocardial perfusion imaging. Int J Cardiol 1990;27:272–4.

119. Rogers EW, Feigenbaum H, Weyman AE, Godley RW, Vakili ST. Evaluation of left coronary artery anatomy in vitro by cross-sectional echocardiography. Circulation 1980;62:782–7.

120. Meaney TF, Weinstein MA, Buonocore E, et al. Digital subtraction angiography of the human cardiovascular system. Am J Roentgenol 1980;135:1153–60.

121. Block M, Bahn RC, Bove AA, Harris LD, Robb RA, Ritman EL. Measurement of coronary artery dimensions and blood flow with the dynamic spatial reconstructor (DSR) (abstract). J Am Coll Cardiol 1983;1:690.

122. Whiting JS, Nivatpumin T, Pfaff M, et al. Assessing the coronary circulation by digital angiography: bypass graft and myocardial perfusion imaging. In: Heintzen PH, Brennecke R, editors. Digital imaging in cardiovascular radiology. Stuttgart: Thieme, 1983;205–11.

123. Brundage BH, Lipton MJ, Herfkens RJ, et al. Detection of patent coronary bypass grafts by computed tomography. A preliminary report. Circulation 1980;61:826–31.

124. Eichstaedt H, Kraemer R, Dougherty FC, Schneider R, Felix R, Schmutzler H. Darstellung von Hypertrophieregression unter chronischer Betablockade mit Hilfe der quantitativen Schichtszintigraphie. Z Kardiol 1983;72:69–74.

PART I

Single photon emission computed tomography
(SPECT): Technical aspects

2. Reconstruction and filtering methods for quantitative cardiac SPECT imaging

BENJAMIN M.W. TSUI

Summary

Cardiac SPECT has become an important imaging tool for the diagnosis of cardiac diseases. In order to obtain the best image quality for clinical diagnosis, it is necessary to understand factors which affect reconstructed images. The understanding allows us to devise image reconstruction and filtering methods which provide quantitative cardiac SPECT images. In this paper, we demonstrate individual and collective effects of major factors which degrade cardiac SPECT images obtained using conventional reconstruction and il-tering methods with 180° and 360° projection data. We also present recc n-struction methods which provide accurate compensation for the image degrading factors. The improved reconstructed images are compared with those obtained from conventional methods in terms of artifacts, distortions, spatial resolution, contrast, noise and quantitative accuracy. Data from a simulation study using a realistic cardiac-chest phantom and from a clinical Tl-201 study are used in the investigation.

1. Introduction

Cardiac imaging using Tl-201 is widely used for assessing regional myocardial perfusion and evaluating coronary artery disease. Conventional planar imaging techniques suffer from poor contrast due to overlying and underlying radionuclide activity distribution. With the advance of single-photon emission computed tomography (SPECT), an imaging method is now available which provides increased image contrast compared with the planar method [1]. The improved clinical efficacy of Tl-201 SPECT over the planar method has also been confirmed in initial evaluation studies [2,3]. This has led to the emergence of Tl-201 SPECT as the favorite radionuclide imaging technique for the diagnosis of myocardial disease and dysfunction.

Cardiac SPECT imaging, however, is affected by a number of image degrading factors. These include statistical fluctuations in photon detection, attenuation of photons through the body before detection, the spatial response function (or spatial resolution) of the collimator-detector system, and

Johan H.C. Reiber & Ernst E. van der Wall (eds.), Cardiovascular Nuclear Medicine and MRI, 29–45.
© 1992 *Kluwer Academic Publishers.*

scatter radiation. If these factors are not properly compensated for or the image data are not appropriately filtered, the reconstructed image will exhibit undesirable artifacts and distortions, poor spatial resolution, low image contrast, or inaccurate quantitative information as compared to the true radionuclide distribution which the reconstructed images are supposed to represent.

In this paper, we first investigate the effects of major factors on cardiac SPECT image quality. The purpose is to understand the characteristics and extent of these effects. A realistic cardiac-chest phantom is constructed based on an x-ray CT study of a normal patient. The phantom closely mimics the anatomy of the thoracic region and the Tl-201 uptake distribution. Simulated projection data are generated from the phantom that include individual and combined effects of the image degrading factors. Reconstructed images are obtained using different reconstruction and filtering methods including conventional and quantitative methods. The results demonstrate the effects of the image degrading factors on the reconstructed images and the effectiveness of various compensation and reconstructed methods in providing good reconstructed image quality.

2. Image degrading factors

There are a number of physical factors which have significant influence on cardiac SPECT imaging. Among these factors attenuation is the most important. Photons emitted from deep inside the patient are less likely to be detected than those emitted from regions close to the surface. This is due to the higher probability of attenuation from intervening tissues. If attenuation is not compensated for, the quantitative accuracy of the reconstructed image will be severely degraded. Also non-uniform attenuation distribution such as that found in the thoracic region will generate undesirable artifacts and distortions.

Another factor is the response function of the imaging system which is largely determined by the geometric response of the collimator. Its primary effect is degradation of spatial resolution in the reconstructed image. Also, the broadening of the collimator response function as a function of distance from the collimator results in variation of spatial resolution throughout the SPECT reconstructed image.

Due to Compton scattering, photons emitted from the radioactive source may experience scattering in the patient before detection. In the process the direction of travel and the energy of the scattered photon vary from that of the emitted photon. These result in misregistration of the position of the photon and reduction of contrast in the detected image. The effects of scatter can be characterized by the scatter fraction, defined as the ratio of the amount of scattered to unsheltered photons, and the scatter response function which describes the spatial extent of scatter radiation from a point source. Both the scatter fraction and scatter response are complex functions of photon energy, energy resolution of the detector and energy window used in data acquisition. In SPECT imaging, the scatter response function is spatially variant throughout the reconstructed image and its shape becomes increasingly asymmetric at positions closer to the edge of the scattering medium.

Cardiac SPECT data especially from Tl-201 studies are affected by low counting statistics leading to a high level of image noise. The presence of image noise has important effects on the detection of image features and clinical diagnosis.

Quantitative cardiac SPECT imaging has been a topic of much research and many investigations in recent years. However, the criterion for quantitation has usually been relative in nature. In our study, we are interested in absolute quantitation where the goal is to obtain a reconstructed image which accurately represents the radioactivity distribution in vivo and without image artifacts and distortions. With proper calibration, the quantitative reconstructed image allows accurate determination of volume, radioactivity concentration and total radioactivity of selected regions of interest for clinical diagnosis. This important goal can only be achieved with proper compensation for the physical factors described earlier.

3. Conventional reconstruction and filtering methods

The filtered backprojection (FB) algorithm is a powerful method for image reconstruction and has been widely used in SPECT imaging. However, the simple FB algorithm assumes an idealized imaging process without any degradation factors. When it is applied to realistic SPECT data, the resultant reconstructed images are less than desirable.

Filtering is usually included as part of the conventional FB reconstruction method for noise smoothing to improve SPECT image quality [4]. Smoothing filters such as the Han filter are considered inadequate because of too much loss of spatial resolution in return for noise smoothing. Filters such as the Butterworth filter have the ability to preserve low spatial frequency image features by selectively smoothing out high frequency noise. Restoration filters, such as the Metz and Wiener filters, attempt to restore image features degraded by the modulation transfer functions (MTF) of the imaging system [5–7] and scatter [8] in the lower spatial frequency region. Although these filters tend to restore spatial resolution in the image, they also have the potential to enhance undesirable noise structures if they are not designed properly. In SPECT imaging, due to the spatially variant imaging and scatter response functions, average MTFs are assumed for use with the restoration filters. The abilities of these filters to improve detection in SPECT images have been investigated [8].

In cardiac SPECT imaging, it has been found that reconstruction from projection data spanning 180° from 45° LPO to 45° RAO around the front side of the patient produces higher image contrast in the myocardial region as compared with 360° reconstruction [9,10]. This is due to the poorer projection data obtained from the posterior side of the patient, as a result of more attenuation, as compared to that obtained from the anterior side. However, it has also been shown that image artifacts and distortions may result from 180° reconstruction [11,12]

A number of attenuation compensation methods have been proposed for situations where the attenuation coefficient is constant throughout the reconstructed image slice. These methods can be grouped into the intrinsic techniques [13,14], techniques which preprocess the projection data [15,16], and techniques which postprocess the reconstructed image [17]. However, these compensation methods for uniform attenuation are inadequate for cardiac SPECT imaging where the attenuation coefficients of various tissues in the thoracic region are very different. Here, compensation methods which incorporate information about the attenuation distribution must be used.

4. Quantitative reconstruction methods

In order to obtain quantitative cardiac SPECT images, accurate compensation for the image degrading factors must be achieved. As described earlier, conventional compensation techniques and reconstruction and filtering methods are inadequate because they have to make certain approximations to the imaging process and as a result compromise the accuracy of quantitation.

An effective method for attenuation compensation in cardiac imaging is the Chang algorithm modified to include the non-uniform attenuation distribution [18–20]. In the modified algorithm, the attenuation correction factor for each reconstructed image pixel is calculated using the known attenuation map. The attenuation compensation method has proven effective in quantitative cardiac SPECT imaging [21].

A new class of reconstruction methods has been studied for use in SPECT imaging. These methods employ iterative reconstruction algorithms which are derived from statistical criteria and estimate the reconstructed image from the measured projection data using parameter estimation techniques. A projector and backprojector pair is required in the iterative reconstruction method. The iterative process continues until the difference between the measured projection data and the projection of the current estimate of the reconstructed image is less than a predetermined value. That current estimate of the reconstructed image is considered to be the solution of the reconstruction problem. Examples of iterative reconstruction algorithms include the ML-EM (maximum likelihood with expectation-maximization) [22,23], WLS-CG (weighted least squares with conjugate gradient) [4] and MAP-EM (maximum a posteriori with expectation-maximization) [24] algorithms.

The projector and backprojector pair used in the iterative reconstruction method models the process of SPECT data acquisition. It is where various image degrading factors can be incorporated into the reconstruction. By doing so, the iterative algorithm compensates for the degrading factors during reconstruction. For example, the exact attenuation map through the patient can be incorporated into the projector and backprojector pair for accurate compensation of non-uniform attenuation in cardiac SPECT imaging [25,21]. By modeling the detector response function in the projector and backprojector pair, one can compensate for the spatially variant detector response [20]. A projector and backprojector pair which model both attenuation and detector response has been shown to provide improved quantitative accuracy, spatial resolution and decreased noise in the reconstructed image [26].

The iterative reconstruction methods are inherently computationally intensive as compared to the conventional reconstruction and filtering methods. Each iteration consisting of a projection and a backprojection step requires about twice as many computations as the FB algorithm. Projectors and backprojectors which model the imaging process require even more calculations. Furthermore, multiple iterations are necessary to achieve satisfactory reconstructed image quality. The exact number of iterations required depends on the convergence properties of the particular iterative algorithm in use [26].

5. Experimental study

The experimental study has two specific aims. First, it is designed to demonstrate the individual and combined effects of image degrading factors on cardiac SPECT images obtained from conventional reconstruction and filtering methods. We are particularly interested in the artifacts, distortions, spatial resolution, contrast and quantitative accuracy of the reconstructed image. The second aim is to demonstrate the effectiveness of quantitative reconstruction methods in compensating for image degrading factors and in providing quantitative cardiac SPECT images.

5.1. *Simulated phantom*

In order to investigate the individual and combined effects of the image degrading factors, a realistic phantom is needed in the simulation study. We have developed a cardiac-chest phantom which is derived from an x-ray CT study of a normal patient [27]. The phantom models the anatomy of the human thorax. An image slice through the center of the myocardium is chosen for use in the study (Fig. 1a). From the CT image, the non-uniform attenuation distribution of the chest region can be derived. The CT image also allows identification of the myocardium and other tissue organs such that the uptake of Tl-201 can be simulated from known biodistributions in

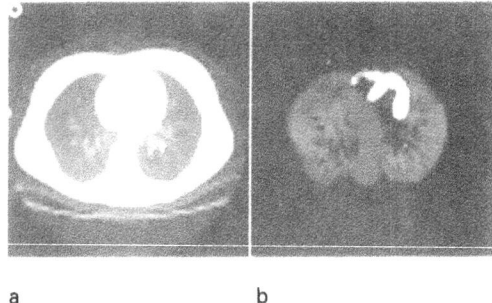

a   b

Figure 1. Cardiac-chest phantom used in the experimental simulation study. (a) A section of attenuation distribution through the center of the myocardium. The data are derived from an X-ray CT study of a normal patient. (b) Simulated distribution of Tl-201 uptake.

humans (Fig. 1b). In the phantom, the ratio of average Tl-201 radioactivity concentrations in the myocardium to the lung is set to be 6:1.

Using the emission phantom shown in Fig. 1 alone, we simulated projection data from 128 views over 360° around the patient without any image degradation. The projection data are reconstructed, using the conventional filtered backprojection (FB) algorithm, into a 64 × 64 reconstructed image matrix. The top and bottom images in Fig. 2a are reconstructed images

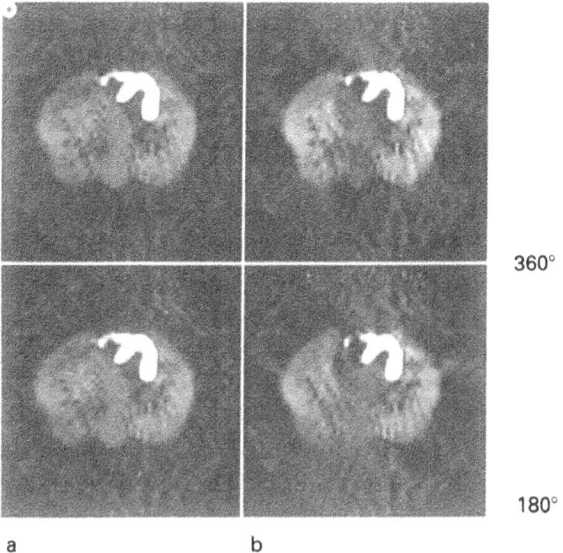

360°

180°

a   b

Figure 2. Transaxial reconstructed images of the cardiac-chest phantom obtained using the FB algorithm. Images in the upper and lower rows are from 360° and 180° reconstructions, respectively. The simulated projection data used in the reconstructions include (a) no image degrading factors and (b) the non-uniform attenuation distribution shown in Fig. 1a.

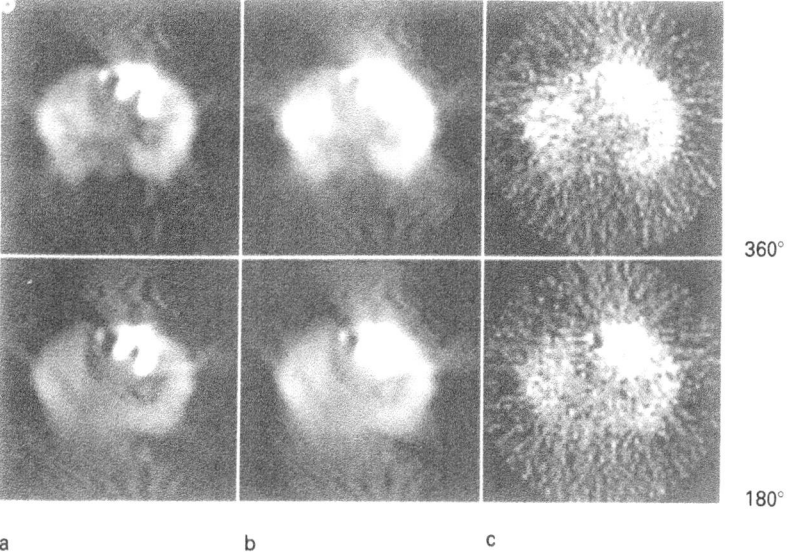

360°

180°

a   b   c

Figure 3. Transaxial reconstructed images of the cardiac-chest phantom obtained using the FB algorithm. Images in the upper and lower rows are from 360° and 180° reconstructions, respectively. The projection data used in the reconstruction include the effects of non-uniform attenuation shown in Fig. 1a. Also included are the effects of (a) the response function of a LEGP collimator, plus (b) the scatter response function, and plus (c) Poisson noise.

obtained using the complete 360° and a section of 180° (from 45° LPO to 45° RAO) projection data, respectively. The images demonstrate the generally good reconstructed image quality that can be obtained from the FB algorithm in the absence of image degrading factors. There are little differences between the 180° and 360° reconstructions. The small artifacts in the reconstructed image are due to the digitization of the image data and the finite number of projection views.

5.2. *Effects of image degrading factors*

To study the effects of photon attenuation, the emission projection data were generated by incorporating the non-uniform attenuation map shown in Fig. 1b. The top and bottom images in Fig. 2b show the 360° and 180° reconstructions, respectively. In general, both images show decreased intensity in the mid-portion of the reconstructed image. There is a distinct pattern of intensity artifacts emanating from the apex region of the myocardium. Also the 180° reconstruction exhibits more distortions in the posterior portion of the image than the 360° reconstruction.

In Fig. 3, the images in the top and bottom rows are from 360° and

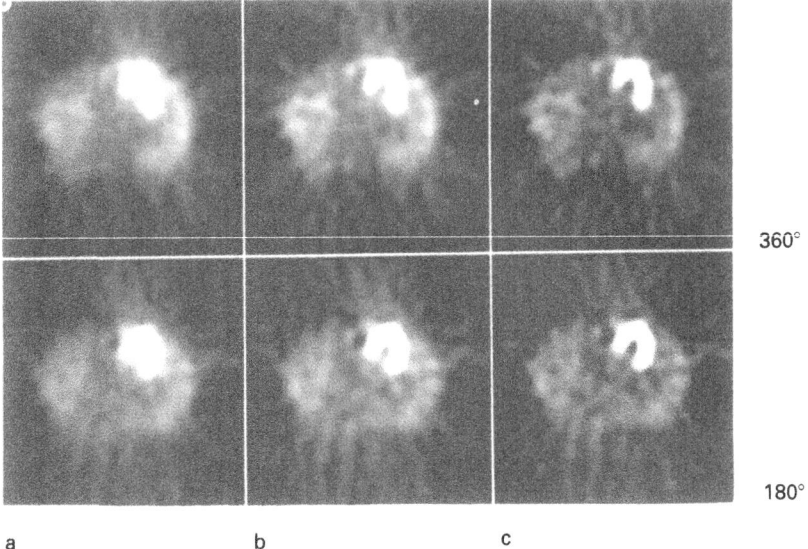

Figure 4. Transaxial reconstructed images of the cardiac-chest phantom obtained using the FB algorithm. Images in the upper and lower rows are from 360° and 180° reconstructions, respectively. The projection data used in the reconstruction are the same as those used in generating the images in Fig. 3c except that the reconstructed images are filtered with (a) a Han filter with fc = 0.3 cycles/pixel, (b) a Butterworth filter with fc = 0.22 cycles/pixel and order of 8, and (c) a Metz filter which includes the average MTFs of the LEGP collimator and scatter and a power of 10.

180° reconstructions, respectively. The images in Fig. 3a are reconstructions from projection data which include, in addition to attenuation, the effects of the spatially variant response function of a low energy general purpose (LEGP) collimator which is fitted on the SPECT imaging system. Four adjacent image slices were included in the simulation to model the three-dimensional effects of the detector response function. When compared to Fig. 2b, similar patterns of image artifacts and distortions are found except for smoothing by the imaging system. The contrast in the myocardial region is found to be higher for the 180° than the 360° reconstruction.

Figure 3b shows results of the reconstructions when scatter radiation is added to the projection data. The general decrease in image contrast is apparent. However, the pattern of image artifacts and distortions described earlier persists. Reconstructed images with Poisson noise fluctuations added to the projection data are shown in Fig. 3c. The level of noise fluctuations is consistent with that found in clinical Tl-201 studies where the average total counts of the projection data are about 150,000. To simulate acquisitions with the same imaging time, the total counts of the projection data used in the 180° reconstruction are twice the total counts of projection data summed over the same projection angles in the 360° reconstruction. The images shown in Fig. 3c show that the noise fluctuations mask details of image artifacts and

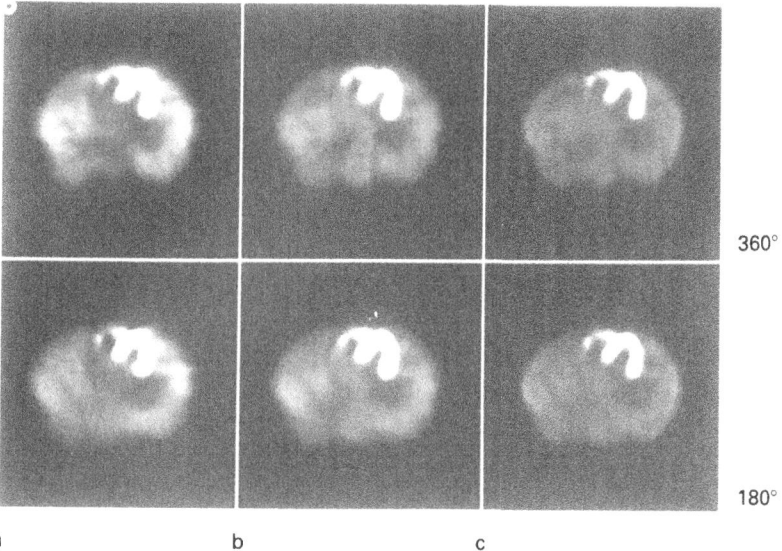

360°

180°

a   b   c

Figure 5. Transaxial reconstructed images of the cardiac-chest phantom obtained using the modified Chang algorithm which utilizes the attenuation map shown in Fig. 1a in calculating the attenuation correction factors. Images in the upper and lower rows are from 360° and 180° reconstructions, respectively. The projection data used in the reconstruction are the same as those used in generating the images in Fig. 3a. The reconstructed images are filtered using (a) a Butterworth filter with fc = 0.3 cycles/pixel and order of 8, (b) a Metz filter which includes the collimator MTF and power of 10, and (c) a Metz filter which includes the MTFs of both the collimator and scatter and power of 10.

distortions shown in the noise-free situation (Fig. 3b). However, the general pattern of artifacts and distortions remains discernible at close examination.

The images in Figs. 4a, b and c are results from filtering the reconstructed images in Fig. 3c using the Han, Butterworth and Metz filters, respectively. The Metz filter utilizes the MTFs of the LEGP collimator and scatter at a source distance equal to the radius-of-rotation of 22.5 cm. The reconstructed images exhibit image quality consistent with the expected performance of the filters. However, they do not eliminate the image artifacts and distortions described earlier.

5.3. *Performance of quantitative reconstruction methods*

To evaluate the performance of various quantitative reconstruction methods, we assume that the attenuation coefficient map about the patient (Fig. 1a) is available. The images in Fig. 5a show the 180° and 360° reconstructions, respectively, from the same projection data used in Fig. 3a but with the modified Chang algorithm which utilizes the attenuation map. The 360° reconstruction shows excellent image quality while the 180° reconstruction

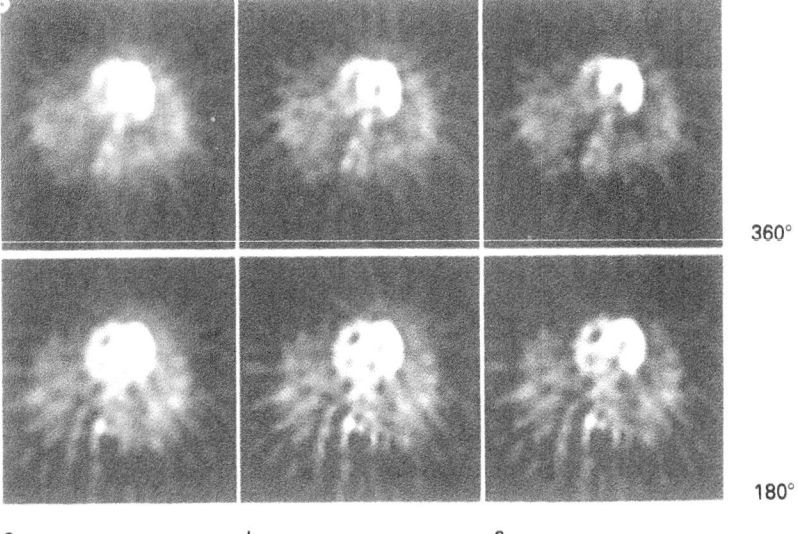

360°

180°

a   b   c

Figure 6. Same as Fig. 5 except that the projection data used in the reconstruction are the same as those used in generating the images in Fig. 3c.

exhibits a distinctive pattern of artifacts and distortions in the noise-free situation. The images in Figs. 5b and c are the same as those in Fig. 5a, except after postprocessing using the Metz filter to incorporate the average collimator MTF and additional scatter MTF, respectively. The sharpened features and increased contrast in the images are apparent.

Similar to Fig. 5, the images shown in Fig. 6 were obtained using the modified Chang algorithm and the same postprocessing filters, except that the projection data in reconstructing the images in Fig. 3c were used. The filtered images demonstrate the effects of the various filters on noisy data.

To demonstrate the performance of the iterative reconstruction methods, Fig. 7 shows reconstructed images obtained from the iterative ML-EM algorithm. The images in Fig. 7a were obtained with a projector and backprojector pair which assumes idealized imaging process, i.e. without any image degrading factors. For the reconstructed images in Fig. 7b, the projector and backprojector pair include the non-uniform attenuation distribution and for the reconstructed images in Fig. 7c, both the attenuation and collimator response function. By comparing the images in Figs. 3a and 7a, we see little difference between the FB and the iterative reconstruction algorithms when no compensation was incorporated.

The reconstructed images shown in Fig. 8 are obtained using the same reconstruction method as in Fig. 7. However, the noisy projection data used are the same as those used in generating the reconstructed images in Fig. 3c. Figure 9 shows the same reconstructed images after postprocessing with a Butterworth filter with a cut-off frequency of 0.25 cycles/pixel and an order

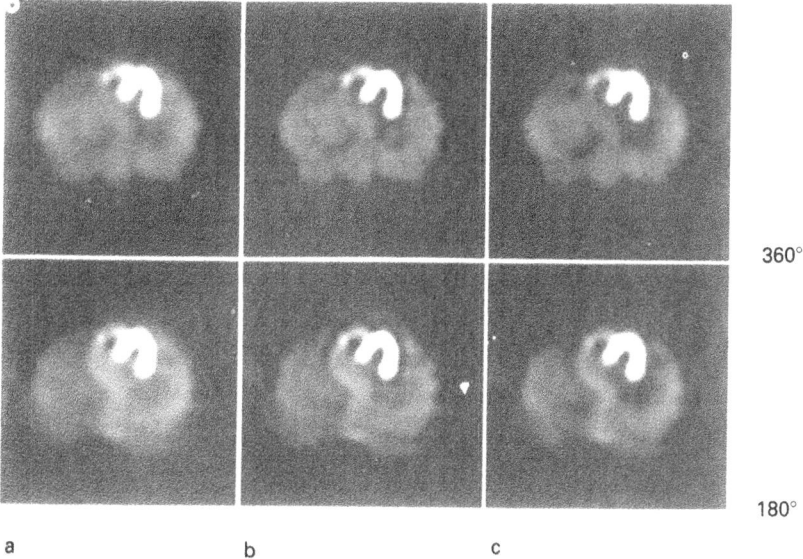

360°

180°

a   b   c

Figure 7. Transaxial reconstructed images of the cardiac-chest phantom obtained using the iterative ML-EM algorithm. Images in the upper and lower rows are from 360° and 180° reconstructions, respectively. The projection data used in the reconstruction are the same as that used in generating the images in Fig. 3a. The projector and backprojector pair used in the iterative method (a) assumes idealized imaging process, (b) incorporates the non-uniform attenuation distribution shown in Fig. 1a and (c) incorporates both the attenuation distribution and response function of the LEGP collimator. All reconstructed images result from 100 iterations.

of 8. The images in Figs. 8 and 9 show the improved image quality and quantitative accuracy obtained using the iterative reconstruction methods.

The quantitative accuracy of the reconstruction methods is assessed using the normalized mean-squared-error (NMSE) calculated from the difference between the reconstructed image and the emission phantom. Figure 10a shows a plot of NMSE as a function of iteration number for the iterative ML-EM reconstruction methods in comparison with the conventional reconstruction methods in the noise-free case. The results show the higher accuracy of the quantitative reconstruction methods.

For noisy data the image noise in the reconstructed images was evaluated by the normalized standard deviation calculated over a 33–pixel region-of-interest placed over the flat area of the background in the phantom image. The results shown in Fig. 10b support the observations found in Fig. 9 that at a low iterative number, with both attenuation and detector response compensation, the image noise is lower than that obtained without any compensation or with attenuation compensation alone. Also, the level of noise fluctuations is lower for the iterative ML-EM compared with the conventional reconstruction methods.

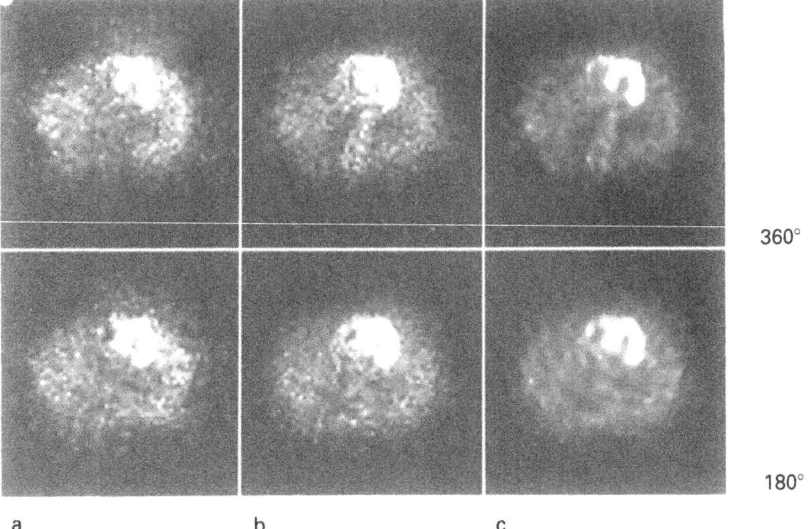

360°

180°

a   b   c

Figure 8. Same as Fig. 7 except that the noise projection data used in the reconstruction are the same as those used in generating the images in Fig. 3c.

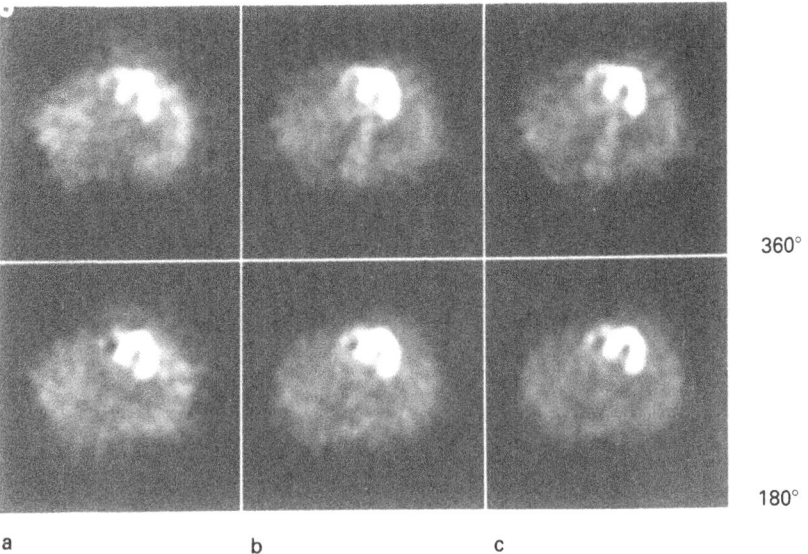

360°

180°

a   b   c

Figure 9. Same as Fig. 8 except that the reconstructed images are postprocessed using a Butterworth filter with cut-off frequency of 0.25 cycles/pixel and order of 8.

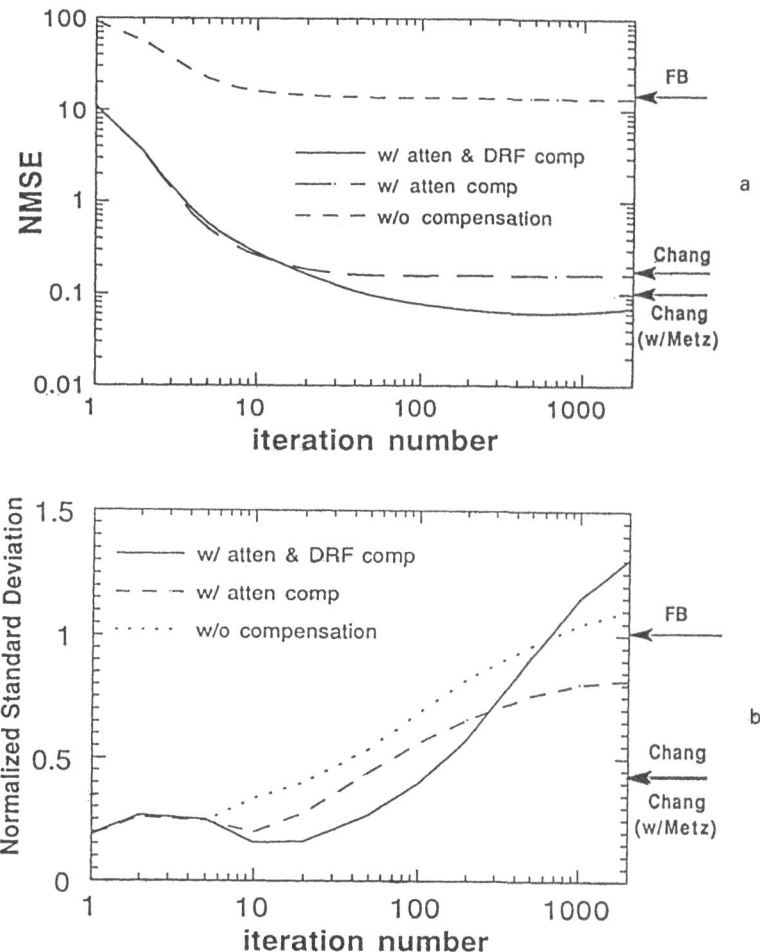

Figure 10. (a) Plot of the normalized mean-square-error (NMSE) between the phantom and the reconstructed images obtained using the iterative ML-EM algorithm with different projector and backprojector pairs as a function of iteration number. The NMSE from images obtained using the conventional reconstruction methods are also plotted for comparison. (b) Plot of the normalized standard deviation of images obtained from the same reconstruction methods.

5.4. Clinical study

The performance of the conventional and quantitative reconstruction methods were compared using data from a Tl-201 patient study. The attenuation distribution of the patient, information necessary for the quantitative reconstruction methods, was derived from transmission CT data acquired using a sheet source mounted on the GE SPECT system [21]. Figures 11a and b show a slice of the original and filtered transmission CT image. In Fig. 12, we show the emission reconstructed images at the same level as the transmis-

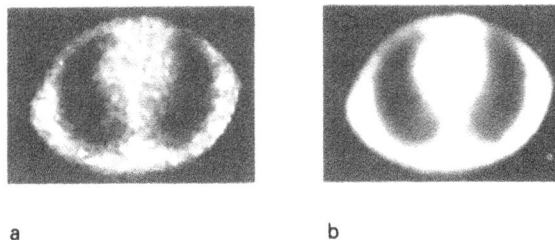

a   b

Figure 11. Transmission CT image through the myocardium from a patient study (a) before and (b) after filtering.

sion CT slice from the FB algorithm without any compensation (Fig. 12a), followed by filtering with a Metz filter which includes the collimator MTF (Fig. 12b) and from the Chang algorithm, which assumes that the attenuation distribution is uniform throughout the chest region (Fig. 12c). The image quality obtained with the conventional reconstruction and filtering methods is similar to that found in the simulation study.

In Fig. 13, the reconstructed image from the FB algorithm is compared with those obtained from the iterative ML-EM reconstruction method without any compensation, with compensation for attenuation by using the attenuation distribution map shown in Fig. 9b and with compensation for both

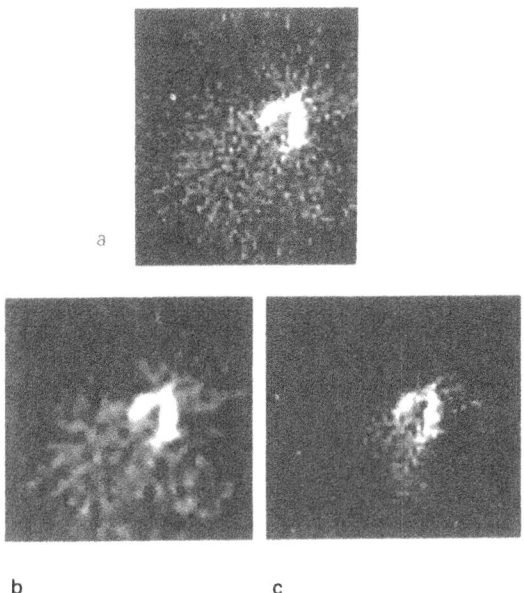

b   c

Figure 12. Transaxial reconstructed images from a clinical Tl-201 SPECT study. The images were reconstructed using the FB algorithm without any compensation (a) before and (b) after filtering with a Metz filter which incorporates the collimator MTF, and (c) using the Chang algorithm which assumes uniform attenuation throughout the body.

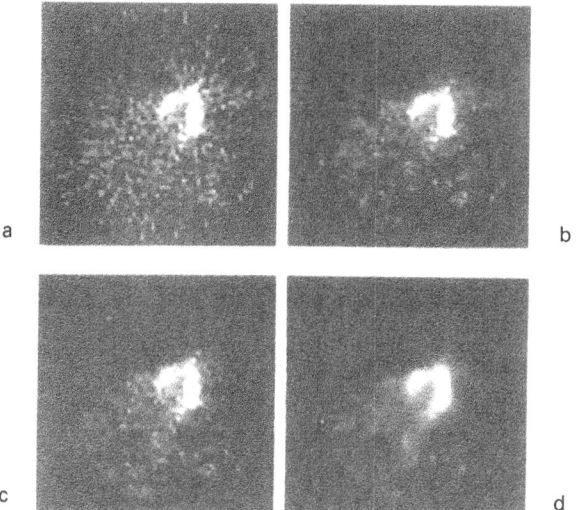

Figure 13. Transaxial reconstructed images from a clinical Tl-201 SPECT study. The images were reconstructed using (a) the FB algorithm without any compensation, and the iterative ML-EM algorithm using a projector and backprojector pair which (b) assumes idealized imaging process, (c) incorporates the attenuation distribution shown in Fig. 11b, and (d) incorporates both attenuation and collimator response function. The reconstructed images in (b) and (c) are results after 30 iterations and (d) after 50 iterations.

the non-uniform attenuation and detector response function. It is shown that without any compensation, the performance of the iterative reconstruction method is very similar to that of the conventional FB method. However, when compensation for attenuation and detector response is included, the iterative methods provide improved image quality not achievable by the conventional techniques.

6. Discussion

By using a realistic cardiac-chest phantom, we demonstrated the individual and combined effects of major image degrading factors on cardiac SPECT imaging. In particular, the non-uniform attenuation distribution of the thoracic region is the single most important image degrading factor. If not compensated, grossly inaccurate quantitative information, severe artifacts and distortions in the reconstructed image will result. The detector response function degrades the spatial resolution, and scatter radiation is responsible for lowering the contrast of the reconstructed image.

Conventional reconstruction and filtering methods only approximately compensate for the image degrading factors. In cardiac SPECT imaging, they are not effective in removing image artifacts and distortions, or in providing accurate quantitative information. Also, although 180° reconstruction gives better image contrast in the myocardial region, it generates more image artifacts and distortions as compared to 360° reconstruction.

Quantitative reconstruction methods, especially those using iterative algorithms, are effective in compensating for the non-uniform attenuation distribution in the chest region and the spatially variant detector response function. They also provide better noise smoothing without the expense of degradation in spatial resolution. The main disadvantage of iterative reconstruction methods is the large amount of computations involved. However, with advances in the development of iterative algorithms and computer hardware, implementation of these methods in clinical environments will be increasingly likely in the near future.

Acknowledgements

The author would like to acknowledge Mr. XiDe Zhao for his assistance in data analysis. This work was supported by the U.S. Public Health Grant #CA39463 and a research contract from the General Electric Medical Systems.

References

1. Jaszczak RJ, Coleman RE. Single photon emission computed tomography (SPECT): Principles and instrumentation. Invest Radiol 1985;20:897–910.
2. Fintel DJ, Links JM, Brinker JA, Frank TL, Parker M, Becker LC. Improved diagnostic performance of exercise thallium-201 single photon emission computed tomography over planar imaging in the diagnosis of coronary artery disease: a receiver operating characteristic analysis. J Am Coll Cardiol 1989;13:600–12.
3. Kiat H, Berman DS, Maddahi J. Comparison of planar and tomographic exercise thallium-201 imaging methods for the evaluation of coronary artery disease. J Am Coll Cardiol 1989;13:613–6.
4. Huesman RH, Gullberg GT, Greenberg WL, Budinger TF. User manual: Donner algorithms for reconstruction tomography. California: Lawrence Berkeley Laboratory, University of California, 1977.
5. Metz CE. A mathematical investigation of radioisotope scan image processing [dissertation]. [s.l.]: Univ. of Pennsylvania, 1969.
6. King MA, Schwinger RB, Doherty PW, Penney BC. Two-dimensional filtering of SPECT images using the Metz and Wiener filters. J Nucl Med 1984;25:1234–40.
7. King MA, Schwinger RB, Penney BC. Variation of the count-dependent Metz filter with imaging system modulation transfer function. Med Phys 1986;13:139–49.
8. Gilland DR, Tsui BM, McCartney WH, Perry JR, Berg J. Determination of the optimum filter function for SPECT imaging. J Nucl Med 1988;29:643–50.
9. Tamaki N, Mukai T, Ishii Y, Fujita T, Yamamoto K, Minato K, et al. Comparative study of thallium emission myocardial tomography with 180 degrees and 360 degrees data collection. J Nucl Med 1982;23:661–6.
10. Maublant JC, Peycelon P, Kwiatkowski F, Lusson JR, Standke RH, Veyre A. Comparison

between 180 degrees and 360 degrees data collection in technetium-99m MIBI SPECT of the myocardium. J Nucl Med 1989;30:295–300.

11. Go RT, MacIntyre WJ, Houser TS, Pantoja M, O'Donnel JK, Feiglin DH, et al. Clinical evaluation of 360 degrees and 180 degrees data sampling techniques for transaxial SPECT thallium-201 myocardial perfusion imaging. J Nucl Med 1985;26:695–706.

12. Knesaurek K. Comparison of 360 degrees and 180 degrees data collection in SPECT imaging. Phys Med Biol 1987;32:1445–56.

13. Tretiak OJ, Metz CE. The exponential Radon transform. SIAM J Appl Math 1980;39:341–54.

14. Gullberg GT, Budinger TF. The use of filtering methods to compensate for constant attenuation in single-photon emission computed tomography. IEEE Trans Biomed Eng 1981;28:142–57.

15. Kay DB, Keyes JW. First order corrections for absorption and resolution compensation in radionuclide Fourier tomography (abstract). J Nucl Med 1975;16:540–1.

16. Budinger TF, Gullberg GT, Huesman RH. Emission computer tomography. In: Herman GT, editor. Image reconstruction from projections: implementation and applications. Berlin: Springer 1979:147–246.

17. Chang LT. A method for attenuation correction in radionuclide computed tomography, IEEE Trans Nucl Sci 1978;25:638–42.

18. Manglos SH, Jaszczak RJ, Floyd CE, Hahn LJ, Greer KL, Coleman RE. Nonisotropic attenuation in SPECT: phantom tests of quantitative effects and compensation techniques. J Nucl Med 1987;28:1584–91.

19. Manglos SH, Jaszczak RJ, Floyd CE. Weighted backprojection implemented with a nonuniform attenuation map for improved SPECT quantitation. IEEE Trans Nucl Sci 1988;NS-35:625–8.

20. Tsui BM, HU HB, Gilland DR, Gullberg GT. Implementation of simultaneous attenuation and detector response correction in SPECT. IEEE Trans Nucl Sci 1988;35:778–83.

21. Tsui BM, Gullberg GT, Edgerton ER, Ballard JG, Perry JR, McCartney WH, et al. Correction of nonuniform attenuation in cardiac SPECT imaging. J Nucl Med 1989;30:497–507.

22. Shepp LA, Vardi Y. Maximum likelihood reconstruction for emission tomography. IEEE Trans Med Imaging 1982;MI-1:113–22.

23. Lange K, Carson R. EM reconstruction algorithms for emission and transmission tomography. J Comput Assist Tomogr 1984;8:306–16.

24. Levitan E, Herman GT. A maximum *a posteriori* probability expectation maximization algorithm for image reconstruction in emission tomography. IEEE Trans Med Imaging 1987;6:185–92.

25. Gullberg GT, Huesman RH, Malko JA, Pelc NJ, Budinger TF. An attenuated projector-backprojector for iterative SPECT reconstruction. Phys Med Biol 1985;30:799–816.

26. Tsui BM, Zhao XD, Frey EC, Gullberg GT. Comparison between ML-EM and WLS-CG algorithms for SPECT image reconstruction. IEEE Trans Nucl Sci. In press.

27. Gilland DR. An investigation of maximum likelihood-EM image reconstruction in single photon emission computed tomography. [dissertation]. Chapel Hill: Univ. of North Carolina, 1989.

3. Volume and activity quantitation in SPECT

MICHAEL A. KING and DAVID T. LONG

Summary

This chapter reviews some of the factors which influence the quantitation of volume and activity with SPECT imaging. For volume quantitation we first compare seven methods of volume quantitation, and then illustrate the bias caused to the measurement of volume by the blurring of the objects inherent in imaging. For activity quantitation, we discuss the influence of attenuation, scatter, and spatial resolution on the accuracy of activity estimation.

1. Introduction

One of the major advantages of single photon emission computed tomography (SPECT) over planar imaging is that SPECT results in a true three-dimensional (3D) image of the radionuclide distribution. As a result, quantitative analysis of SPECT images is possible because overlying structures, which can impede true quantitative analysis of planar images, are separated into their true 3D spatial relationships. As compared with visual assessment, quantitative analysis of nuclear medicine images offers the advantages of reduced inter- and intra-observer variability, and use of numerical criteria for separating normal from abnormal studies. Quantification of the volume of, or activity within, an organ, anatomical structure, or lesion plays a crucial role in quantitative analysis, and is the topic of this review.

2. Volume quantitation

2.1. *Planar imaging vs SPECT*

The volume of a source distribution can be estimated from single or multiple planar images given a geometrical model of the source. An example of this is the use of a prolate ellipsoid model for the cardiac ventricles [1,2]. With the assumptions that the concentration of activity is constant within the volume, and that locations within the volume are counted with approximately

Johan H.C. Reiber & Ernst E. van der Wall (eds.), Cardiovascular Nuclear Medicine and MRI, 47–60.
© 1992 *Kluwer Academic Publishers.*

the same sensitivity, changes in the background corrected counts are proportional to changes in the volume of the activity distribution. This has been used with planar imaging to quantitate changes in the relative volumes of the cardiac chambers as a function of time [3,4]. Non-geometric determination of the absolute volume of the ventricles has been accomplished by obtaining a blood sample from the patient and the use of either a regression relation obtained by comparison to contrast angiographic volumes [5], or attenuation correction of the counts from the ventricular regions of interest (ROIs) [6]. Geometric models have also been combined with use of the counts to obtain absolute volumes [7]. The determination of the volume occupied by a source distribution is, in principle, easier in SPECT slices than in planar images. This is because the third dimension, which is lacking in planar images, is provided in SPECT slices.

2.2. *Methods of SPECT volume quantitation*

The methods of SPECT volume quantitation can be broken up into either geometrical or count based methods. With geometrical methods, a definite 3D surface boundary is determined in some manner, and the volume is estimated as the sum of the voxels within the 3D boundary times the unit volume of a single voxel. The geometrical methods which have been used to determine the boundary location in SPECT can be classified as: 1) operator-determined regions of interest (ROI) [8,9], 2) fixed and adaptive count thresholding techniques [10–13], or 3) methods based on edge-detection using derivative operators [14,15]. With count based methods, the volume is calculated as the product of the volume of a voxel and the ratio of the total number of counts within the region determined by a geometrical method to the maximum count per voxel [16]. Count based methods assume that the concentration of activity is constant within the source volume. They provide estimated volumes which are less dependent on the boundary definition than the geometrical methods for high contrast objects.

Recently, a comparison of a number of methods of image segmentation for volume quantitation in SPECT was conducted [17]. The specific methods evaluated included: 1) operator drawn ROIs, 2) count-based correction of these ROIs, 3) fixed 50 %, 40 %, and 25 % count thresholds with interpolative correction for surrounding activity, 4) an adaptive thresholding technique based on gray-level histograms [14], 5) a two-dimensional (2D) gradient-based edge detection method, and 6) a 3D gradient-based edge detection method. Simulated SPECT images of six Tc-99m filled spheres in an elliptical cross-sectional attenuator were used to study volume quantitation with these methods. The diameters of the spheres were 6.0, 5.0, 4.0, 3.0, 2.0, and 1.5 cm, respectively, resulting in ideal sphere volumes of 113.1, 65.5, 33.5, 14.1, 4.2, and 1.8 cc, respectively. Simulated images were generated using a 3D

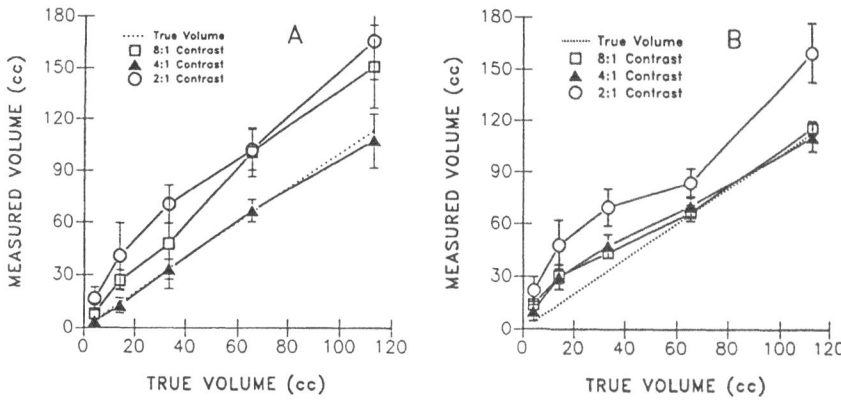

Figure 1. Plots of measured vs true volume for (a) Operator-drawn ROIs, and (b) Count-based correction of operator-drawn ROIs (reproduced with permission from ref. 17).

analytical, non-stationary simulation of SPECT for object to background activity contrast ratios of 8:1, 4:1, and 2:1. Poisson noise was introduced into the projection images, and five independent noise realizations were made for count levels of 100,000 counts per projection image. Pixel size was set at 0.58 cm.

Volume estimation results are shown in Figs. 1–3. In each figure, the average measured volume for the five noise realizations of each sphere are plotted on the ordinate axis with the true volume plotted on the abscissa. The error bars indicate the standard deviation. Volume data are shown for the 6.0, 5.0, 4.0, 3.0, and 2.0 cm diameters spheres. The dotted line indicates the line of identity between the true and measured volumes.

The results for the operator-drawn and count-based methods are shown in Fig. 1. The operator was given knowledge of the true shape of the objects, and encouraged to mark the regions with care. It can be seen that this resulted, on occasion, in excellent results (4:1 contrast Fig. 1A). However, the volumes were more commonly significantly overestimated and there was a very large standard deviation between the five noise realizations. Use of the count-based correction resulted in good agreement between the measured and true volumes for the 8:1 and 4:1 contrast spheres (Fig. 1B). However, as the contrast decreased to 2:1 the measured volumes were significantly larger than the true volumes. The results of Fig. 1B were obtained with the operator redefining his ROIs at the full extent of the spheres. When the original ROIs used to quantitate volume (Fig. 1A) were corrected by the count-based method, the volumes of the 6.0, 5.0, and 4.0 cm diameter spheres were consistently underestimated for the 8:1 and 4:1 contrast levels. Similarly, without the count-based correction, the volumes of the spheres drawn for use with count-based quantitation of volume overestimated the volumes consistently.

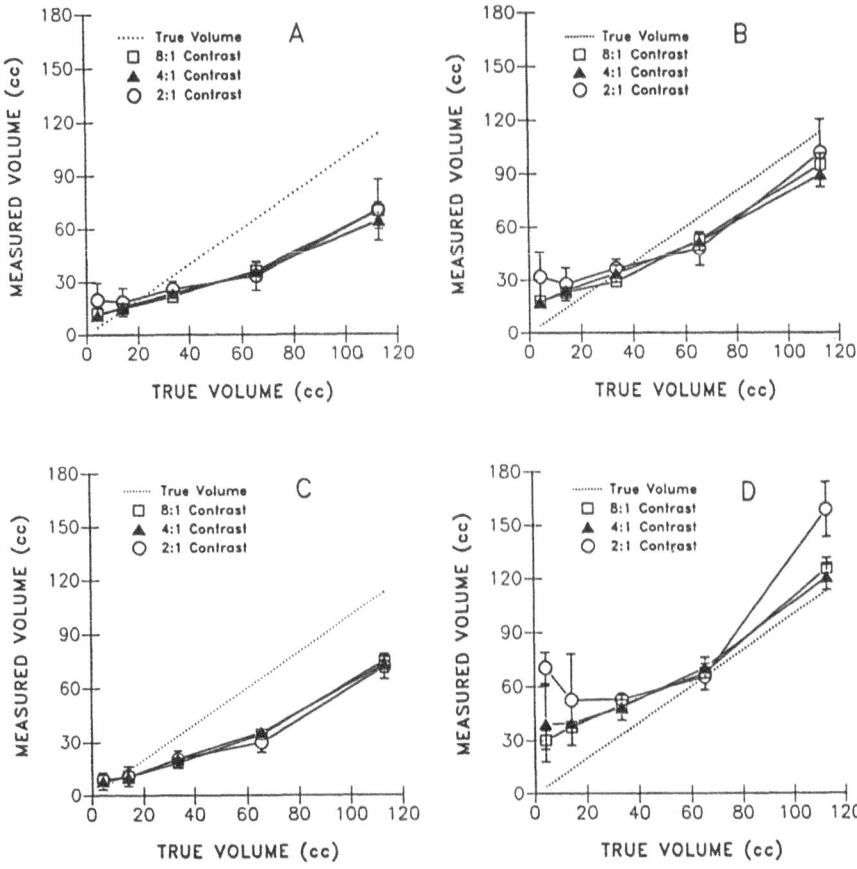

Figure 2. Plots of measured vs true volume for (a) fixed 50 % threshold, (b) fixed 40 % threshold, (c) fixed 25 % threshold with boundary voxels weighted by one-half, and (d) adaptive count threshold for each subregion (reproduced with permission from ref. 17).

The measured volumes by the thresholding methods are plotted in Fig. 2. Figure 2A shows the measured volumes underestimate the true volume of all but the smaller spheres when a 50 % threshold is employed. The volumes measured with 40 % and 25 % thresholds are also shown in Fig. 2 to illustrate what happens as the threshold changes. The volumes for the 25 % threshold would have been overestimated except for the inclusion of weighting the boundary voxels by one half [13]. The usefulness of the trilinear interpolative correction for surrounding activity is shown in Fig. 2 by the close agreement in the results with the different contrasts. Also shown in Fig. 2D are the results for an adaptive threshold method [11]. It was necessary to include trilinear interpolative correction with this method since without it the method was found to be very sensitive to contrast. Even with this correction, the method was found to produce a systematic overestimation of the volume of

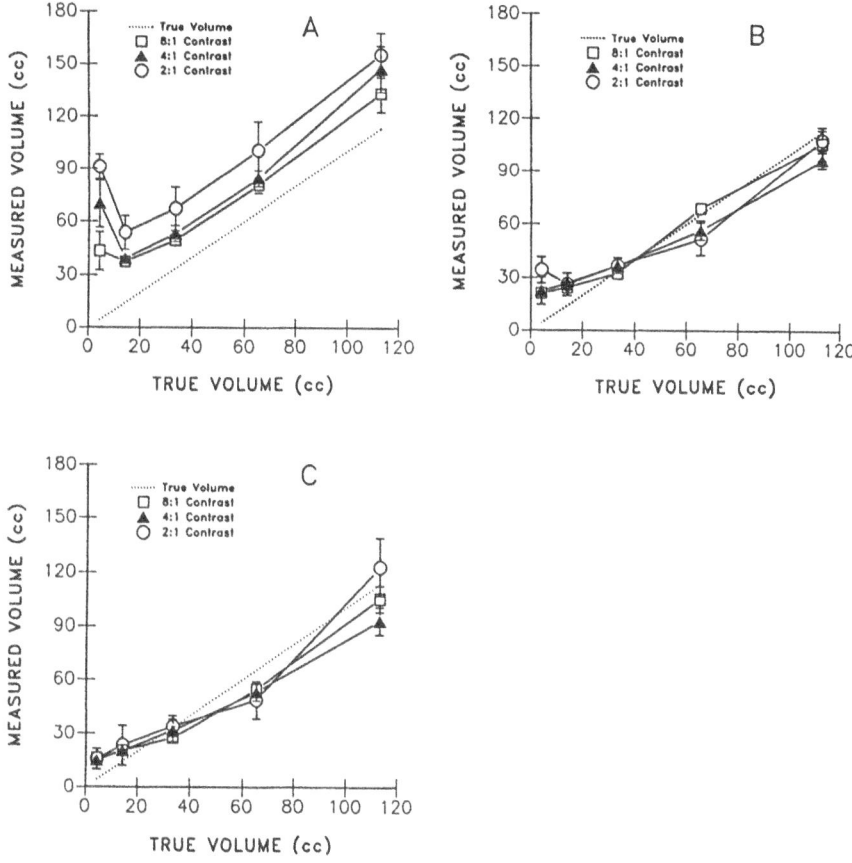

Figure 3. Plots of measured vs true volume for (a) 2D gradient-based edge detection, (b) 3D gradient-based edge detection, and (c) 3D zero crossing of directional second derivative (reproduced with permission from ref. 17).

the spheres which became worse with a decrease in contrast or size of the spheres.

The measured volumes for the gradient-based methods are shown in Fig. 3. Figure 3A shows that with the 2D method there is a consistent overestimation of sphere volume which seems to increase with decreased contrast. The 3D method (Fig. 3B) shows a small underestimate of sphere volume with the larger spheres which is independent of sphere contrast. The 3D gradient operator calculates the gradient as the maximum change in count in 3D normal to the surface of the spheres. Note that at the top of the spheres, the gradient direction is aligned with the Z axis, or perpendicular to the transverse slices. The 2D gradient operator applied to the transverse slices calculates the gradient based on the 2D disks which compose the individual tomographic slices. The inclusion of the Z axis or interslice component to the 3D gradient results in edges which 'close up' as the object boundary is resolved in the third dimension. Thus, for the 2D gradient method, object boundaries will be detected that extend beyond the range of those detected by the 3D gradient method. This causes an over-estimation of volume as shown in Fig. 3A.

At low object contrast levels and high noise levels the boundaries determined by the 3D gradient based method are not always closed [15]. When the region is determined by the zero-crossings of the second directional derivative operator, a closed boundary is determined each time [18,19]. The results for a 3D extension of the second directional derivative method are shown in Fig. 3C, and can be compared to the results for the 3D gradient with non-maximum suppression shown in Fig. 3B. Although second directional derivative operators are related to non-maximum suppression, the second directional derivative operator produces significantly more accurate volume quantitation than use of non-maximum suppression with the 3D gradient operator [19].

Of the methods compared, we believe the 3D second directional derivative method to be the most useful. This is because it diminishes the reproducibility, subjectivity, and tedious time consuming user-interaction problems associated with operator drawn boundaries, while producing a method which is reasonably accurate and consistent across changes in object contrast and volume.

2.3. *Influence of spatial resolution, and source size and shape on SPECT volume quantitation*

A number of factors influence the accuracy of estimation of source volume with SPECT. One of the most influential of these is the source size and shape relative to the system spatial resolution. In a recent investigation [20], a rectangular parallelepiped (bar), a right cylinder, and a sphere were mathematically modeled as being imaged with a SPECT system by calculating the 3D convolution of them with symmetric Gaussian functions. The resulting activity profiles were analyzed to determine the location of the edges as a function of the source size relative to the system full width at half-maximum (FWHM). The edge definition criteria studied were: 1) the location of the 50 % count threshold, and 2) the maximum in the local gradient. In addition, the threshold which yielded the correct edge location was also determined.

Figure 4 shows a plot of the percent error in the location of the edge determined by the 50 percent count threshold criterion along the x-axis of each of the three sources as a function of the ratio of the source width along the x-axis to the FWHM of the system blur. For the bar source, the estimated location of the edge is essentially equal to the actual location of the edge until the width of the object has decreased below 2 times the FWHM. Using a 50 % threshold to determine the location of the edge along the x-axis of

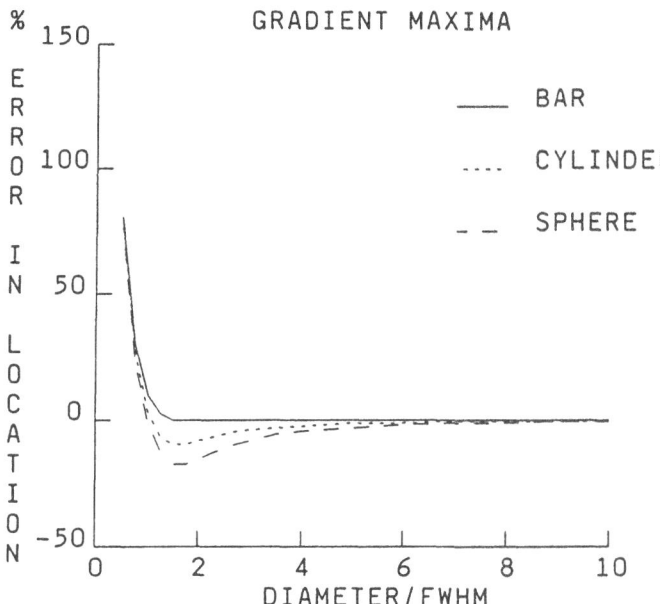

Figure 4. Plot of percent error according to 50 percent count threshold criterion in location of edge along x-axis of three source distributions as a function of the ratio of source width or diameter to spleen FWHM (reproduced with permission from ref. 20).

the cylindrical and spherical sources leads to an underestimate of the source volume even with large ratios of the diameter of the source to FWHM. Once the ratio decreases below 2.0, the edge starts to move back out, and eventually the volume is overestimated as the ratio increases further. The result is that the direction and amount of the error in the volume estimation depends on the shape of the source, and the ratio of the width of the source to the FWHM of the system.

A plot of the count threshold required to yield the correct location of the edge along the x-axis of each of the source distributions is presented in Fig. 5. There it can be seen that the threshold required for accurate edge location is a function of the source size and shape relative to the system FWHM.

Plots of the percent error in the location of the edge determined by the maximum local gradient criterion vs object width along the x-axis are given in Fig. 6 for the three source distributions. The results are similar to that of using the 50 percent threshold (Fig. 4) except that the negative errors display a greater maximum magnitude and continue negative to lower ratios. Also, the overestimation of source size is slightly less with the maximum gradient than it would be with the 50 percent threshold criterion for very small sources (diameter equal to FWHM or less). The pattern of under- and overestimation of source size is similar to that seen with the 3D gradient, and 3D directional

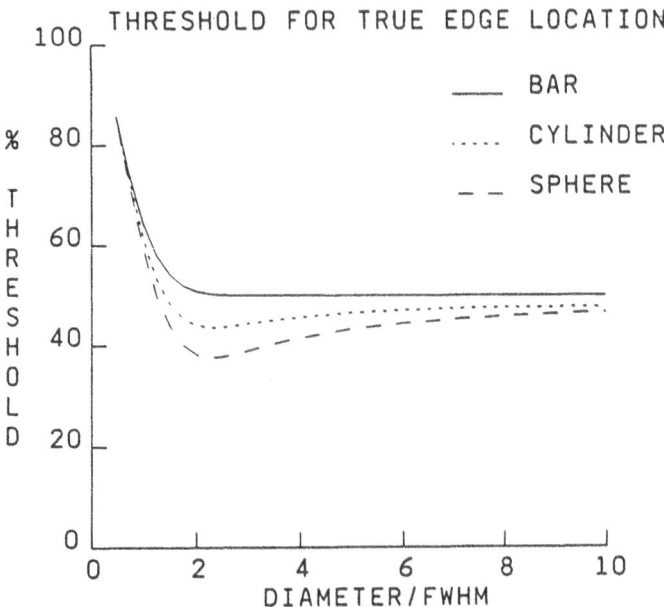

Figure 5. Plot of count threshold required to obtain the correct edge location as a function of the ratio of source width or diameter to septum. FWHM for three source distributions (reproduced with permission from ref. 20).

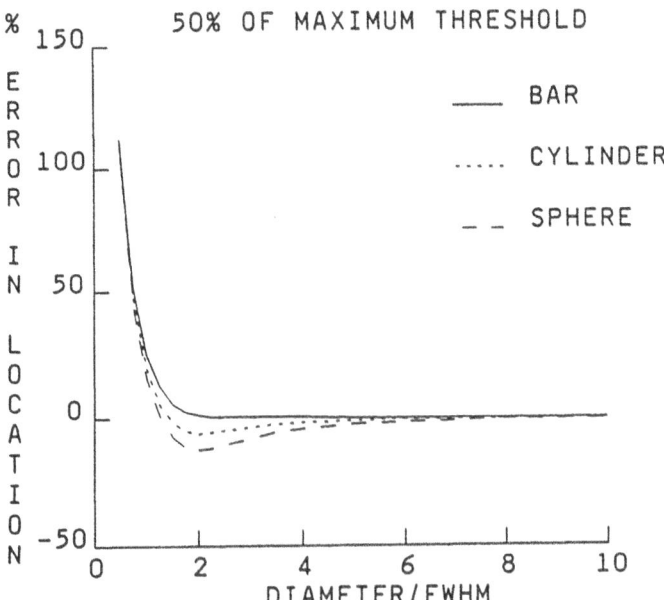

Figure 6. Plot of percent error according to maximum gradient criterion in location of edge along x-axis of three source distributions as a function of the ratio of source width or diameter to system FWHM (reproduced with permission from ref. 20).

second derivative methods of Fig. 3, and thus explains the biases observed with these methods.

3. Activity quantitation

3.1. *Planar imaging vs SPECT*

Methods which estimate activity from planar images have to address the problems of correcting for attenuation and the imaging of scattered photons, correcting for the contribution of counts from surrounding activity, identification of boundaries, and possibly correction for camera nonuniformity. Correction for attenuation and scatter is typically performed by using some combination of the counts from conjugate views [21–23]. One of the major problems with such methods is the correction of counts from over- or underlying tissues and organs. This, in principle, also is easier with SPECT, and thus is one of the advantages of SPECT quantitation over planar imaging.

3.2. *Attenuation correction of SPECT studies*

One of the major factors which must be addressed with activity quantitation is attenuation [24]. A number of attenuation correction methods have been developed for use with filtered backprojection. These include pre-reconstruction [25], post-reconstruction [26], and intrinsic methods [27–31]. Intrinsic methods solve explicitly for attenuation by inverting the Radon transform. In a comparison of a number of intrinsic correction methods for the case of uniform attenuation [32], the methods of Bellini, et al. [30], and Hawkins, et al. [31], were observed to yield the least positionally dependent three-dimensional modulation transfer function. Both of these methods are exact solutions for uniform attenuation within a convex body, and both make use of the frequency-distance relationship [33,34] to provide improvement in the signal-to-noise ratio of the reconstructions obtained with intrinsic attenuation compensation.

To perform attenuation correction for the case of non-uniform attenuation some estimate of the variation in the attenuation coefficient throughout the body is required. This can be obtained by using a planar source [35,36], or moving line source [37] with a parallel hole collimator, a point source with a cone beam collimator [38], or from CT images [39]. It has been noted that small errors in determining the body outline can significantly influence the accuracy of activity quantitation [40]; therefore, it would seem that simultaneous acquisition of the emission and transmission images is the desired approach. With filtered backprojection, both an iterative Chang post-correction [41], and a correction based upon simulated build-up functions [42] have been shown to improve the accuracy of quantitation. Alternatively, full iterative reconstruction can be used [43].

3.3. *Correction of scatter with SPECT imaging*

The interaction of the primary photons in the patient's body not only leads to a loss of counts for which attenuation correction is required; it also leads to the inclusion of misplaced or scattered events within the image. The inclusion of these events leads to a loss of contrast, and necessitates numerical compensation for them with attenuation correction. The best way to compensate for scatter would be to not include it in the image in the first place by using a camera system with excellent energy resolution. However, most SPECT systems available employ NaI (Tl) with its finite energy resolution. A number of scatter compensation techniques have been developed. These include: 1) decreasing the value of the linear attenuation coefficient used with attenuation correction to account for the additional scattered photons being images [44], 2) use of an average scatter fraction (SF) to numerically correct for scatter [44], 3) use of convolution methods to estimate the amount and spatial distribution of scatter [44–51], 4) use of an asymmetric energy window to decrease the amount of scatter imaged to begin with [44], 5) use of a fraction of the counts from a second (or multiple) lower energy window(s) to estimate scatter in the primary window [44,48,50,52,53], use of holospectral imaging [54], and 7) prediction of the number of scatter counts in each pixel by use of information from the energy spectrum of each pixel [55–57].

In Monte Carlo simulated energy spectra for NaI(Tl) [50,55], it was noted that scattered photons contribute more to the lower energy portion of the photopeak than the high energy side. It was, therefore, hypothesized that if the photopeak was divided into two non-overlapping energy windows, a regression relation could be obtained between the ratio of counts within these windows and the scatter fraction (SF) for counts within the total region [58]. This idea was tested by dividing the standard 20 % energy window used for Tc-99m imaging into two 10 % windows, and acquiring planar acquisitions of a point source at a number of locations in a 30×23 cm tub phantom. From these and acquisitions of the same source at the same locations in air, a regression between the SF and the window ratio was determined. When it was applied to correct the acquisitions of the point source in the tub on a pixel by pixel basis, the residual SF was reduced below 0.05. SPECT acquisitions were made of a 5 cm diameter sphere at the center of a tub phantom and a 5 cm sphere at one fourth, one half, and three fourths the distance from the center along the major axis of the phantom. When the activity at the center of the sphere was determined, a significant improvement in the accuracy of activity quantitation was noted with use of the dual photopeak method of scatter correction [58].

3.4. *Influence of spatial resolution on quantitation of activity*

At the center of small objects (objects whose width is less than 2 to 2.7 times the system FWHM depending on shape [59]), and at the edge of large objects, the finite spatial resolution of the system blurs the counts out such that the counts per voxel are distorted [59]. Since the FWHM varies with location and direction in SPECT, this can cause a variation in the maximal counts determined in extended thin objects [60,61]. A number of methods have been tried to diminish the influence of spatial resolution on quantitation. These include: 1) the use of recovery coefficients [59,60], 2) the use of restoration filters [62], and maximum-likelihood estimation from the projection data [63,64] and in the slices themselves [65].

Acknowledgements

The authors would like to acknowledge many useful conversations with and several presentations of Ernest V. Garcia, Ph.D. and Benjamin M.W. Tsui, Ph.D., on the topic of SPECT volume and activity quantitation. We would also like to acknowledge our past and present colleagues whose work forms the basis for much of this manuscript. This work was supported in part by the National Cancer Institute under PHS Grants CA 42165 and CA 50641.

References

1. Strauss HW, Zaret BL, Hurley PJ, Natavajan TK, Pitt B. A scintiphotographic method for measuring left ventricular ejection fraction in man without cardiac catheterization. Am J Cardiol 1971;28:575–80.
2. Seldin DW, Easer PD, Nichols AB, Ratner SJ, Alderson PO. Left ventricular volume determined from scintigraphy and digital angiography by a semi-automated geometric method. Radiology 1983;149:809–13.
3. Parker JA, Secker-Walker R, Hill R, Siegel BA, Potchen EJ. A new technique for the calculation of left ventricular ejection fraction. J Nucl Med 1972;13:649–51.
4. Reiber JH, Lie SP, Simoons ML, et al. Clinical validation of fully automated computation of ejection fraction from gated equilibrium blood-pool scintigrams. J Nucl Med 1983;24:1099–107.
5. Dehmer GJ, Lewis SE, Hillis LD, et al. Nongeometric determination of left ventricular volumes from equilibrium blood pool scans. Am J Cardiol 1980;45:293–300.
6. Links JM, Becker LC, Shindledecker JG, et al. Measurement of absolute left ventricular volume from gated blood pool studies. Circulation 1982;65:82–91.
7. Massardo T, Gal RA, Grenier RP, Schmidt DH, Port SC. Left ventricular volume calculation using a count-based ratio method applied to multigated radionuclide angiography. (published erratum appears in J Nucl Med 1990;31:1449). J Nucl Med 1990;31:450–6.
8. Keyes JW Jr, Brady TJ, Leonard PF, et al. Calculation of viable and infarcted myocardial mass from thallium-201 tomograms. J Nucl Med 1981;22:339–43.

9. Lee KH, Liu HT, Chin DC, Siegel ME, Ballard S. Volume calculation by means of SPECT: analysis of imaging acquisition and processing factors. Radiology 1988;167:259–62.

10. Tauxe WN, Soussaline F, Todd-Pokropek A, et al. Determination of organ volume by single-photon emission tomography. J Nucl. Med 1982;23:984–7.

11. Strauss LG, Cloris JH, Frank T, Van Kaick G. Single photon emission computerized tomography (SPECT) for estimates of liver and spleen volume. J Nucl Med 1984;25:81–5.

12. Mortelmans L, Nuyts J, Van Pamel G, Van den Maegdenbergh V, De Roo M, Suetens P. A new thresholding method for volume determined by SPECT. Eur J Nucl Med 1986;12:284–90.

13. Mut F, Glickman S, Marciano D, Hawkins RA. Optimum processing protocols for volume determination of the liver and spleen from SPECT imaging with technetium-99m sulfur colloid. J Nucl Med 1988;29:1768–75.

14. Kircos LT, Carey JE Jr, Keyes JW Jr. Quantitative organ visualization using SPECT. J Nucl Med 1987;28:334–41.

15. Long DT, King MA, Penney BC. 2D vs 3D edge detection as a basis for volume quantitation in SPECT. In: Ortendahl DA, Leacer J, editors. Information processing in medical imaging. New York: Wiley-Liss, 1991:457–71.

16. Caputo GR, Graham MM, Brust KD, Kennedy JW, Nelp WB. Measurement of left ventricular volume using single-photon emission computed tomography. Am J Cardiol 1985;56:781–6.

17. Long DT, King MA, Sheehan J. Comparative evaluation of image segmentation methods for volume quantitation in SPECT. Med Phys. In press.

18. Canny J. A computational approach to edge detection. IEEE Trans Patt Anal Mach Intell 1986;8:679–98.

19. Gennert MA, Gosselin DR, King MA, Long DT. A comparison of 3D methods for volume quantitation in SPECT. Information Processing in Medical Imaging. In press.

20. King MA, Long DT, Brill AB. SPECT volume quantitation: influence of spatial resolution, source size and shape, and voxel size. Med Phys. In press.

21. Graham LS, Neil R. In vivo quantitation of radioactivity using the Anger camera. Radiology 1974;112:441–2.

22. Wu RK, Siegel JA. Absolute quantitation of radioactivity using the buildup factor. Med Phys 1984;11:189–92.

23. Doherty P, Schwinger R, King M, Gionet M. Distribution and dosimetry of indium-111 labeled F(ab')$_2$ fragments in humans. In: Schlafke-Stelson A, Wetson E, editors. Fourth international radiopharmaceutical dosimetry symposium: Oak Ridge, Tenessee: Dept of Energy, 1985:464–76.

24. Jaszczak RJ, Coleman RE, Whitehead FR. Physical factors affecting quantitative measurements using camera-based single photon emission computed tomography (SPECT). IEEE Trans Nucl Sci 1981;28:69–80.

25. Larsson SA. Gamma camera emission tomography. Development and properties of a multi-sectional computed tomography system. Acta Radiol Suppl. (Stockh) 1980;363:1–75.

26. Chang LT. Method for attenuation correction in radionuclide computed tomography. IEEE Trans Nucl Sci 1978;25:638–43.

27. Tretiak O, Metz C. The exponential radon transform. SIAM J Appl Math 1980;39:341–54.

28. Gullberg GT, Budinger TF. The use of filtering methods to compensate for constant attenuation in single-photon emission computed tomography. IEEE Trans Biomed Eng 1981;28:142–57.

29. Tanaka E, Toyama H, Murayama H. Convolutional image reconstruction for quantitative single photon emission computed tomography. Phys Med Biol 1984;29:1489–500.

30. Bellini S, Piacentini M, Cafforio C, Rocca F. Compensation of tissue absorption in emission tomography. IEEE Trans Acou Speech Signal Process 1979;27:213–8.

31. Hawkins WG, Leichner PK, Yang N. The circular harmonic transform for SPECT recon-

struction and boundary conditions on the Fourier transform of the sinogram. IEEE Trans Med Imaging 988;7:135–48.

32. Glick SJ, Hawkins WG, King MA, et al. Choice of intrinsic attenuation correction method and the three-dimensional transfer function of SPECT. Med Phys. In press.

33. Edholm PR, Lewitt RM, Lindholm B. Novel properties of the Fourier decomposition of the sinogram. Proc SPIE 1986;671:8–18.

34. Hawkins WG, Yang N, Leichner PK. Validation of the circular harmonic transform (CHT) algorithm for quantitative SPECT. J Nucl Med 1991;32:141–50.

35. Malko JA, Van Heertum RL, Gullberg GT, Kowalsky WP. SPECT liver imaging using an iterative attenuation correction algorithm and an external flood source. J Nucl Med 1986;27:701–5.

36. Bailey DL, Hutton BF, Walker PJ. Improved SPECT using simultaneous emission and transmission tomography. J Nucl Med 1987;28:844–51.

37. Tan P, Bailey DL, Hutton BF, et al. A moving line source for simultaneous transmission/emission SPECT (abstract). J Nucl Med 1989;30:964.

38. Manglos SH, Bassano DA, Duxbury CE, Capone RB. Attenuation maps for SPECT determined using cone beam transmission computed tomography. IEEE Trans Nucl Sci 1990;37:600–8.

39. Fleming JS. A technique for using CT images in attenuation correction and quantification in SPECT. Nucl Med Commun 1989;10:83–97.

40. Hosoba M, Wani H, Toyama H, Murata H, Tanaka E. Automated body contour detection in SPECT: effects on quantitative studies (see comments). J Nucl Med 1986;27:1184–91. Comment in: J Nucl Med 1989;30:266–7.

41. Manglos SH, Jaszczak RJ, Floyd CE, Hahn LJ, Greer KL, Coleman RE. Nonisotropic attenuation in SPECT: phantom tests of quantitative effects and compensation techniques. J Nucl Med 1987;28:1584–91.

42. Ljungberg M, Strand SE. Attenuation correction in SPECT based on transmission studies and Monte Carlo simulations of build-up functions. J Nucl Med 1990;31:493–500.

43. Tsui BM, Gullberg GT, Edgerton ER, et al. Correction of nonuniform attenuation in cardiac SPECT imaging. J Nucl Med 1989;30:497–507.

44. Jaszczak RJ, Floyd CE, Coleman RE. Scatter compensation techniques for SPECT. IEEE Trans Nucl Sci 1985;32:786–93.

45. Axelsson B, Msaki P, Israelsson A. Subtraction of Compton-scattered photons in single photon emission computerized tomography. J Nucl Med 1984;25:490–4.

46. Floyd CE Jr, Jaszczak RJ, Greer KL, Coleman RE. Deconvolution of Compton scatter in SPECT. J Nucl Med 1985;26:403–8.

47. Msaki P, Axelsson B, Dahl CM, Larsson SA. Generalized scatter correction method in SPECT using point scatter distribution functions. J Nucl Med 1987;28:1861–9.

48. Gilardi MC, Bettinardi V, Todd-Pokropek A, Milanesi L, Fazio F. Assessment and comparison of three scatter correction techniques in single photon emission computed tomography. J Nucl Med 1988;29:1971–9.

49. Frey EC, Tsui BM. Parameterization of the scatter response function in SPECT imaging using Monte Carlo simulation. IEEE Trans Nucl Sci 1990;37:1308–15.

50. Ljungberg M, Msaki P, Strand SE. Comparison of dual window and convolution scatter correction techniques using the Monte-Carlo method. Phys Med Biol 1990;35:1099–110.

51. Ljungberg M, Strand SE. Scatter and attenuation correction in SPECT using density maps and Monte Carlo simulated scatter functions. J Nucl Med 1990;31:1560–7.

52. Jaszczak RJ, Greer KL, Floyd CE Jr, Harris CC, Colenian RE. Improved SPECT quantification using compensation for scattered photons. J Nucl Med 1984;25:893–900.

53. Koral KF, Swailem FM, Buchbinder S, et al. SPECT dual-energy window Compton correction: scatter multiplier required for quantitation. J Nucl Med 1990;31:90–8.

54. Gagnon D, Todd-Pokropek A, Arsenault A, Dupras G. Introduction to holospectral imag-

ing in nuclear medicine for scatter subtraction. IEEE Trans Med Imaging 1989;8:245–50.

55. Koral KF, Wang XQ, Rogers WL, Clinthorne NH, Wang XH. SPECT Compton-scattering correction by analysis of energy spectra. J Nucl Med 1988;29:195–202.

56. Rosenthal MS, Henry LJ. Evaluation and comparison of two scatter correction techniques (abstract). J Nucl Med 1990;31:873.

57. Logan KW, McFarland WD. Single photon scatter compensation by photopeak energy distribution analysis. IEEE Trans Nucl Sci. In press.

58. King MA, Ljungberg M, Hademenos G, Glick SJ. A dual photopeak window method for scatter correction (abstract). J Nucl Med. In press.

59. Kessler RM, Ellis JR Jr, Eden M. Analysis of emission tomographic scan data: limitations imposed by resolution and background. J Comput Assist Tomogr 1984;8:514–22.

60. Galt JR, Garcia EV, Robbins WL. Effects of myocardial wall thickness on SPECT quantification. IEEE Trans Med Imaging 1990;9:144–50.

61. Maniawski PJ, Morgan HT, Wackers FJ. Orbit related variation in spatial resolution as a source of artifactual defects in Tl-201 SPECT (abstract). J Nucl Med 1990;31:718.

62. King MA, Coleman M, Penney BC, Glick SJ. Activity quantitation in SPECT: A study of pre-reconstruction Metz filtering and use of the scatter degradation factor. Med Phys. In press.

63. Huesman RH. A new fast algorithm for the evaluation of regions of interest and statistical uncertainty in computed tomography. Phys Med Biol 1984;29:543–52.

64. Carson RE. A maximum likelihood method for region-of-interest evaluation in emission tomography. J Comput Assist Tomogr 1986;10:654–63.

65. Muller SP, Kijewski MF, Moore SC, Holman BL. Maximum-likelihood estimation: a mathematical model for quantitation in nuclear medicine. J Nucl Med 1990;31:1693–701.

4. Computer techniques for quality control in planar imaging and SPECT

L. STEPHEN GRAHAM, KITHSIRI B. HERATH and
JUDY NEGRETE

Summary

The sophistication of modern imaging instruments requires a comprehensive quality control program. The spread of differential uniformity and the Uniformity Index is known to be a sensitive measure of field uniformity but should be supplemented with a visual display of nonuniform areas. Spatial resolution can be quantitated by Fourier techniques that appear to be sensitive to small changes with time. SPECT imaging systems require additional calibrations and quality control. Periodic calibration of the Center-of-Rotation will prevent loss of spatial resolution in clinical studies. High count floods are needed for studies that involve high count density but may not be required for low count density imaging (e.g. Tl-201). On a quarterly basis two additional studies should be done with phantoms. Reconstructions of a line source is useful for monitoring system spatial resolution. Reconstructions of a Jaszczak phantom provide information on image noise, contrast, the presence of artifacts, and the accuracy of attenuation correction.

Introduction

The sophistication of modern imaging instruments demands a comprehensive quality control (QC) program for planar imaging and Single-Photon-Emission-Computed-Tomography (SPECT). The presence of automatic tuning and energy and linearity correction circuits on most state-of-the-art cameras does not obviate the need for quality control. It has been documented that a lack of uniformity can be a serious problem in the interpretation of scintillation images [1]. It was found that overall accuracy of interpretation decreases with increasing nonuniformity. In addition, it must be noted that nonuniformities that are not visible in ordinary flood field QC images can produce ring artifacts in SPECT studies. Although analog techniques are useful for evaluating the performance of scintillation cameras, computer techniques provide more sensitive and objective measures and facilitate the appreciation of temporal changes. They also provide the potential for automated evaluation and the use of action levels.

Johan H.C. Reiber & Ernst E. van der Wall (eds.), Cardiovascular Nuclear Medicine and MRI, 61–74.
© 1992 *Kluwer Academic Publishers.*

Planar flood field uniformity

When a distant point source of radiation is used to expose the uncollimated detector of an Anger scintillation camera, the resultant image will show variations in the number of detected photons per cell. Some of the variation is expected since each cell in the image is a Poisson random variable. In addition, variations will be caused by spatial distortions and changes in point-source sensitivity across the detector [2–4]. Uniformity is often judged by looking at images recorded on x-ray film. Although it has been suggested that some quantitative statements can be made after viewing these images, it is generally agreed that this method cannot distinguish subtle variations in field uniformity.

Data acquisition

For a comprehensive quality control program it is important that techniques be available for the quantitation of field uniformity. From the standpoint of camera setup, the first decision must be to determine the number of counts to be collected. Quality control flood field images typically contain 1.25 million (small field-of-view), 2.5 million (large field-of-view), or 4 million (rectangular large field-of-view) counts [5]. Flood field images that are to be used for acceptance testing contain counts ranging from 14 million to 20 million [6]. The former has the advantage of requiring less time; the latter provides images that are less subject to statistical errors. As will be discussed below, some indices of uniformity can be used on images containing a relatively small number of counts; others require many more counts.

A decision must also be made as to whether intrinsic or system uniformity is to be measured. Intrinsic methods expose the technologist to less radiation and are useful for testing field uniformity for different photon energies [5,7]. However, they are more time consuming because the collimator must be removed. System methods are faster and test for collimator damage, but produce higher personnel exposure. In addition, if liquid-filled phantoms are used, extra care is required to thoroughly mix the solution of Tc-99m.

Data analysis

Over the years several numerical methods have been suggested for measuring uniformity when the Anger scintillation camera is interfaced to a computer. A study by Sharp and Marshall was carried out to investigate the effectiveness of four indices for measuring image uniformity: 1) Integral nonuniformity; 2) Differential nonuniformity; 3) Coefficient of variation of the counts per element; 4) The width of the frequency distribution of the contrast between neighboring elements (spread of differential uniformity) [8]. Spearmans rank correlation coefficient was used to see how well the subjective impression of uniformity agreed with the values provided by each of the objective measures [9]. Further, the sensitivity (i.e., the degree of change of each of the four indices that indicates a significant subjective change in image uniformity) of each index in assessing uniformity was investigated.

A significant correlation (r = 0.4–0.87) was found between the objective measures of uniformity and subjective assessments, except between the integral uniformity values and the black and white analog images (r < 0.4). For both analog and digitized images, the mean correlation coefficients for measure four (the spread of differential uniformity) were highest, while integral uniformity had the lowest correlation. In general, the correlation for color images were higher than black and white ones.

In their estimations the sensitivity of each measure of uniformity was about 10 %. If a change of two standard deviations indicates a significant difference, they conclude that a 20 % change in the uniformity measure would be needed to produce visually perceptible differences in uniformity.

A subsequent study by Hughes and Sharp revealed that all four indices showed a marked dependence on count density over a range of 1–30 million counts per image [10]. The four indices for the smoothed (9 point smoothing according to NEMA specifications) 10M count images were significantly smaller than those for the 30M count images for all the three cameras (t-test, p < 0.05).

The daily variability of the indices as a function of count density was also measured. At higher count densities the indices were sensitive to variations in detector response rather than Poisson noise which indicates that a genuine change in camera performance would cause a significant alteration in the indices. With the exception of the smoothed images, a large part of the daily variability of the two indices specified by NEMA (indices 1 and 2) was shown to be due to the poor reproducibility of the indices themselves, whereas the indices 3 and 4 were only responsible for approximately half of the variation observed from day to day. A fifth index, the 'Uniformity Index' derived by Cox and Diffey, was also estimated [11,12]. It is based on the total variance of all the pixels in the flood, minus the Poisson variance of each pixel, and hence it is much less dependent on the count density than the spread of differential uniformity. The Poisson variance is estimated by the average pixel count.

The sensitivity of the indices to the presence of a computer simulated cold spot as a function of count density was also quantitated by them. Of all, the most effective for detecting the presence of the cold spot artifact, the spread of differential uniformity, had displayed the greatest sensitivity at all count densities. The authors of this paper have found that for low count images (2.5 million), the weekly change in the uniformity index was more sensitive than integral or differential uniformity.

Either the spread of differential uniformity which requires on the order of 30 million counts, or the uniformity index which requires 5–10 million counts, can be profitably supplemented by a different measure. Keyes et al. proposed measuring the number of pixels in the computer image where the counts fell within an acceptable range [13]. A computer image was then generated with pixels outside the acceptable range highlighted. The acceptable range was centered around the average pixel count and was a specified percent of the average pixel count. Extending the acceptable range by twice the square root of the average pixel count was intended to compensate for the Poisson nature of each pixel count.

Computer images produced by the method of Keyes et al. [13] provide an indication of focal nonuniformity based on the highlighted locations of the pixels outside the acceptable range. Overall uniformity can be measured with the Keyes method using the number of pixels in the acceptable range.

Hence the conclusion is that the indices specified by NEMA to measure camera nonuniformity do not appear to be very sensitive. A more acceptable alternative appears to be to use those indices calculated using all the pixels in the images and to supplement these data with an image showing the location of nonuniformities.

An interesting alternative for evaluating uniformity was proposed in 1986 by Grossman et al. [14]. Their method was designed to separate stochastic and non-stochastic effects by calculating the noise power spectrum which carries information about the patterns of noise in flood field images. In their initial implementation only small regions in the center of the field were utilized. Borm and Busemann-Sokole recently described a similar technique for checking A/D and D/A artifacts [15]. They evaluated the entire field-of-view. However, it seems unlikely that this method would be useful for routine quality control by the technical staff.

Action levels

A logical extension of the calculation of numerical indices is the use of action levels. The IAEA recommends that action levels be set at 20 % for most scintillation camera performance parameters [16]. Unfortunately, TECDOC-317 [16] does not describe the logic behind selection of 20 % as an action level. However, it is interesting to note that Sharp and Marshall had found that a 20 % change in the uniformity measure was needed to produce visually perceptible differences in uniformity as described above. On the other hand, Kasal et al. had reported that a functional change in FWHM of approximately 10 % produced a perceptible change in image quality over a considerable range of values of the full-width-at-half-maximum (FWHM) [17]. More work needs to be done in this area.

Expert systems

Slomka and Todd-Pokropek are currently developing an expert system for use in quality control [18]. Highly automated quality control protocols seem appropriate for busy departments and/or centers where experience in imaging with a scintillation camera is limited. The system will provide intelligent responses in cases of abnormal function. It compares observed features in flood field images with predefined configurations. The data base will include different types of cameras, results from many cameras, tolerance limits, and recommend actions to be taken.

Spatial resolution

Properly exposed four quadrant bar pattern analog images can be useful for evaluating camera intrinsic spatial resolution. The same is true of digital images provided there is adequate spatial sampling. The general rule-of-thumb is that the full-width-at-half-maximum is approximately 1.8 times the minimum bar pattern spacing that can just be resolved [5]. To sample the entire field in both dimensions eight images are needed. If a PLES phantom with small bar spacing (FWHM/1.8) can be found, only two images are needed. Of course it must be kept in mind that the display system and/or the formatter may produce a loss of spatial resolution independent of the camera.

Although the FWHM of line spread functions can be used to quantitate spatial resolution, it only provides information about one region and is probably inappropriate for routine quality control measurements. We have investigated the feasibility of analyzing bar pattern images using Fourier analysis. Profiles automatically drawn perpendicular to the bars of a four quadrant pattern are processed using a FFT algorithm to output the dominant frequency and its amplitude. The amplitude can be expressed as a percent of a benchmark amplitude measured at the time of acceptance testing or by comparison with the DC value. By using three profiles oriented radially, the change in resolution across a quadrant can be evaluated.

Preliminary work by the authors of this manuscript indicates the method shows promise. A 25 % loss of spatial resolution caused by a noisy computer ADC produced a 25 % decrease in the amplitude of the dominant frequency of 3.5 mm bars (Table 1). Analysis of bar pattern images on an older camera revealed poor linearity as an increase in the dominant frequency from the center of the field to the edge (Table 2). Although there are potential problems, rotation of the bars relative to the camera/computer axes, a loss of resolution due to 'grid cutoff,' and inadequate digital sampling on some computer systems, only the latter appears to be a significant limitation in the use of this technique.

Table 1. Change in amplitude of dominant frequency (Siemens Orbiter 75)

Amplitude*		
Stationary bar pattern	Bar pattern rotated	Loss of amplitude
13.6 %	18.2 %	25 %
12.8 %	13.1 %	–
3.4 %	6.8 %	50 %
2.0 %	1.7 %	–

*Calculated as percent of DC value.

Table 2. Change of dominant frequency as a function of radial distance from center

ROI location	Dominant frequency (cycles/cm)			
	Quadrant 1		Quadrant 2	
	Tech S420	Siem Orb 75	Tech S420	Siem Orb 75
Center	1.42	1.24	2.27	2.17
Middle	1.42	1.24	2.27	2.17
Outside	1.71	1.24	2.56	2.17

SPECT

Although the value of quality control for planar imaging must not be underestimated, it is of even more critical importance in SPECT. A camera may be operating at the peak of its ability as a planar imaging instrument but give SPECT images that contain no more, or perhaps even less, information than can be obtained from a planar study. More seriously, artifacts can be present that will produce incorrect diagnoses. The goal of quality control tests must be to provide the highest level of confidence that all components, hardware and software, are working properly, not just to provide information for the quality control file.

Spatial Resolution

Because of the importance of spatial resolution in SPECT studies it is important to periodically verify that the software for performing the center-of-rotation correction is working properly, especially after any modification of software [19,20]. Verification is also needed after service on the interface and/or analog-to-digital converter (ADC).

The best method for measuring spatial resolution in tomographic images involves use of the phantom described in the 1986 edition of Performance Measurements of Scintillation Cameras, section 4.4.3 [6]. At the present time, performance values measured in accordance with this document have been published by only two vendors. The phantom is commercially available

(Nuclear Associates, Carle Place, NY) and consists of a lucite cylinder 20 cm in diameter which contains three line sources. When all three lines are filled with Tc-99m, streak artifacts sometimes interfere with calculation of the full-width-at-half-maximum (FWHM), especially if less than 180 views are used. This problem is not present if only the central line is filled with radioactivity.

A simpler procedure can be used to determine the extent to which resolution is lost when tomography is performed [21]. The camera should be set with a 15 or 20 % symmetrical window (whichever is used clinically) and the count rate should not exceed 20000 cps. A general purpose collimator should be used for this study and the phantom must be parallel to the axis of rotation. A circular orbit of radius 200 mm is appropriate for most cameras.

The AAPM and NEMA recommend use of 256 × 256 matrices [22,6]. As an alternative, a 128 × 128 matrix can be used with a two-fold zoom. In the author's experience a 128 × 128 matrix without zoom is satisfactory. For a single line source, adequate angular sampling can be obtained with 120 (128) views. Each view should contain at least 100,000 counts. The highest resolution filter that is available, preferably a ramp or its equivalent, must be used for reconstruction. Both attenuation and uniformity correction can be applied but this is not necessary.

Two different transverse sections, each 10 ± 3 mm in thickness, should be used for evaluating spatial resolution. Each should be located near the end of the line source, but partial volume effects must be avoided.

Visual inspection can be used to evaluate the reconstructed images. If the COR correction software is working properly, and there has been no shift of the COR since calibration, the reconstructed sections will appear as a Gaussian shaped point. Large COR errors will produce a doughnut shaped image.

A more sensitive technique involves calculating the FWHM for single pixel straight line profiles that pass through the maximum point in both the horizontal (X) and vertical (Y) directions. All computer systems provide some means for listing these data. Linear interpolation can be used to calculate the FWHM. FWHM values expressed in pixels can be converted to mm if the pixel size is known but that is not required.

To compare the planar spatial resolution with that obtained in a SPECT study, the same phantom must be used. The distance from the collimator face to the center line must be 200 mm. FWHM values can be calculated from 10 mm wide profiles drawn across the line source in the same positions that were used for the SPECT analysis. The FWHMs (X and Y direction) calculated from the SPECT study should be within ± 10 % of the FWHM calculated from the planar image. Table 3 presents a summary of the results for 24 systems.

Loss of resolution in the reconstructed sections as compared to that which is present in the planar image may be due to an incorrect COR calibration value or an improperly applied COR correction [23–26]. If a significant error

Table 3. Loss of spatial resolution in SPECT line phantom study*

Magnitude of spatial resolution loss in SPECT relative to planar	Percent of FWHM measurements
<5 %	66.1
5–<10 %	19.5
10–<15 %	10.2
>15 %	4.2

*$128 \times 128 \times 16$ matrix; 120 views; 100K cts/view; Ramp filter with 1 Nyquist cutoff; radius of rotation = 200 mm; General purpose collimator.

is detected, the first step would be to perform a new center of rotation calibration and repeat the study.

Field uniformity

Nonuniformities that are not apparent in planar images can produce significant errors in reconstructed tomographic sections [27,28]. These may be due to true detector nonuniformities or may be due to damaged septa in the collimator that look like 'cool' photomultiplier tubes. Nonuniformities in individual views produce full or partial rings in the reconstructed images [28,29].

Evaluation of uniformity

Although it is essential to display the image that is to be used for flood correction and carefully inspect it, quantitative evaluation of the flood is preferred if the appropriate software is available [30]. Vendors do not publish specifications for system uniformity but the sensitive indices described earlier would be the most appropriate choices for quantitation. In general, all images will exhibit some nonuniformity, mostly due to the collimator, but ADC nonlinearities should not be seen with 30M counts [31].

One important fact must be kept in mind. Flood field correction cannot be used as a substitute for poor camera uniformity or collimator damage. Flood correction can significantly change the appearance of artifacts in an image taken with a camera that has poor system uniformity but does not necessarily eliminate them.

System performance

The existence of a current COR calibration and high count flood does not guarantee optimum operation of a SPECT system. Changes in analyzer window size and a loss of energy resolution will produce a loss in image

Table 4. Measured uniformity and RMS noise for Jaszczak phantom study[*]

Parameter	Average (%)	±1 SD (%)	Range
Integral uniformity			
No flood correction	13.9	9.3–18.5	4–29
Flood corrected	14.7	10.2–19.2	7–24
Root-Mean-Square (RMS) noise			
No flood correction	5.15	4.4–5.9	4–6
Flood corrected	5.08	3.3–6.8	3–9

[*]64 × 64 × 16 matrix; 64 views; 500K cts/view; Hann/Hamming filter with 1 Nyquist cutoff; radius of rotation = 200 mm; General purpose collimator; attenuation correction applied.

quality that will not be evident from any of the tests that have been described so far.

One of the primary advantages of SPECT imaging is the improvement in contrast, which determines the detectability of small lesions [32]. On the other hand, statistical and reconstruction noise produce artifacts and can reduce apparent contrast. These parameters can be quantitated with a 'Jaszczak' or 'Carlson' phantom. Phantoms are also useful for assessing the accuracy of field uniformity and attenuation corrections [23].

Data acquisition

The phantom should be filled with 8 to 10 mCi of a uniformly mixed solution of Tc-99m. For comparison with the data presented below, a general purpose collimator should be used. However, the individual user may choose to use the collimator that is most commonly used for SPECT studies. If this is the high resolution collimator a larger amount of activity can be used (approximately 15 mCi). Position the phantom on the end of the ECT table and tape it firmly in place. Care must be taken to be sure that the central axis of the phantom is parallel to the axis of rotation. Adjust the detector so the average radius of rotation is 200 mm. Set the pulse height analyzer window to 20 % if it is desired to compare the results of these tests with the values shown in Tables 4 and 5.

Before acquisition is initiated, images that are taken through the ECT couch should be checked. Some tables have metal plates near the end and these should be avoided if possible. Move the detector to a position directly above the phantom and determine the time required to collect 500K counts. Set the computer for acquisition of a 64 × 64 matrix, 64 (or 60) views, 360 degrees, and the time for 500K counts per view as determined above. Do not apply zoom unless a jumbo or large rectangular field camera is used. When either of these camera types is used, a zoom factor that gives a pixel size between 0.6 and 0.7 cm for a 64 × 64 matrix should be selected.

At the completion of data acquisition, reconstruct the images with a Hann

Table 5. Measured contrast for Jaszczak phantom study* (no high count flood correction)

Parameters	Measured values		
Sphere size (mm)	Mean sphere contrast (%)	Sphere contrast (1 SD) (%)	Range
31.8	64.1	54.9–73.3	43–79
25.4	44.8	34.5–55.1	27–69
19.1	29.1	20.0–38.2	13–56
15.4	19.3	11.4–27.2	3–37

*64 × 64 × 16 matrix; 64 views; 500K cts/view; Hann/Hamming filter with 1 Nyquist cutoff; radius of rotation = 200 mm; General purpose collimator; attenuation correction applied.

filter using a one Nyquist cutoff. Apply an attenuation correction using 0.12/cm as the linear attenuation coefficient, or its equivalent.

Analysis of data

Display a transverse section from a uniform part of the phantom (e.g. above the spheres in the Jaszczak phantom). Draw a six pixel wide horizontal profile across the center of the phantom and verify that it is flat. A profile that is flat but which is higher on one side than the other indicates that the boundary drawn for attenuation correction is closer to the edge of the object on one side than the other. If the profile shows over- or under-correction, the data set should be reconstructed again with a different attenuation coefficient and/or a new pixel size calibration should be performed. This process should be repeated until the appropriate attenuation coefficient is found.

On the same slice draw a 15 × 15 pixel square region-of-interest (ROI) centered on the reconstructed image. A 60 × 60 pixel ROI must be used for ADAC systems. Record the mean counts per pixel, the maximum and minimum pixel counts within the ROI, and the standard deviation, if provided. Carefully examine the images for the presence of any ring artifacts. If both the maximum and minimum pixel counts within the ROI are available, calculate the reconstructed image uniformity by the equation:

$$\text{Image Uniformity (\%)} = 100 \times \frac{(\text{maximum pixel ct} - \text{minimum pixel ct})}{(\text{maximum pixel ct} + \text{minimum pixel ct})}$$

Image uniformity values obtained with a Jaszczak phantom on a small number of cameras [23] are presented in Table 4.

When standard deviation values are output by the ROI program, the root-mean-square (RMS) noise can be calculated by the equation

$$\text{RMS Noise (\%)} = (\text{Standard Deviation} \times 100)/\text{Mean pixel value}$$

The calculated value should fall within the range shown in Table 4.

Table 6. Measured contrast for Jaszczak phantom study* (high count flood correction applied)

Parameters	Measured values		
Sphere Size (mm)	Mean sphere contrast (%)	Sphere contrast (1 SD) (%)	Range
31.8	63.4	42.9–78.0	43–78
25.4	45.5	34.5–56.5	27–68
19.1	29.6	20.4–38.8	15–54
15.4	20.3	12.7–27.9	7–34

*64 × 64 × 16 matrix; 64 views; 500K cts/view; Hann/Hamming filter with 1 Nyquist cutoff; radius of rotation = 200 mm; General purpose collimator; attenuation correction applied.

Next, select the transverse section where the cold spheres are most clearly defined. Note the number of spheres that can be visualized. For each sphere, determine the number of counts in the 'coolest' pixel. In some software a ROI the size of the sphere can be drawn and the program will list the number of counts in the 'coolest' pixel. In other software packages it may be necessary to mark multiple individual pixels for each 'sphere' until the one with the smallest number of counts is located. Record the lowest pixel value for each sphere that can be visualized. Calculate the contrast for each sphere using the equation

$$\text{Contrast} = \frac{(\text{Average pixel cts from uniform section} - \text{min pixel cts}) \times 100}{\text{Average pixel cts from uniform section}}$$

Calculated values should fall within the average plus or minus one standard deviation range shown in Tables 5 and 6. If a Hamming filter is used the contrast values generally fall at the upper end of the range. Keep in mind that head tilt, gantry flexing, and tilt of the phantom relative to the axis of rotation will produce a loss of contrast in the section that contains the spheres.

Although the sample size for the data shown in Tables 5 and 6 is relatively small, systems that produce values below the limit of plus or minus one standard deviation are probably not operating properly. When larger radii of resolution are used, the contrast values will be slightly lower. On the other hand, if 15 % pulse height analyzer window widths are used the contrast values will generally be higher.

Summary and conclusions

A comprehensive quality control program is an essential ingredient of high quality planar and SPECT imaging. The spread of differential uniformity and the uniformity index have been found to be sensitive indicators of flood field nonuniformity and these indices correlate well with observer studies.

However, for maximum effectiveness a larger number of counts is required for the latter (approximately 30 million). Display of the uniformity as a function of time greatly enhances the value of quantitation. Expert systems which are under development require quantitative measures and should be helpful for busy departments and those which utilize personnel with limited experience in the use of scintillation cameras. A method for quantitating camera spatial resolution has been proposed which uses Fourier analysis of bar pattern images. A preliminary study suggests that method may be useful for evaluating changes in spatial resolution as a function of time. Studies of SPECT system performance using a Jaszczak phantom can also provide quantitative information concerning uniformity, noise, attenuation correction, and contrast. Data collected on a number of different SPECT systems are provided.

It seems appropriate to conclude with the following quotation: "Certainly, the need for careful quality assessment, and thoughtful quality assurance will grow with instrument complexity if new performance capabilities are to be translated into clinical gain." (Herrera NE et al.: Medical Radionuclide Imaging, Vol II, 177–187, IAEA, Vienna, 1981.)

Acknowledgements

We would like to acknowledge the assistance of the Research Service of the Department of Veteran's Affairs of the United States of America in this study. The involvement of Kithsiri Herath was made possible through his appointment as Fellow by the International Atomic Energy Agency (IAEA), Vienna, Austria. Judy Negrete participated through the Department of Energy, Associated Western University (AWU) – Minority Access to Energy Related Careers (MAERC) Student Fellowship Program directed by Dr. Donald E. Biachi of the California State University at Northridge, Northridge, CA.

References

1. Van Tuinen RJ, Kruger JB, Bahr GK, Sodd VJ. Scintillation camera nonuniformity: effects on cold lesion detectability. Int J Nucl Med Biol 1978;5:135–7, 139–40.
2. Soussaline F, Todd-Pokropek AE, Raynaud C. Quantitative studies with the gamma-camera: correction for spatial and energy distortion. In: Brill AB, Price RR, editors. Review of information processing in medical imaging. Oak Ridge: Oak Ridge National Laboratory, 1977:360–75.
3. Todd-Pokropek AE, Erbsmann F, Soussaline F. The non-uniformity of imaging devices and its impact in quantitative studies. In: Ericson A, editor. Medical radionuclide imaging. Vienna: International Atomic Energy Agency, 1977: Volume 1, 67–84.
4. Wicks R, Blau M. Effect of spatial distortion on Anger camera field uniformity correction: concise communications. J Nucl Med 1979;20:252–4.

5. Graham LS. Quality assurance procedures. In: Simmons GH, editor. The scintillation camera. New York: Society of Nuclear Medicine, 1988:79–98.
6. Publication/No. NU1 (NEMA NU 1–1986). National Electrical Manufacturers Association, Washington, D.C. (1986).
7. La Fontaine R, Graham LS, Behrendt D, Greenwell K. Personnel exposure from flood phantoms and point sources during quality assurance procedures. J Nucl Med 1983;24:629–32.
8. Sharp P, Marshall I. The usefulness of indices measuring gamma camera non-uniformity. Phys Med Biol 1981;26:149–53.
9. Maxwell AE. Analysing Qualitative Data. London: Griffin, 1970.
10. Hughes A, Sharp PF. Factors affecting gamma-camera non-uniformity. Phys Med Biol 1988;33:259–69.
11. Cox NJ, Diffey BL. A numerical index of gamma-camera uniformity (letter). Br J Radiol 1976;49:734–5.
12. Cahill PT, Knowles RJ, Becker DV. Scintillation camera field uniformity: visual or quantitative? IEEE Trans Nucl Sci 1980;27:509–12.
13. Keyes JW Jr, Gazella GR, Strange DR. Image analysis by on-line minicomputer for improved camera quality control. J Nucl Med 1972;13:525–7.
14. Grossman LW, Anderson MP, Jennings RJ, et al. Noise analysis of scintillation camera images: stochastic and non-stochastic effects. Phys Med Biol 1986;31:941–53.
15. Borm JJ, Busemann-Sokole E. The use of Fourier techniques for the evaluation of A/D and D/A converter performance in scintillation cameras (abstract). Eur J Nucl Med 1990;16:442.
16. International Atomic Energy Agency. Quality control of nuclear medicine instruments. Vienna: International Atomic Energy Agency, 1984.
17. Kasal B, Sharp PF, Dendy PP. Gamma camera image quality: A comparison of subjective and objective measurements. In: Mould RF, editor. Quality control of nuclear medicine instrumentation. London: The Association, 1983.
18. Slomka P, Todd-Pokropek AE. A general purpose micro-computer based quality assurance package designed to be used under an expert system shell (abstract). Eur J Nucl Med 1990;16 Suppl:S83.
19. Hoffman EJ, Huang SC, Phelps ME. Quantitation in positron emission computed tomography: 1. Effect of object size. J Comput Assist Tomogr 1979; 3: 299–308.
20. Kircos LT, Carey JE Jr, Keyes JW Jr. Quantitative organ visualization using SPECT. J Nucl Med 1987;28:334–41.
21. Graham LS. A rational quality assurance program for SPECT instrumentation. In: Freeman LM, Weissmann HS, editor. Nuclear medicine annual 1989. New York: Raven Press, 1989: 81–108.
22. American Association of Physicists in Medicine. Rotating scintillation camera SPECT acceptance testing and quality control. New York: American Institute of Physics, 1987.
23. Greer KL, Coleman RE, Jaszczak RJ. SPECT: A practical for users. J Nucl Med Tech 1983;11:61–5.
24. Harkness BA, Rogers WL, Clinthorne HN, Keyes JW Jr. SPECT: Quality control procedures and artifact identifications. J Nucl Med Tech 1983;11:55–60.
25. Farrell TJ, Cradduck TD, Chamberlain RA. The effect of collimators on the center of rotation in SPECT (letter). J Nucl Med 1984;25:632–3.
26. Todd-Pokropek A: Quality control, detection and display. In Kuhl DE, editor. Radionuclide imaging. Paris: Pergamon Press, 1982: 27–76.
27. Woronowicz RL, Eisner RL, Gullberg GT, et al. Factors affecting single photon emission computed tomography image quality and recommended QC procedures. S.L.: General Electric Company, 1982.
28. Rogers WL, Clinthorne HN, Harkness BA, Koral KF, Keyes JW, Jr. Flood-field requirements for emission computed tomography with an Anger camera. J Nucl Med 1982;23:162–8.
29. Nowak DJ, Gullberg GT, Eisner RL, Malko JA, Woronowicz EM. An investigation to

determine uniformity requirements for rotating gamma camera tomography (abstract). J Nucl Med 1982;23:P52–3.

30. Halama JR, Henkin RE. Quality assurance in SPECT imaging. Appl Radiol 1987;16:41–2,44,46,49–50.

31. English RJ, Brown SE: SPECT: single-photon emission computed tomography: a primer. New York: Society of Nuclear Medicine, 1986.

32. Jaszczak RJ, Murphy PH, Huard D, Burdine JA. Radionuclide emission computed tomography of the head with 99mCc and a scintillation camera. J Nucl Med 1977;18:373–80.

PART II

SPECT: New developments

5. Myocardial ischemia detection by expert system interpretation of thallium-201 tomograms

MARK D. HERBST,* ERNEST V. GARCIA, C. DAVID COOKE, NORBERTO F. EZQUERRA, RUSSELL D. FOLKS and E. GORDON DePUEY

Summary

The accuracy of interpreting tomographic nuclear medicine images of the heart varies depending on the expertise of the diagnostician. This variability is a problem at some community hospitals or private imaging centers where expertise is limited due to the small number of studies performed. In order to standardize image interpretation at an expert's level, we developed a totally automated rule-based expert system for interpreting three-dimensional myocardial perfusion distributions obtained from stress and delayed thallium-201 perfusion tomograms. The rules of the expert system determine the presence, location, and certainty of each fixed or reversible coronary lesion, combining certainty factors according to the MYCIN algorithm. Computer consultations were compared with interpretations of a human expert for a pilot group of 20 patients. The expert system interpreted myocardial perfusion distributions with artifacts, coronary territory overlap and multiple defects at a level approaching that of the human expert.

Introduction

Quantitative tomographic imaging of stress/delayed thallium-201 (Tl-201) three-dimensional (3D) myocardial perfusion distributions has attained widespread clinical use for the non-invasive assessment of coronary artery disease (CAD) [1,2]. At present, identifying myocardial hypoperfusion involves visual detection of myocardial regions with relatively lower count density from Tl-201 tomograms. However, unaided visual detection of defects is subject to observer variability, is not standardized, and requires a significant degree of nuclear cardiology experience. Previously, we developed a prototype computerized expert system to overcome this problem [3]. The reports generated by this prototype knowledge base, which handled multiple stress defects,

*This work was supported in part by grant RM29–LMO4692 from the National Library of Medicine.

Johan H.C. Reiber & Ernst E. van der Wall (eds.), Cardiovascular Nuclear Medicine and MRI, 77–88.
© 1992 *Kluwer Academic Publishers.*

considered age- and gender-related artifacts, and provided certainty factors for its conclusions, compared favorably to the interpretations of the same data by human experts and to the results of coronary arteriography [3]. Nevertheless, this preliminary approach was limited since the users were required to describe perfusion defects subjectively and enter the information manually, and the system did not utilize data from delayed scans to assess perfusion defect reversibility. Investigators have documented and used the visual finding of "normalization" or "reversal" of a stress-induced perfusion defect several hours after stress as a reliable marker of myocardial ischemia [4], not previously assessed by the prototype expert system. In order to overcome these limitations, we have implemented an automated process of systematically describing the perfusion defects to the expert system. Importantly, we also have incorporated new rules which use information from delayed myocardial tomograms to draw specific inferences regarding the degree of perfusion defect reversibility associated with coronary lesions. This report describes in detail the new features and the performance of this expert system in interpreting myocardial perfusion studies.

Methods

Exercise, imaging and standard processing procedures

Our procedure for standard quantitative single photon emission computed tomography (SPECT) thallium studies has been previously described in detail [2]. A patient undergoes stress on the treadmill according to the Bruce protocol. At peak exercise, a dose of 3.5 mCi of Tl-201 is injected and exercise continues for approximately 60 sec. Each patient is then imaged using a 400 mm field of view gamma camera six to ten minutes after exercise (stress) and three to five hours later (delayed). The acquisition is performed using a circular orbit over a 180° range starting at the 45° right anterior oblique projection and ending at the 45° left posterior oblique projection. Each of 32 projections is acquired using a 64 × 64 matrix at 40 sec per image. Each projection is corrected for nonuniformity using a 30 million count Co-57 flood source. Each projection is then filtered using a 2–dimensional Hanning filter with a cut-off frequency of 0.83 cycles/cm. Filtered back-projection is then applied to these preprocessed projections using a Ramp filter in order to generate transaxial slices. No scatter or attenuation correction is used. From these transaxial images the long axis of the left ventricle is identified and oblique angle images are generated in the short axis, vertical long axis, and horizontal long axis orientations. Maximal count circumferential profiles are generated on each of the short axis slices in forty 9° arcs and ranging from apex to base. These count profiles are then interpolated to the equivalent of 15 slices and stored in two 15 × 40 arrays, one for the stress and one for the delayed distribution. For display purposes, these arrays are then transformed into a polar plot known as the "raw bull's-eye map." See Fig. 1.

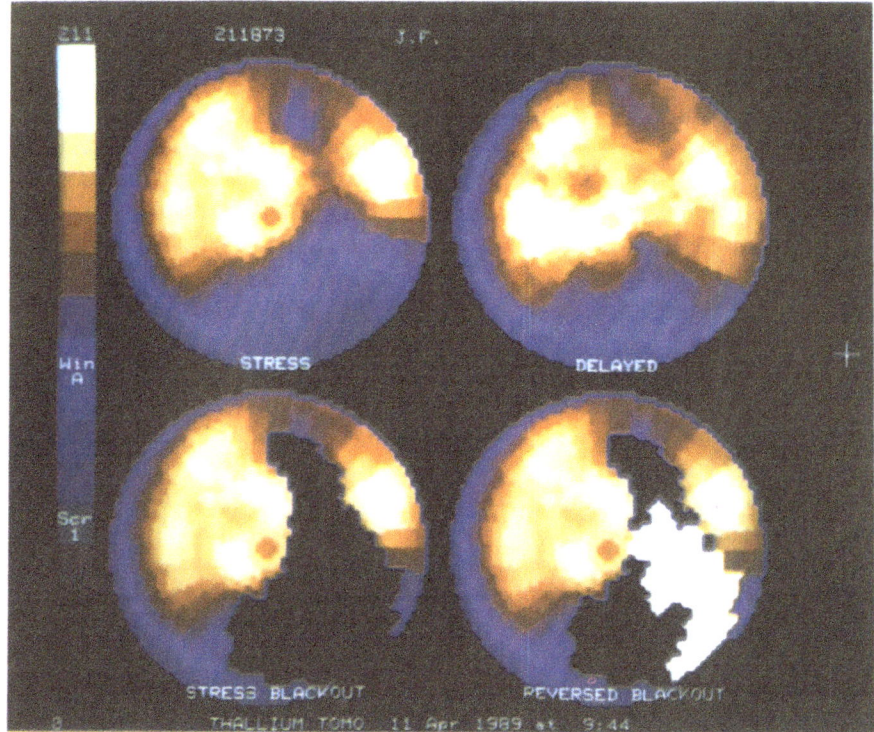

Figure 1. Bull's-eye polar representations of stress/delayed three-dimensional thallium-201 myocardial distributions. Raw stress and delayed data are depicted on the top row, and the blackout and white-out representations are on the bottom row. This example shows reversible perfusion defects. See text for further explanation.

In order to identify stress perfusion defects objectively, each patient's profiles are compared with gender-matched normal files. The normal files were developed using individuals with <5% probability of CAD based on Bayesian analysis of age, gender, chest pain history and exercise treadmill performance. Previously, we established the profile curves representing 2.5 standard deviations (SDs) below the mean normal response as our threshold for stress perfusion defect detection. The clustered profile points falling below this established normal limit are identified as the "extent" of the defect. Subsequently these abnormal points are transformed to polar coordinates and plotted in a "blackout" bull's-eye in which the black region within the bull's-eye plot defines the extent of the stress perfusion abnormality.

Quantification of defect reversibility

Our procedure for quantification of defect reversibility has been described previously [4]. Using the 15×40 array representing the stress myocardial

Tl-201 distribution, the 5 × 5 pixel area with the greatest counts is identified as the most normal area and used for normalization so that this area has a maximal count of 1000. Using the delayed array, the same 5 × 5 pixel region location is used to normalize the maximal counts to 1000. Each point in the normalized stress array is subtracted from the corresponding point in the normalized delayed array resulting in an new 15 × 40 array representing improvement from stress to rest or defect reversibility. For display purposes, these arrays are transformed into a polar plot known as a "reversibility bull's-eye." In order to identify defect reversibility objectively, each patient's reversibility array is compared with gender-matched normal files developed from the low likelihood of CAD group in which the mean values and SD were established from the pooled reversibility arrays of these normal patients. Previously, we established the points representing 1.5 SDs above the mean normal response as our threshold for detecting reversibility in regions already identified to exhibit a stress perfusion defect [4]. The clustered array points falling above this established normal limit are identified as the "extent" of the reversibility. We also established that if a stress defect was considered visually reversible by experts, in general, the extent of reversibility was at least 15 percent of the extent of the stress perfusion defect, although regions as small as 5 percent were perceived by the experts as having partial reversibility. Therefore a 5 percent threshold has been used as the cut-off point in interpreting reversibility. In order to display the relation of the region which reverses to the stress perfusion defect extent, the points which reverse in the black region (perfusion defect) of the stress blackout bull's-eye are set to white, generating what is known as a "reversibility whiteout bull's-eye." Examples of the stress, delayed, blackout and whiteout bull's-eyes are shown in Fig. 1.

Feature extraction and certainty factor assignment

The automatic feature extraction program on the nuclear medicine computer [5] uses as input the 15 × 40 blackout and whiteout bull's-eyes and their associated standard deviation arrays. To identify the first perfusion defect, it searches through the blackout array for any pixel that has been set to zero (blacked out as abnormal) and performs edge-hugging operations to isolate all other pixels set to zero that are also connected to the first blackout pixel. This procedure repeats for each perfusion defect. The location of each defect is expressed in the form of 32 possible descriptor pixels or "dixels." The perfusion defect dixels are defined as coordinates of both depth (basal, medial, apical) and angular location (subsets of septal, anterior, inferior, and lateral myocardial walls). The values from the corresponding dixels in the standard deviation array are used to determine a certainty factor (CF) associated with the dixel and are measures of both the extent and severity of the perfusion defect. The range of values assigned to certainty factors follows the system designed for the MYCIN expert system developed at Stanford [6]. In this system, a CF of 1 corresponds to a "definitely abnormal" state, -1 corresponds to "definitely normal." Most values fall somewhere between, depending on how abnormal or normal the perfusion distribution is. Dixels having all of their pixels in the normal range are set to a certainty factor of -1. Abnormal dixel CF values are calculated according to the following formula:

$$CF = 0.145 \ SD - 10.163 \tag{1}$$

where SD is the average number of standard deviations below the mean normal response for the abnormal pixels. Equation [1], which was derived empirically, provides a linear relation between the CF and the SD such that a dixel whose SD was at the threshold level of 2.5 standard deviations below mean normal would result in a borderline equivocal CF of 0.2. If the dixel averages 8 standard deviations it would result in a CF of 0.99 (almost definitely abnormal). A similar procedure is used on the reversibility data, using the following equation to convert SD to CF:

$$CF = 0.229 \ SD - 10.145 \tag{2}$$

Thus, the feature extraction program generates a descriptor file which is used to specify to the expert system the number of perfusion defects detected in the stress distribution, the dixels occupied by each defect, the dixels within the perfusion defect which showed reversibility, and the certainty factors for each abnormal and each reversed dixel.

Expert system implementation

The IBM Expert System Development Environment running on an IBM 3090 supercomputer was used for this project. The inference engine of the expert system uses our knowledge base to determine automatically the location and shape of each of the perfusion defects from the features extracted from bull's-eye polar maps. The knowledge-base makes these determinations based on the firing or execution of about 200 heuristic rules to produce new facts or draw new inferences. These rules were initially based on a review of 291 patient studies with angiographic correlation [3]. For each input parameter and for each rule, a certainty factor is assigned (between -1 to $+1$) that is traced to infer the certainty of each conclusion reached during the consultation. A diagram depicting how information flows in and out of the expert system is shown in Fig. 2.

The automatic consultation procedure is initiated by the IBM expert system by using the PASCAL interface to request the output files of the feature extraction program. Each file provides the following: patient's name, age, sex, the number of perfusion defects, the number of abnormal dixels per defect, a set of 32 CF values for each defect corresponding to the 32

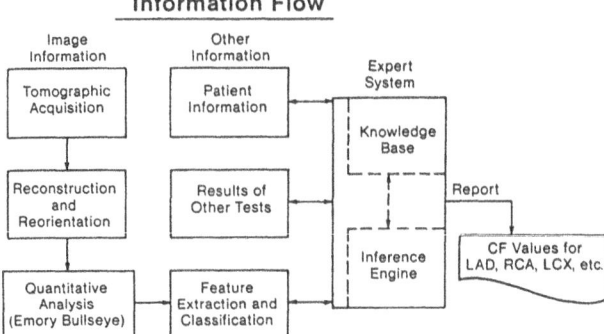

Figure 2. Information flow in the knowledge-based expert systems for interpreting thallium-201 myocardial distribution. CF = certainty factors, LAD = left anterior descending, RCA = right coronary artery, LCX = left circumflex.

descriptors of the defect, the number of reversible defects, the number of reversible dixels per defect and the corresponding 32 descriptors CF values. A simple example of how two heuristic rules use the values from these input parameters to infer a conclusion is as follows:

RULE ILM_LOCATION
FIF DEFECT_DESCRIPTOR IS 'ilm'
THEN DEFECT_LOCATION IS 'infero_lateral.'

RULE RCA_INFEROLATERAL
FIF DEFECT_LOCATION IS 'infero_lateral'
THEN THERE IS STRONG EVIDENCE THAT DISEASED_CORON-
ARIES IS 'RCA.'

The rules are composed of a premise and an action or conclusion following the format: IF premise THEN action or conclusion. FIF stands for a "fuzzy if" operator which uses the certainty of the premise to update the certainty of the action. Rule ILM_LOCATION states that if the certainty that the input parameter defect descriptor ilm (infero-lateral-medical location) is greater than 0.2 then the rule should fire and affirm that the location of the defect is in the infero-lateral wall. Rule RCA_INFEROLATERAL states that if the location of the defect is in the infero-lateral wall with a certainty greater than 0.2, then the rule should fire and affirm that the RCA (right coronary artery) is diseased. The certainty factors of the affirmed statements are derived according to MYCIN algorithms [6] which combine the certainty of the premise, the certainty of the rule (strong evidence = 0.7), and any prior certainty of the affirmed statement (from previously fired rules).

Knowledge Base Configuration

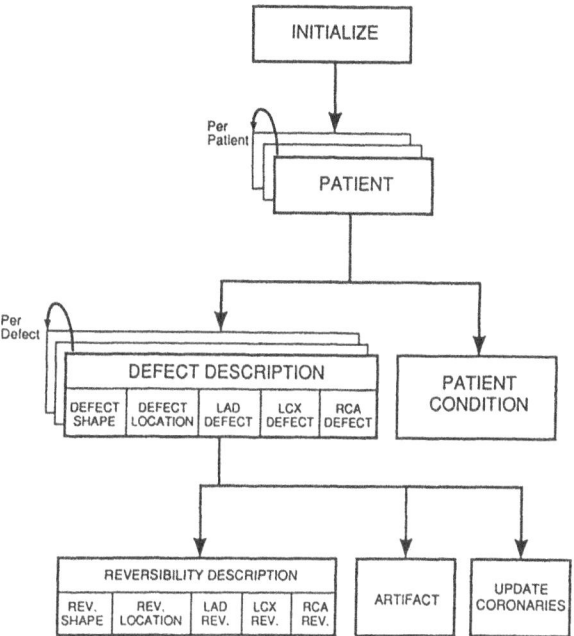

Figure 3. Frame configuration of the knowledge-based expert system.

Knowledge base configuration

Figure 3 illustrates how the current knowledge-based expert system, which contains approximately 200 heuristic rules, was structured into six major subsets of rules known as frames (or focus control blocks). These six major frames have been defined as follows: (a) "PATIENT" in which patient-specific information is obtained; (b) "DEFECT DESCRIPTION" which uses the symbolic descriptors to determine the shape and location of each stress perfusion defect in a medically useful representation to assign incremental evidence that the perfusion defect corresponds to disease in the left anterior descending (LAD), left circumflex (LCX), and right coronary artery (RCA); (c) "REVERSIBILITY DESCRIPTION" which emulates part of the rule base in b above using the reversibility descriptors to determine whether the defect is consistent with ischemia or scar; (d) "ARTIFACT" which uses patient information such as sex and age coupled with the defect shape and location to determine if this defect is a possible artifact; (e) "UPDATE CORONARIES" which combines the incremental evidence of coronary artery disease from all defects and (f) "PATIENT CONDITION" which draws conclusions regarding the overall condition of the patient.

Inference engine

The inference engine (inferencing mechanism) searches through the knowledge base to evaluate pertinent rules and to produce new facts. The strategy used in the search is backward chaining, a goal-oriented control strategy. A goal, or set of goals, is usually associated with each frame such that the system can reach specific, near-term goals as it moves toward achieving its overall objective. For example, the goal of the frame "DEFECT_DE-SCRIPTION" is to ensure that the defect's shape and location have been determined, and to determine the degree to which evidence has been found for the presence or absence of disease in the vascular territories.

Reversibility rules

The rules in the prototype knowledge base which assessed the size, shape, and certainty of perfusion defects in stress blackout bull's-eyes provided the framework for a set of new rules which assessed the certainty of reversibility within stress defects from the delayed whiteout bull's-eyes. These rules produced certainty factors regarding the presence or absence of disease and/or reversibility in each of the three coronary vascular territories: LAD, LCX, and RCA. New rules utilized these inferences as input to characterize the coronary lesions, as shown in the following examples:

RULE LAD_LESION_NOT_PRESENT
FIF PT_DISEASED_CORONARIES IS NOT 'LAD'
THEN PT_LESIONS_PRESENT IS NOT 'LAD'

RULE LAD_LESION_PRESENT
FIF PT_DISEASED_CORONARIES IS 'LAD'
THEN PT_LESIONS_PRESENT IS 'LAD'

RULE LAD_LESION_REVERSIBLE
FIF PT_REVERSED_CORONARIES IS 'LAD'
THEN PT_LESIONS_REVERSIBLE IS 'LAD'
AND PT_LESIONS_PRESENT IS 'LAD'

RULE LAD_LESION_FIXED
FIF PT_DISEASED_CORONARIES IS 'LAD'
AND PT_REVERSED_CORONARIES IS NOT 'LAD'
THEN PT−LESIONS_FIXED_AT-4HRS IS 'LAD'

The first two rules determine whether or not a lesion is present in the LAD, based on the conclusions drawn from rules fired previously and influenced by the perfusion defect's size and severity. The third rule determines whether the LAD lesion is reversible, and if it is, the action statement of this rule also reaffirms that there is a lesion present in the LAD. The MYCON algorithm increments the certainty factor of the 'LAD' value of the parameter PT_LESIONS_PRESENT, just as a human expert might increase his or her confidence that a lesion is present if reversibility is demonstrated in the same region of myocardium. The fourth rule infers that a lesion is fixed if it lacks reversibility.

Pilot study

To compare the interpretations of the expert system to those of a human expert (EGD), a set of 20 tomographic thallium studies (from 13 males and 7 females, 52–79 years old) were chosen for the pilot group. There were no strict inclusion criteria for this group other than a desire to challenge the computer expert system with thallium scans from patients with single fixed defects, single reversible defects, multiple vessel disease, imaging artifacts, and normal scans. The human expert, whose opinions were considered the gold standard in this study, was asked to examine the stress, blackout, delayed, and whiteout bull's-eyes. His interpretations were constrained to the following information: normal or abnormal, identification of possible artifacts if present, and reversible or fixed lesions in each of the three vascular territories.

Results

According to the human expert, whose interpretations were considered the gold standard of this study, 4 of the 20 patients' studies were normal and 16 were consistent with CAD, eight with fixed lesions only (consistent with scar) and eight with at least one reversible lesion (consistent with ischemia). One of the normal studies was said to exhibit a count reduction in the anterior wall due to breast attenuation, but was still probably normal. In three of the studies interpreted as CAD, two were also interpreted to exhibit a probable breast artifact, and one an anteroapical count reduction due to an anatomic variant. The computer expert system identified all 16 abnormal studies of patients with CAD. The expert system also identified all four of the artifacts correctly, but called the one normal study with breast artifact probably abnormal. The computer agreed with the human expert in 7 of 8 patients with ischemia and all 8 patients with scar (and no ischemia). All of the 28 abnormal vascular territories identified by the human expert were correctly localized by the expert system (although the expert system incorrectly identified an additional 10 abnormal vascular territories). Of the 28 abnormal vascular territories, the expert system correctly classified 12 of 16 as reversible (ischemic) and 11 of 12 as fixed (infarcted).

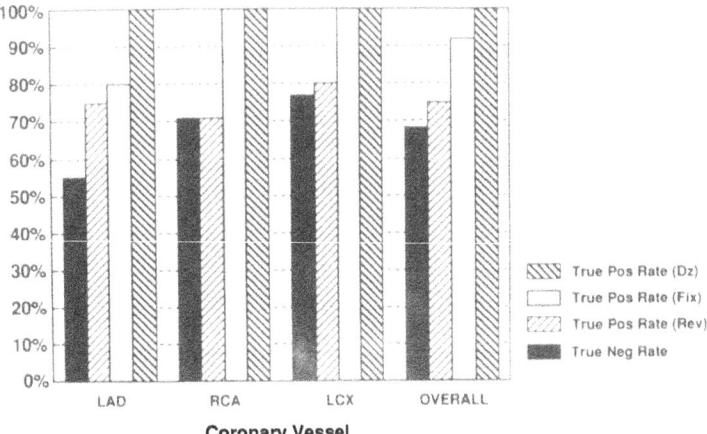

Figure 4. Performance of the computer expert system compared with a human expert.

Results for individual vascular territories

Six of 11 LAD territories identified as normal were correctly classified by the expert system for a 55 % true negative rate. The true positive rate for identification of LAD ischemia (reversible perfusion defects) was 3/4 or 75 %, for LAD scar (fixed at four hours) 4/5 or 80 %, and for LAD disease without regard to reversibility 9/9 or 100 %. For RCA territories, the true negative rate was 5/7 or 71 %, and the true positive rates for ischemia, scar and disease were 5/7 (71 %), 6/6 (100 %) and 13/13 (100 %) respectively. For LCX territories, the true negative rate was 10/13 or 77 %, and the true positive rates for ischemia, scar and disease were 4/5 (80 %), 2/2 (100 %) and 7/7 (100 %) respectively. These data are illustrated in Fig. 4.

Example

Figure 1 shows a study from a 79 year old male with a large anterior, lateral, and inferior stress perfusion defect with inferolateral redistribution. The polar maps were interpreted as ischemia in the LAD and in the RCA-or-LCX vascular territories by the human expert. The computer identified disease in the LCX (CF = 0.993), RCA (CF = 0.889) and LAD (CF = 0.478) vascular territories, but characterized only two of them as reversible: LCX (CF = 0.886) and RCA (CF = 0.879). The presence of reversibility in the LAD territory was equivocal, so it was not identified as either fixed or reversible.

Discussion

How good is the computerized expert system? Compared to the human expert, the computer was equally able to identify the abnormal patients and equally able to identify artifacts which could affect the readings. It was nearly as good as the human expert in distinguishing patients with some ischemia from those with fixed lesions only. It called more abnormal vascular territories than the human expert, but did not mistakenly call any abnormal territories normal. Using bull's-eye maps to identify CAD, agreement among experienced readers exceeded 90 % [2]. In this pilot group, the computer expert described correctly 50 or 60 vascular territories, or 83 %. This difference may not be significant, since the test groups were not the same. We showed previously that the reversibility plot could identify 73 % [7] or 82 % [4] of the reversible lesions and 80 % [7] or 81 % [4] of the fixed lesions compared with a panel of human experts. Kiat and coworkers [8] reported 72 % and 83 % agreement rates between reversibility plots and human experts for reversible and fixed lesions respectively, using a different approach to their reversibility polar maps. Our results show that the computer expert system using the reversibility plots can identify reversible lesions at a 75 % rate and fixed lesions at a 92 % rate compared to a single human expert. Although these results indicate that the computer could be close to the human expert in proficiency, further evaluations are needed to determine the true accuracy of the method on a large prospective patient population.

Conclusion

Noninvasive cardiovascular nuclear medicine screening is becoming widespread. However, the human task of interpreting stress and delayed quantitative myocardial thallium-201 scans is complex. It requires visual recognition of differences in myocardial radionuclide activity and awareness of coronary artery distributions. For readings to be clinically useful, the diagnostician must compare the patient's scan with known normal limits, consider the patient's age and gender, and distinguish between real abnormalities and artifacts. The complexity of the task, the large number of studies performed yearly, and the resultant relative shortage of available human experts make myocardial thallium-201 imaging a good candidate for application of artificial intelligence methods. While the finer points of interpretation will probably always require a human expert, the essential skills and knowledge can be analyzed, simulated by computerized feature extraction and a knowledge-based system, and automated.

Previous efforts have laid the groundwork for the advances described here [9]. Quantitative bull's-eye maps and automatic feature extraction programs portray three-dimensional data in a convenient two-dimensional format. Comparison with gender-matched control files allows detection of abnormal myocardial radionuclide activity. A successful prototype rule-based expert system was limited, but promising. The ability of the current expert system to consider reversibility of myocardial perfusion defects and its automation are additional advances. The current implementation of the expert system can be used as a training tool for residents and fellows. A new version of the expert system is being implemented on a workstation computer using NEXPERT environment where it may eventually provide expert interpretation of Tl-201 scans to novice readers.

References

1. Garcia EV, Van Train K, Maddahi J, et al. Quantification of rotational thallium-201 myocardial tomography. J Nucl Med 1985;26:17–26.
2. DePasquale EE, Nody AC, DePuey EG, et al. Quantitative rotational thallium-201 tomography for identifying and localizing coronary artery disease. Circulation 1988;77:316–27.
3. Ezquerra NF, Garcia EV. Artificial intelligence in nuclear medicine imaging. Am J Card Imaging 1989;3:130–41.
4. Klein JL, Garcia E, DePuey EG, et al. Reversibility bull's eye: A new polar map to quantify reversibility of stress induced SPECT Tl-201 myocardial perfusion defects. J Nucl Med 1990;31:1240–6.
5. Hise HL, Steves AM, Klein JL, Ezquerra NF, Garcia EV. Feature extraction as a means for consistent Tl-201 image interpretation. (Abstract) J Nucl Med 1987;28(4):618.
6. Shortliffe EH. Computer-based medical consulations: MYCIN. New York: North Holland, 1976.
7. Garcia EV, DePuey EG, Sonnemaker RE, et al. Quantification of the reversibility of stress induced Tl-201 myocardial perfusion defects: a multicenter trial using bull's-eye polar maps and standard normal limits. J Nucl Med 1990;31:1761–5.
8. Kiat H, Van Train K, Berman D, et al. Quantitative analysis of SPECT thallium-201 reversibility: development and preliminary validation of an objective method (abstract). J Nucl Med 1989;30:739.
9. DePuey EG, Garcia EV, Ezquerra NF. Three-dimensional techniques and artificial intelligence in thallium cardiac imaging. AJR 1989;152:1161–8.

6. Three-dimensional display in SPECT imaging: Principles and applications

JEROLD W. WALLIS

Summary

Tomographic studies may be viewed in several forms: orthogonal slices, oblique slices, mappings (projections of curved surfaces onto two dimensions), surface rendering, and volume rendering. The best form of display varies depending on the type of tomographic study; the display should be chosen so as to best preserve the information needed for study interpretation. Cardiac perfusion studies are best viewed as oblique slices or polar (Bull's-eye) maps, optionally with the information from the Bull's-eye display mapped onto a perspective view of the myocardium. In 'hot-spot' imaging, volume rendering utilizing maximum activity projection from multiple angles is preferred. Surface rendering may have some role in 'cold-spot' imaging, but surface rendering is of limited value overall in display of SPECT images. Regardless of the form of three-dimensional display used, slice data should be reviewed in addition to the rendered images.

Introduction

As tomography is employed to a greater degree in Nuclear Medicine, there is increasing interest in three-dimensional displays. Three-dimensional displays can combine the many sagittal, coronal, and transverse slices into a single unified image, with the goal of aiding in image interpretation and providing enhanced perception of continuity of structures across slices. A given display technique can either enhance or obscure diagnostic information; knowledge of the methods used in constructing each three-dimensional display is essential in choosing the appropriate display method for a particular type of tomographic image.

Johan H.C. Reiber & Ernst E. van der Wall (eds.), Cardiovascular Nuclear Medicine and MRI, 89–100.
© 1992 *Kluwer Academic Publishers.*

Three-dimensional display techniques

Conventional techniques

The most common form of displaying three-dimensional data is in the format of multiple slices. While the data are typically reconstructed in the form of transaxial slices, the degree of axial sampling readily allows reformatting the data into coronal and sagittal slices. In cases where the structure being evaluated lies obliquely with respect to the axis of the body (such as cardiac imaging), the cube of data may be rotated to produce oblique slices. The major disadvantages of slice display are the number of images that need to be reviewed and the difficulty in integrating information about structures that do not lie entirely in a single plane.

When the three-dimensional object being represented approximates a curved surface, standard cartographic techniques may be employed. Polar and Mercator maps have been used for many years to depict the curved surface of the earth; although they introduce distortions, such techniques are quite effective. These types of maps have been extensively used in nuclear cardiology, since at typical imaging resolutions the thin myocardium can be considered to be a curved surface.

Surface rendering

Rendering is the process of converting a three-dimensional data set into two dimensions, usually for viewing on a two-dimensional computer display. One of the most commonly used forms of rendering is surface rendering. The process of surface rendering can be divided into several steps: (1) surface definition, (2) selection of viewing perspective, with elimination of hidden structures, and (3) addition of depth cues. The first step, surface definition, distinguishes this technique from volume rendering. In surface definition, some segmentation process is performed to convert the grey scale image into a binary image; all voxels within the background are set to zero, and all voxels within the organ or structures being imaged are set to one. This segmentation process can be based upon several factors, including voxel intensity (thresholding), rate of change of voxels in the image (gradient-based edge detection), or voxel location with respect to manually drawn regions on each slice.

The next step is to determine which voxels will be visible from a given viewing perspective. As interior voxels will not be seen, all interior voxels can be set to zero, leaving only the surface voxels for further processing. A viewpoint is then chosen, and rays are traced from the chosen viewpoint through the cube of data; either diverging rays (a viewing point) or parallel rays (a viewing plane) may be employed. The first non-zero voxel found along each ray will determine the pixel value in the final rendered image. It is useful to note the depth of the first non-zero voxel from the viewpoint; this information is frequently stored in a 'Z-buffer', so-called because it records the depth in the Z direction with respect to the final rendered image.

If the image were displayed at this point, it would still be a binary image with only two colors: black and white. Grey scale or color information is then added back to the image in order to provide the perception of a third dimension; the coloring provides depth cues to the viewer. The simplest depth cue is depth coding or depth weighting, in which distant objects in the image are displayed at a lesser intensity than near objects. The depth information is readily available directly from the Z-buffer, described above. However, rendered images using only depth coding appear rather crude. Fine surface detail is not shown, since the extent in the Z direction of variations on the object surfaces is small with respect to the total Z dimensions of the image. For this reason simulated illumination is typically added as a second depth cue.

In computer illumination, the first step is to choose the position of the light source with respect to both the cube of data and the viewpoint. The next step is to calculate the angulation of the surface at each point in which the surface is visible. Where the surface forms a 45 degree angle with respect to both the light and the viewer, light will 'bounce' off the surface and reach the viewer at maximum intensity; these highlights are referred to as spectral illumination. At other angles, a lesser degree of light reaches the viewer. If desired, a diffuse illumination component may be added as well, which is independent (or less dependent) on the surface angle. Various illumination/shading models have been employed [1,2]; typically the final illumination value depends on the light source vector, the illumination vector, the surface normal, and the settings for the amount of spectral and diffuse reflection to be used in the rendering. Approximate surface normals can be computed quickly from the Z-buffer information, but it is more accurate to calculate them from gradients in the original data set.

If desired, other depth cues can also be added. Additional depth cues include stereoscopic display (in which an image from a slightly different viewpoint is produce for each eye), use of simulated illumination from multiple angles (possibly with different colored light sources), and production of a sequence of images from successive angles to be viewed in a cine format (simulating rotation of the three-dimensional object).

It is important to keep in mind that no matter how realistic the depth cues, the underlying data being depicted is still binary; grey scale information from the original data was discarded at the initial segmentation step.

Volume rendering

Volume rendering differs from surface rendering in that there is no initial segmentation step. Instead, the voxel intensities are retained, and utilized

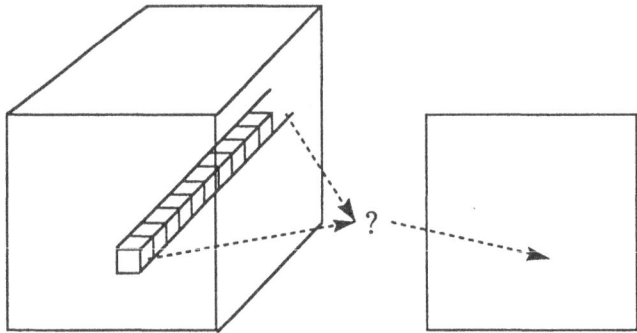

Figure 1. For each column of data in the tomographic study, intensities are combined using the chosen rendering operation. The resulting value is placed in the corresponding location in the rendered image. In this example the chosen viewpoint is a plane located in front of the cube.

throughout the rendering process. The volume rendering operation consists of combining voxel intensities along columns to produce a value for the corresponding pixel in the rendered image, as shown in Fig. 1. This process is done for each column of data, resulting in the two dimensional rendered image. Various mathematical techniques have been proposed for the combining or compositing operation, and are described below.

Summation

The simplest compositing operation is summation, optionally with distance weighting. This results in a volume rendered image that is quite similar to a planar projection, as the process mimics addition of gamma rays from various depths during planar acquisition. Summation has been proposed for use in nuclear medicine [3,4], but results in loss of the enhanced contrast gained during tomographic acquisition [5].

Volumetric compositing

Another form of compositing, sometimes referred to as volumetric compositing, is frequently used in X-ray computed tomography and magnetic resonance imaging [6,7]. This technique is illustrated in Fig. 2. Each voxel in the image is assigned a color (C_i) and an opacity (α). For each column, colors are accumulated from the back to the front, relative to the viewing direction. The color entering a voxel (C_{in}) will be decreased in proportion to the voxel's opacity (α); this color will then be combined with the color of the voxel itself, resulting in the exiting color (C_{out}).

$$C_{out} = C_i + (1 - \alpha_i)\, C_{in}$$

Opacities and colors are assigned in a classification step based on the voxel intensities. For example, on a CT scan, bone densities could be assigned

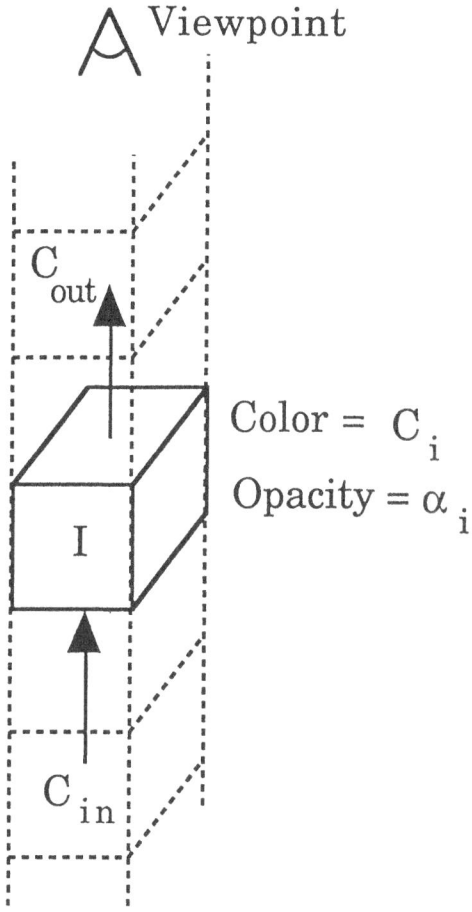

Figure 2. Each voxel in the image is assigned a color and and an opacity. After choosing a viewing direction (top), intensities are combined from farthest to nearest. The entering color (C_{in}) is diminished by the opacity of voxel I, and the result is combined with the voxel's color (C_i) to form the exiting color (C_{out}).

'white/opaque' and water density assigned 'red/translucent.' Intermediate densities are assigned intermediate values (e.g. 'pink/partially translucent'). This differs from the thresholding process used in surface rendering, as the classification is not binary. This multi-valued classification reduces the potential for artifacts in the image, although it makes the computation more complex.

Optionally, opacity can be a function of gradients in the image, so that the uniform interior of each object is transparent and only object surfaces are portrayed [6]. Calculation of surface normals from the gradients allows use of simulated illumination, as described above in the section on surface display. If illumination is employed, the color (C_i) at each voxel is determined by the tissue classification and the amount of light reflection off a surface oriented with respect to the gradient at that voxel. The above equation can then be modified so that the contribution of a voxel to the output color is also a function of its opacity, since a transparent voxel would not be expected to reflect light well.

$$C_{out} = \alpha_i C_i + (1 - \alpha_i) C_{in}$$

Maximum activity projection

Another compositing technique is to select the maximum voxel along each column, and record this value in the rendered image. This technique of maximum activity projection was independently developed for nuclear medicine tomography by our group at Washington University [5,8,9] and by other investigators for magnetic resonance angiography [10,11]. Maximum activity projection results in substantially greater image contrast than present in either planar imaging or summed projection, and results in contrast nearly equal to that present in the tomographic slices [5]. Furthermore, the final image depicts relative intensity values, rather than light reflection from surfac.s, thus preserving diagnostic information.

Since illumination is not employed as a depth cue, other depth cues need to be incorporated into the rendering process to provide the three dimensional effect. Given the computational simplicity of the algorithm, it is feasible to produce rendered images from a series of angles about the patient. Subsequent display in cine form conveys a strong three-dimensional effect, and likely increases the ability of the viewer to discern subtle abnormalities [12]. If no depth weighting is employed, there is ambiguity regarding the direction of rotation [13]. Addition of depth weighting prior to choosing the maximum voxel eliminates this ambiguity, and allows the closer structures to be examined with less interference from distant structures as the rotated images are viewed. Any decreasing function can be used for depth weighting; we have found exponential weighting with attenuation coefficients of 0.024 to 0.049 cm^{-1} to be useful for most tomographic acquisitions.

The result of application of the different rendering methods can be seen in Fig. 3, which shows a liver with a metastatic lesion in the dome of the liver, imaged using sulfur-colloid and rendered from several angles. The surface rendered images in the top row were produced with a simulated light source in the upper left of the image. The lesion can be clearly seen at the dome of the liver as it is on the surface of the liver; an interior lesion would not be visible. The second row illustrates summed projection; the result is similar to planar images, with fewer counts at the thin inferior margin. The third row shows images produced utilizing volumetric compositing with illumination, as described above. The net effect is similar to that of surface rendering, however the margins are slightly smoother than seen with surface rendering and the effect of transparency can be seen at the thin inferior

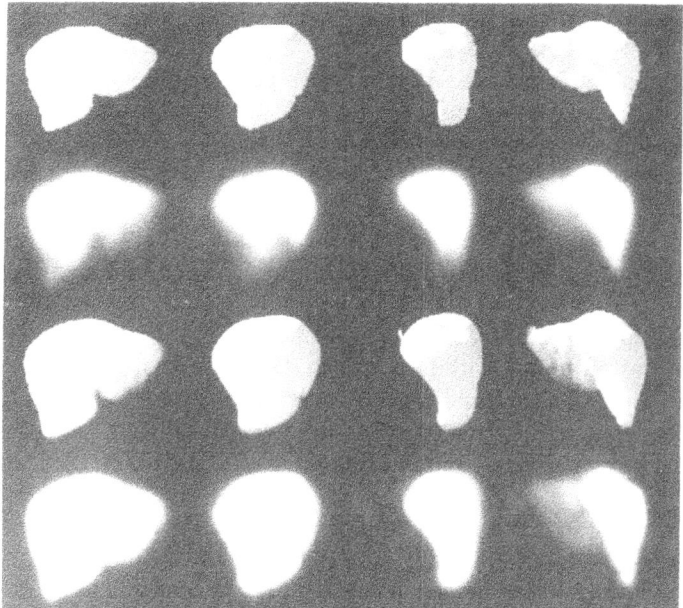

Figure 3. Images from a tomographic sulfur-colloid liver-spleen scan, rendered from several angles. A metastatic lesion is present in the dome of the liver. Row 1: surface rendering. Row 2: Summed projection. Row 3: Volumetric compositing with illumination. Row 4: Depth-weighted maximum activity projection. See text for discussion.

margin of the left lobe. The last row of images was created using depth-weighted maximum activity projection. The outline of the liver parenchyma is clearly depicted, but the cold lesion is not shown well in this 'hot-spot' rendering technique.

Applications

Imaging in nuclear medicine can be roughly divided into studies where the primary goal is to detect areas of increased uptake ('hot-spot' imaging) and studies where the diagnostic information is contained in areas of decreased tracer uptake ('cold-spot' imaging). Bone scintigraphy, gallium scintigraphy, and hepatic blood pool imaging are examples of hot-spot imaging, and myocardial perfusion imaging and sulfur-colloid liver/spleen imaging are examples of cold-spot imaging. Both the diagnostic goals and the optimal forms of three-dimensional display are different for these two categories of images, and it is appropriate to examine them separately.

Hot-Spot Imaging

Each of the above rendering methods have been applied to hot-spot SPECT studies. Prior to choosing the best method, it is appropriate to examine the characteristics of hot-spot scintigraphic studies:

1) There can be substantial variation of normal activity within an organ in different anatomic locations (e.g. bone in ribs vs spine), and the degree of uptake varies significantly between patients;
2) There is substantial overlap between normal organ uptake and abnormal uptake (e.g. abnormal uptake in a rib might reach the same intensity as normal uptake in the sacroiliac joint);
3) Variations of uptake within organs contain the majority of the diagnostic information and are important to depict in the rendered image;
4) Surface detail of organs is of little importance, and subtle surface features are not present in the acquired tomographic data due to noise and resolution limitations;
5) The most intense areas of uptake contain the majority of the diagnostic information.

The variation of uptake and overlap between normal and abnormal activity (#1 and #2 above) imply that segmentation using thresholding is not useful, and make any form of automatic segmentation quite difficult. The location of the diagnostic information and the limited usefulness of surface detail (#3 and #4 above) make use of surface displays inappropriate, as surface renderings are essentially binary images with superimposed depth cues. The fact that areas of increased uptake are most important to detect (#5 above) suggests that when regions of moderate/low uptake and regions of increased uptake overlap, the region of increased uptake should be emphasized in the rendered image. These principles suggest that volume rendering using maximum activity projection will be the most useful of the above-described techniques for three-dimensional display in hot-spot imaging.

One major advantage of maximum activity projection is the fact that no arbitrary thresholds need be chosen. This increases reproducibility and permits automatic generation of rendered images as part of the tomographic reconstruction process. Volume rendered images using depth-weighted maximum activity projection have been produced routinely in our clinic for all bone, gallium, and hepatic blood pool studies for several years as an adjunct to review of slice images, and the rendered images have been found to be valuable both in study interpretation and in communicating of information to the referring physician. An example of volume rendering in hepatic blood-pool imaging is shown in Fig. 4.

Several factors should be considered when implementing this algorithm. We have found it most useful to produce renderings from 64 angles about the patient, roughly corresponding to the views that were obtained during the 360 degree tomographic acquisition. Production of renderings from these oblique angles can be achieved either by tracing oblique paths through the

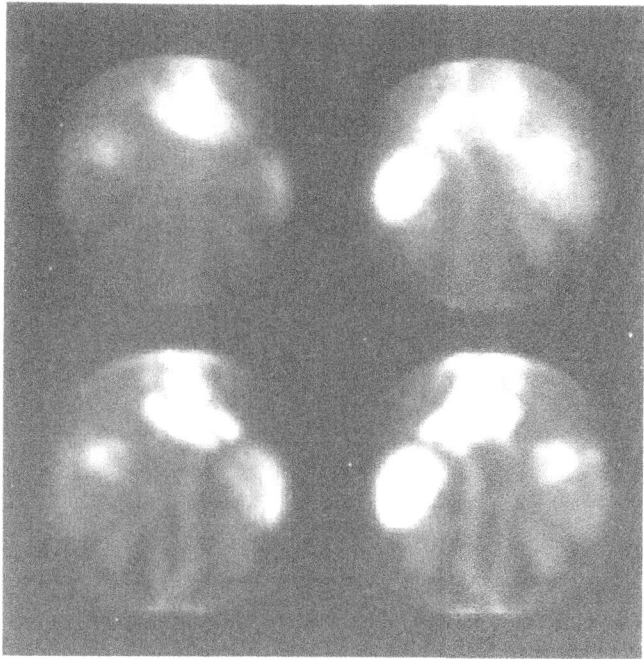

Figure 4. Blood-pool study of the chest and abdomen in a patient with a large hepatic hemangioma and several small hemangiomas; anterior (left) and posterior (right) images are shown. Contrast and image quality are superior in rendered SPECT images (bottom) compared to the planar images (top).

data, or by rotating the cube of data to the desired angle and tracing along rows and columns. The latter has the advantage that one can render from four directions with each rotation of the cube. If speed is critical, nearest neighbor interpolation when rotating the cube yields results that are only slightly inferior to bilinear interpolation. Interpolation of slices from 64×64 up to 128×128 prior to rotation allows use of nearest neighbor interpolation without loss of image quality. Rotation to any angle should always be performed from original (unrotated) cube of data, as successive rotations of the data would accumulate error and introduce additional blurring. As the rotations are typically about the Z axis, they can be performed on a slice-by-slice basis, if needed, to reduce computer memory requirements. It may be appropriate to use a lesser depth weighting factor in studies with a high degree of background activity, in order to maintain image contrast [5]. Careful attention to optimal programming techniques allows a 64 view cine of volume rendered images to be produced in 2–4 minutes on current high-end personal computers and low-end workstations, and processing is substantially faster on current RISC workstations.

Gated tomographic blood-pool imaging is an exception to the principles described above. While maximum activity projection can be employed successfully in this setting [9], principles #2, #3, and #4 are no longer applicable. There is little or no information contained in the interior of the blood pool, and all the diagnostic information is contained in the surface contours. This allows surface displays to be employed in a useful manner [14,15,16]. Due to limited resolution and the partial volume effect (which may change with chamber size during the cardiac cycle), thresholding is still not the optimal method of segmentation for use during production of surface rendered images. More complex gradient based techniques should be employed for detection of chamber boundaries.

Cold-spot imaging

Myocardial perfusion imaging is the most commonly performed form of cold-spot imaging. The myocardium can be considered to be a curved surface as it is thin with respect to the imaging resolution, allowing use of mapping techniques for three-dimensional display. Polar 'Bull's-eye' maps were introduced for thallium tomographic imaging in 1985 [17], and have been demonstrated to be useful in study interpretation [18]. Several methods of producing the Bull's-eye maps have been proposed. The original technique involved construction of each ring of the Bull's-eye map separately from maximal count circumferential profiles on individual short axis slices. As one approaches the apex, the slices are increasingly tangential to the myocardium. For this reason, it becomes difficult to distinguish between a true apical perfusion defect and decreased counts due to partial volume effect involving a slice which includes only a portion of the apex. One approach has been to use information from a long axis slice for the central portion of the Bull's-eye. Another more recent technique is to construct the polar map using a three-dimensional search for maximal wall counts, searching radially outward from the center of the ventricle [15]. Searches perpendicular to the wall have also been proposed.

All of these techniques produce Bull's-eye maps which overemphasize defects near the base of the heart, due to the distortions inherent in Polar maps. This is analogous to the falsely enlarged size of Greenland on maps of North America. Investigators have proposed decreasing the thickness of the rings of the Bull's-eye as one moves from apex to base, in order to compensate for this effect [19,20].

Another approach to minimizing distortion is to portray the maximal myocardial counts in three-dimensional format with cine presentation, analogous to viewing a slowly rotating globe of the earth. The counts may be mapped either onto a standard geometrical form [20,21] or onto the detected myocardial surface [15]. It is interesting to note that this latter method is equivalent to maximum activity projection with searching radially from the ventricular center, as opposed to the front-to-back search used for hot-spot imaging described above.

Surface displays have been employed for detection of cold defects in renal imaging, where the defects can be expected to lie at the cortical surface. It is unclear, however, whether three-dimensional display is needed in these small, relatively homogeneous organs.

Evaluation of the brain is a complex task, since both areas of increased and decreased uptake may be present. Bull's-eye maps have been proposed as a display method [22], however this will result in loss of information regarding the radial position of the abnormalities, and may be misleading if abnormalities do not extend across the full thickness of the brain. Limiting the search to the area between concentric ellipses may improve display accuracy [23]. Surface displays employing thresholding and maximal activity projection have also been employed in display of brain perfusion, however each has limitations in this setting. They may be used for aiding in orientation, but individual slices must be carefully examined as well.

Detection of areas of decreased uptake in large solid organs, such as the liver, require a different approach, and work is in progress in this area at our institution [24].

Future work

Improved methods of display of complex images containing both areas of increased and decrease uptake are needed. Although preliminary experience with three-dimensional displays has been quite encouraging, formal evaluation of the effect of rendered images on accuracy of diagnostic interpretation is necessary. Three-dimensional displays also clearly have a role in communication of information to the referring physician, and in correlation of information between different diagnostic and therapeutic modalities [21,25–28].

References

1. Phong BT. Illumination for computer generated pictures. Comm of the ACM 1975;18:311–17.
2. Goroud H. Continuous shading of curved surfaces. IEEE Trans on Comp 1971;C-20:623–9.
3. Goris ML, Boudier S, Briandet PA. Interrogation and display of single photon emission tomography data as inherently volume data. Am J Physiol Imaging 1986;1:168–80.
4. Silverstein EA, Spies SM, Zimmer AM, Spies WG. Three dimensional visualization of SPECT image data by presentation as stereo pairs. J Nucl Med 1988;29:810 (Abstract).
5. Wallis JW, Miller TR. Volume rendering in three-dimensional display of SPECT images. J Nucl Med 1990;31:1421–30.
6. Levoy M. Volume Rendering: Display of surfaces from volume data. IEEE Comp Graph Appl 1988;8(May):29–37.
7. Drebin RA. Volume Rendering. Comp Graph Appl 1988;22:65–74.

8. Wallis JW, Miller TR, Lerner CA, Kleerup EC. Three-Dimensional Display in Nuclear Medicine. IEEE Trans Med Imaging 1989;8(4):297–303.

9. Miller TR, Wallis JW, Sampathkumaran KS. Three-dimensional display of gated cardiac blood-pool studies. J Nucl Med 1989;30:2036–41.

10. Keller PJ, Drayer BP, Fram EK, Williams KD, Dumoulin CL, Souza SP. MR angiography with two-dimensional acquisition and three-dimensional display. Work in progress. Radiology 1989;173:527–32.

11. Masaryk TJ, Modic MT, Ross JS, et al. Intracranial circulation: preliminary clincal results with three-dimensional (volume) MR angiography. Radiology 1989;171:793–9.

12. Bailey DL. Improved display of SPECT data. J Nucl Med 1991;32:360–1.

13. Foley JD, Van Dam A. Fundamentals of Interactive Computer Graphics. Reading, MA: Addison-Wesley, 1982:545.

14. Gibson CJ. Real time 3D display of gated blood pool tomograms. Phys Med Biol 1988;33:569–81.

15. Miller TR, Starren JB, Grothe RAJ. Three-dimensional display of positron emission tomography of the heart. J Nucl Med 1988;29:530–7.

16. Faber TL, Stokely EM, Templeton GH, Akers MS, Parkey RW, Corbett JR. Quantification of three-dimensional left ventricular segmental wall motion and volumes from gated tomographic radionuclide ventriculograms. J Nucl Med 1989;30:638–49.

17. Garcia EV, Van Train K, Maddahi J, et al. Quantification of rotational thallium-201 myocardial tomography. J Nucl Med 1985;26:17–26.

18. Van Train KF, Maddahi J, Berman DS, et al. Quantitative analysis of tomographic stress thallium-201 myocardial scintigrams: a multicenter trial. J Nucl Med 1990;31:1168–79.

19. Tamaki N, Ohtani H, Yonekur Y, et al. A new bull's eye polar map display of thallium-201 SPECT imaging for quantitative measurement of perfusion defects. J Nucl Med 1990;31:808 (Abstract).

20. Cooke CD, Garcia EV, Folks RD, Peifer JW, Ezquerra NF. Visualization of cardiovascular nuclear medicine tomographic perfusion studies. Atlanta, GA: IEEE Computer Society Press, 1990: 185–189.

21. DePuey EG, Garcia EV, Ezquerra NF. Three-dimensional techniques and artificial intelligence in thallium-201 cardiac imaging. Am J Roent 1989;152:1161–8.

22. Maurer AH, Siegel JA, Comerota AJ, Morgan WA, Johnson MH. SPECT quantification of cerebral ischemia before and after carotid endarterectomy. J Nucl Med 1990;31:1412–20.

23. Links JM, Loats HL, Holcomb HH, Loats SE, Stumpf MJ, Wagner HN. Cortical circumferential profiling: an objective approach to cortical quantification in emission tomography. J Nucl Med 1989;30:816 (Abstract).

24. Wallis JW, Miller TR. Display of cold lesions in volume rendering of SPECT studies. J Nucl Med 1991;32:(Annual SNM abstract issue, in press).

25. Levin DN, Hu XP, Tan KK, et al. The brain: integrated three-dimensional display of MR and PET images. Radiology 1989;172:783–9.

26. Cooke C, Jofre L, Klein L, et al. 3–dimensional reconstruction of arterial structure from biplane angiography. Proceedings of 8th Annual IEEE technicon '87 conference. New York: Institute of Electrical and Electronics Engineers, 1987: 31–34. (Also see AJR 152:1161–1168).

27. Levoy M, Fuchs H, Pizer S, et al. Volume rendering in radiation treatment planning. Atlanta, GA: IEEE Computer Society Press, 1990: 4–10.

28. Jack CR, Marsh WR, Hirshcorn KA, et al. EEG scalp electrode projection onto three-dimensional surface rendered images of the brain. Radiology 1990;176:413–8.

7. New workstations for nuclear medicine

JOSEPH AREEDA and KENNETH VAN TRAIN

Summary

Modern nuclear medicine has benefitted from the recent development of more powerful and easier to use computer systems. The concept of a workstation, a powerful single user machine, has become feasible in recent years with the advent of high performance computers in relatively low cost and small packages. Furthermore local area networks using standard protocols have made the interconnection of multiple workstations from a single manufacturer routine, and soon will allow systems from multiple vendors to be integrated.

Requirements for a new nuclear medicine workstation are best expressed in terms of which studies will it acquire and/or process, and the necessary throughput. In addition acceptance testing for computer equipment, patterned after the gamma camera test, is important. The systems available are mostly full function systems providing acquisition, processing, display and reporting capabilities, with a few providing acquisition only modules. By dedicating workstations to a particular task and thereby reducing the importance of unrelated functions cost can be minimized. The most important factors for stations doing clinical acquisition are image resolution, count rate capabilities, planar as well as SPECT capabilities, gated data acquisition for SPECT and planar studies, and possibly on the fly SPECT reconstruction and ease of operation. For stations assigned to processing studies, ease of operation, speed of the programs, the availability of clinical quantification procedures and SPECT reconstruction are important. Display and reporting stations require the highest image resolution and viewing area. Furthermore they must be optimized for quick review by busy physicians, implying that ease of operation and speed are paramount.

Several current systems are examined and compared in terms of architecture, capabilities, and performance. The Siemens MaxDelta, DeltaManager and the integration of the soon to be released ICON provide an example of a server/client organization with a Digital Equipment VAX as the server. The ADAC Pegasys is based on a Sun workstation with special purpose stations for acquisition that communicate via Ethernet. The Picker Prism system uses a Stardent minisupercomputer based imaging workstation with a separate acquisition module. Several metrics will be presented which will allow the participants to judge aspects of different systems on their own.

Johan H.C. Reiber & Ernst E. van der Wall (eds.), Cardiovascular Nuclear Medicine and MRI, 101–111.
© 1992 *Kluwer Academic Publishers*.

Productivity and indeed the future of nuclear medicine is in a large part controlled by the tools available. The current systems available (or soon to be) are dramatic improvements from the previous generation in the performance available, their graphical user interfaces, and their interconnectivity. Furthermore, the introduction of object oriented software development tools promises long term benefits for the developers by being able to reuse more software, and more effective methods for program design.

New hardware platforms

Trends in the industry are showing us more of a continuum from low cost low performance personal computers, to high performance imaging workstations. The personal computers are increasing in power while traditional high performance systems are coming down in price with a good deal of overlap.

Of the systems we will be looking at, the Siemens ICON and the MedImage produced DeltaManager are based on a Macintosh personal computer. The ADAC is based on a Sun SparcStation and the Picker Prism is based on a Stardent minisupercomputer.

These systems all are based on 32–bit CPUs; the Macintosh is based on the Motorola 68030, a CISC (complex instruction set computer) microprocessor. On the other hand, the Sun uses a SPARC microprocessor and the Stardent uses up to 2 R3000; these are RISC (reduced instruction set computers). These systems provide a large memory address space and significantly improved processing power over previous generations. The Sun SparcStation 1 + used in the ADAC system is rated at 15.8 MIPS (million instructions per second) and 1.7 MFLOPS (million floating point instructions per second), while the Stardent GS-3020 is rated at 32 MIPS and 8.5 MFLOPS. A Macintosh IIfx is rated at about 2.6 MIPS and 1.2 MFLOPS. Compare these figures with previous generation systems in which even large servers such as the Vax 780 used in the Siemens MaxDelta configuration offered about 1 MIPS, while typical minicomputers such as the Digital Equipment PDP-11 and Data General Nova had about 0.7 MIPS.

Even with performance offered by the new systems general purpose CPUs most manufacturers continue to augment the power with special purpose array processors. The Stardent systems, as powerful as they are, cannot match the reconstruction speed of the attached backprojection engine used in tomographic reconstructions. The ADAC systems used proprietary processors, while the Siemens uses dedicated RISC processors to control display and additional array processors for computationally intensive functions such as backprojection, filtering and other image manipulations. In the systems we are considering only the DeltaManager relies on off the shelf hardware, and its functions are limited to display of existing data with no acquisition and minimal processing capabilities.

Large high resolution displays make many functions possible. The new software technologies discussed below rely upon bitmapped (each pixel is directly addressable) display to implement multiple windows with independent controls.

On line storage has not advanced to the same extent as the computing power. While computing power has increased by a factor of 10–20 over the previous generation of 16–bit processors, current disk technology is on the order of 3–5 times the capacity and 2–3 times the speed – a healthy improvement with some networked systems having over a gigabyte (1 billion bytes) of on line magnetic media.

Archival storage using optical disk drives is common. This media provides high capacity, up to 900 MB at each workstation, of reliable long term storage. The cost per megabyte is very reasonable at about US\$ 0.15 for a 900 MB WORM cartridge, compared to US\$ 1.00 per MB for a floppy disk. Thus more and more it is feasible to store all studies which is important for later recall if the patient returns and for potential research purposes.

New software technology

Advances in software have been steady over the years and the current generation is easier to use and to maintain, offering multiple sessions (if not multi-tasking) allowing easier transfer of data between programs, or viewing of complementary data simultaneously. In addition advancements and standardization of networking technology allow independent systems, often from different manufacturers, to communicate freely.

Windowing environment

The most striking difference of the new software is the windowing environment and graphical user interface. Windowing is a metaphor allowing multiple logical terminals to be open at one time. A window is basically a frame for viewing something. The contents are determined by the application. More than one window may be open at a time, and they may overlap. In other words the currently active window may obscure other information on the screen. This arrangement allows the operator to set aside information, yet have easy access to it. It also facilitates easy transfer of information between windows. Using operations such as cut and paste, parts of a document or image may be moved between windows or programs. In a windowing environment actions such as moving windows, resizing them or overlapping them, are done in a consistent system wide fashion, however, the application program must be involved. For example, in most window systems only the applications program knows the contents of its windows; when one window is uncovered by moving an obstructing window, the program must redraw that section of the screen. These operations do not affect the contents of the

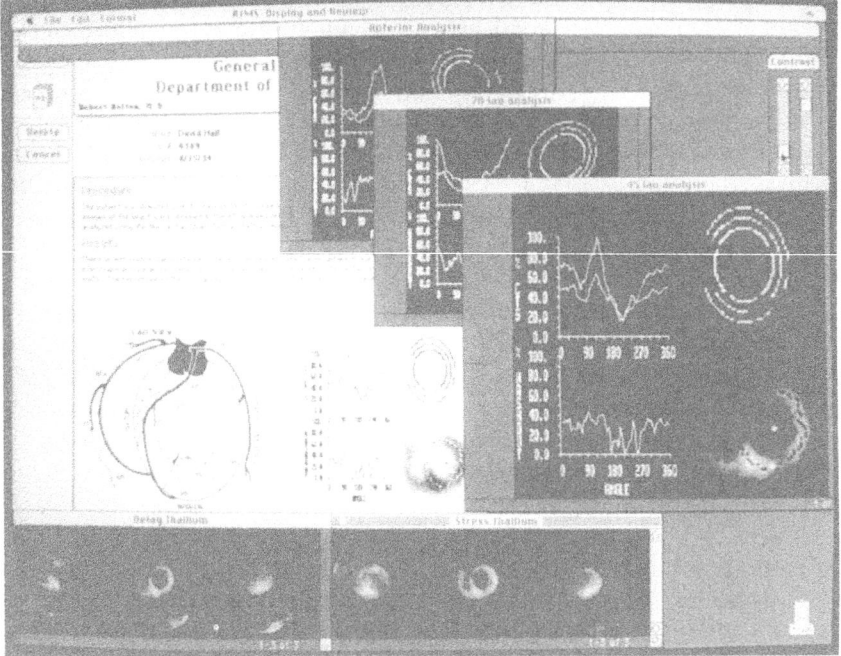

Figure 1. Example of how multiple overlapping windows can be used.

windows, only the user's view of them. Thus the user is able to tailor the work environment without fundamentally changing the elements of the applications.

Figure 1 shows multiple overlapping windows taken from a DeltaManager system. It presents the users with considerable information yet allows them to focus on an individual window and perform related functions. In this example we see six open windows as they may be presented during the diagnosis of a planar thallium study. At the bottom there are 3 views of stress and three views of delayed thallium-201 images. On the right are the results of quantification with circumferential profiles plotted, and ellipses encoding the comparison against normal limits. In the background on the left is the clinician's report. The strong point of the windowing environment is the ease with which the application program context can be changed. If the doctor uses a mouse or other device to activate the report window he may type in his clinical impressions or conclusions. If he wishes to look at the images in detail he selects that window and may adjust contrast.

Graphical user interface

A graphical user interface or GUI is an alternate man-machine interface. All implementations of GUI's to date have been combined with windowing

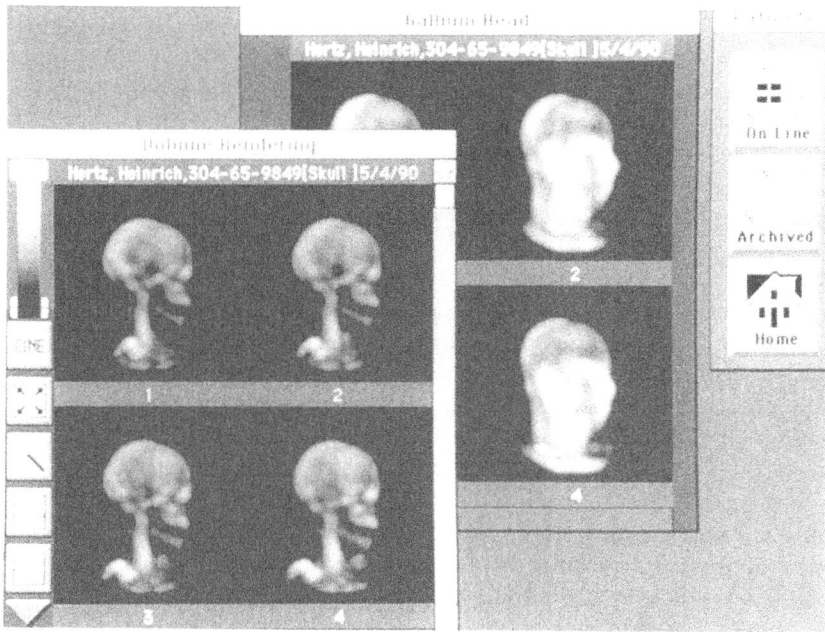

Figure 2. Graphical user interfaces use icons to represent commands available.

to provide a more intuitive user environment. A GUI uses symbols, icons and tools which are meant to represent things people are familiar with (Fig. 2).

These metaphors from the real world give the users a set of expectations which they can apply to the computer [1,2]. In addition, these objects are directly manipulated with a mouse or other pointing device. For example, to delete a file from a disk one will identify the file by pointing to it and clicking the button on the mouse, then dragging it to a trash can icon. In most cases this trash can icon will then change in some way to indicate there is something in it. The file itself is not actually deleted until another action called emptying the trash is performed.

The direct manipulation of objects gives people the feeling they are in charge. In addition, the users are now put in the position of seeing and pointing to what they want to do rather than remembering and typing a command. So the process becomes one of recognition rather than recall. Most programmers, or people who use computers extensively, work efficiently with a command line interface which requires memorization and Boolean logic. However new computer users or occasional users gain impressive increases in productivity from the graphical interface.

When a system is designed around a graphical interface, programs acquire a consistency of operator interaction not seen in other approaches. Both within a single program and across applications this consistency is the key to

GUI effectiveness. A person is thus able to use a general set of skills learned in one program and apply those skills to all others. This consistency is developed in two ways. First of all the system level tools for developing a program interface give a certain look to the objects drawn on the screen, but it is not enough to enforce consistent behavior across applications. This behavioral consistency is demanded by the users and quickly becomes a major standard for judging the quality of a program.

The development of programs which operate under a graphical user interface tend to be more complicated than similar programs in a more traditional environment. This is the result of a subtle concept of user control central to the GUI. In a command line interface the program has control, it gives the users a limited set of options depending on the current context, it gets a command, performs an operation, and prompts for the next action. The user is in the passive position of responding to the computer's prompts. Under a GUI the program has a wider range of events to respond to. The user may pick a choice from a menu, type in characters, use the mouse to select a new tool, or use the mouse to select another window belonging to another application. Because of this wide range of events it is harder to predict what path a user will take to get to any section of the program.

To handle this wide range of events, programs are usually organized into what is called an 'event loop'. The main program is a large case statement. The system provides the program with events, and the main program looks for events it knows how to process. An event may be a mouse click in one of its windows, a menu selection, a character typed, or a network message. If the program does not process an event it may be passed back to the system to try other running applications. This does not mean, however, that a program must be able to perform any command at any time. For example, before a user has opened a file, say, holding images, the commands to save or close the file make no sense. These situations are usually handled by disabling certain menu options until they are applicable.

Networking

Most current systems provide network hardware and software. The most common standard is Ethernet which was developed by Xerox Corp in the 1970s. It defines the low level physical connections but not higher level program to program communications protocols. This means there can be multiple systems using the same Ethernet cable which cannot communicate with each other. For example, Fig. 3 shows a typical Ethernet configuration.

Note that Ethernet is a bus structured network. This means that there is no central node, and the network is not a loop, so there is a 'backbone' cable running through the area with systems simply tapping into it. Some of these systems could be Macintoshes using an Appletalk protocol to send files back and forth, and others could be Sun workstations using TCP/IP. Except

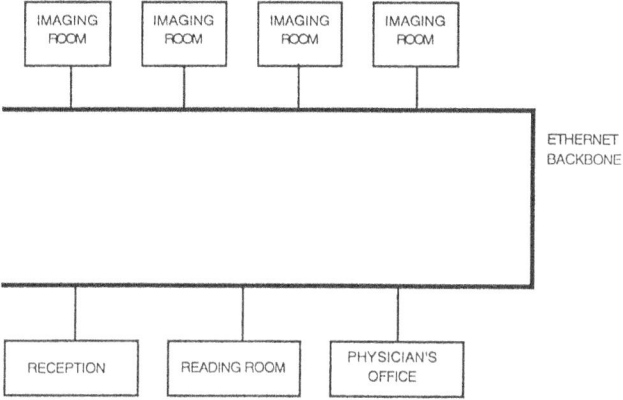

Figure 3. Typical network configuration.

for the availability of the backbone these systems would not know of each other's existence.

There are many protocols in use by the different workstations. Fortunately though, many of these systems can support multiple protocols simultaneously. For example, a Macintosh on a network with other Macintoshes, DEC VAXes, Sun Workstations, and other Unix based systems could easily use different network software to communicate with each type of system. Appletalk would be used for the Macintoshes, DecNet for the VAXes, and TCP/IP for the Unix based systems. This software would allow a Macintosh user to sign onto any system as a terminal, or transfer files to and from the other system, and possibly use part of one of the other systems disks as though it were physically attached to the Mac.

Networks are cost effective because workstations are dedicated to a particular task, yet have access to all the information on other systems in the network. This allows the workstation to be configured to perform its task rather than to be loaded with expensive hardware and software to perform any task. For example, the imaging rooms contain acquisition–only stations, the physician offices and reading rooms, contain display–only stations with a few additional processing stations to analyze the studies. In this way, camera time is maximized, and stations for reading studies are more available.

Networks can extend beyond a department or hospital. Local area networks are usually defined as those which can be wired together, or use low power radio transmitter/receivers. It is often desirable for a Nuclear Medicine department to be connected with remote sites. This often means connecting a hospital with a related outpatient facility, or multiple related facilities. The major alternatives are to use low speed phone line connections to transmit data on demand. These connects vary in speed up to about 2000 bytes per second using current state of the art dial-up modems (V.42).

If higher data rates are needed T1–bridges may be used. These devices use high speed (1.2 million bits per second/150,000 bytes per second) lines leased from the phone company to connect two or more local area networks. When they are operational, data from either site may be accessed at close to normal network speeds. There are solutions with even higher data rates, such as direct fiber optic connections, or even microwave transceivers which are used by businesses which demand highly reliable, high volume data transmission but the need for this kind of equipment in Nuclear Medicine has not been demonstrated.

Object oriented programming

The object-oriented paradigm, or model, is a new approach to analysis, design, and implementation of computer software. It involves abstraction mechanisms developed to address increasing complexity in today's software and also addresses issues regarding the reuse of code as a means of increasing productivity and reliability. There are three concepts basic to the object-oriented approach, they are called encapsulation, polymorphism, and inheritance [3]. Object-oriented languages such as C^{++}, Object Pascal, and Smalltalk provide mechanisms for easily using these concepts but one should not confuse these languages with the methodology which is independent of the implementation. There are many object-oriented ideas currently implemented in operating systems, and user interfaces developed in older procedural languages.

The basic unit in the object-oriented paradigm is not surprisingly called an object. An object is an abstraction encapsulating both data and functions. Finding and creating these objects is a problem of structuring knowledge and activities. This encapsulation takes the structured programming concept of modularity even further.

As a matter of contrast, procedural programming separates functions and data structures. In structured procedural design we first try to define what needs to be done. Then through a process step wise refinement each task is broken into smaller tasks until we reach a point where a unit of code called a module can be written. Thus procedural programming deals with the implementation of a program almost from the beginning. The first question we ask ourselves is how.

Object-oriented programming begins more abstractly. We first look at the intent of the program. We define objects and their connections. These objects model the problem in terms more easily understood by the end user. Objects may be formed of things such as images, studies, or protocols, on the user level, or windows, tools and controls on the interface level. It is important to note that objects are models of the problem space as opposed to programs which are models of the solutions. Thus in object-oriented design the first question we ask is what.

Once an object is defined and its functionality and necessary information are combined and encapsulated a public interface is created. This defines how other objects and parts of the program may access this object. Everything else is hidden. In this way objects may evolve without affecting the other objects which refer to them. Limiting access to a strictly defined interface allows the use of another abstraction called polymorphism. Polymorphism is the ability of two or more objects to respond to the same request, each in its own way. In other words the requesting object does not need to know much about the object it is making a request of. It just needs to know that many different kinds of objects can respond to a particular request.

For example, consider objects called Time-Activity-Curve, Region-of-Interest, Static-Image, and Dynamic-Image. Each type of object has different requirements for data storage, applicable functions, and presentation, however each could respond to a display message (request). Each would implement the display function in a completely different manner but the object requesting this function would only need to know that each could be displayed.

Polymorphism allows us to exploit similarities between different classes of objects. We can recognize that many objects could respond to the same message, each in their own way. The object requesting the function can be indifferent to how the individual classes perform their functions. Similar generality is much more complicated in a procedural environment, although not impossible. It becomes a matter of maintaining the data structure and corresponding routines, at some level, though these must be matched and different procedures called.

Inheritance is another abstraction mechanism which allows one class to define its behavior and data structures as a superset of another class or classes. In other words, we can say that the new class is almost like the old class except that it includes something extra. This is a powerful mechanism to produce code that can be reused many times. We can design groups of classes (all somehow related) which share common behavior and data. The terms superclass and subclass are defined such that the subclass inherits behavior from its superclass.

Figure 4 shows a simple inheritance diagram, or class hierarchy. At the top is a class called Patient-Data. It is the superclass. It could define basic functions common to many of the subclasses such as creating index entries and data files, operator interaction for selection, deletion of files. It may even have some sort of rudimentary display methods. Obviously on this level we don't even know what we are going to display but there may be functions common to all displays, such as opening a window displaying tools for changing color tables.

On the next level down each subclass would use the methods (functions) defined by the superclass but would add methods particular to each object class such as display, read, write. Each would have methods called the same name so polymorphism could take advantage of the similarities between the classes on the same level, while inheritance would take advantage of similari-

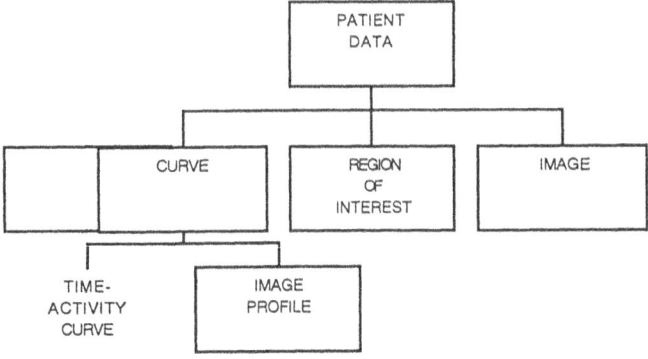

Figure 4. Sample class hierarchy.

ties between superclasses and subclasses. Note that with an inherited display routine each subclass may add functionality specific to its class but use all appropriate methods.

New problems

The new technologies discussed are not without their own problems. The high resolution displays and graphical user interfaces require extensive computing power to be responsive. With bitmapped displays in full color these systems use the power of today's CPUs to the full extent.

Graphical user interfaces are complex to program. This is partially because the user has the freedom to select almost any action at any time. This results in more paths through a program, making it more difficult to test thoroughly. Also because of the advanced display capabilities, programs tend to display full graphics on line. For example, word processors will display a document as it would look when printed, even as text is being entered. There is also a great deal of code which simply deals with the user interface. There is little doubt that this effort is well spent, but these programs may spend 30–50 % of the lines code on the user interface compared with 10–30 % for a command line oriented program. Object-oriented programming with object libraries dedicated to user interaction makes these problems more manageable.

Networking ties different systems together into a distributed department, with each system tailored to a particular task. The whole network may be vulnerable to failure in some new ways. For example, a system could go down in such a way that it overloads the network with spurious messages. While not a major service problem, the network may be unusable until the offending unit is identified and brought off-line for repair. Thus equipment redundancy and emergency planning are more important.

Conclusion

Nuclear Medicine workstations have advanced significantly since the previous generation. This generation is based on commercial image processing systems and has shown improvement in computing power, operator interfaces, display technology, interoperability, and software engineering tools. This paper has examined the hardware and software components involved and has presented the basics of the new technologies.

References

1. Apple Computer, Apple Human Interface Guidelines: The Apple Desktop Interface. Reading, Massachusetts: Addison-Wesley, 1987:3–11.
2. Sun Microsystems, Open Look Graphical User Interface Applications Style Guidelines. Reading, Massachusetts: Addison-Wesley, 1990:2–9.
3. Wirfs-Brock F, Wilkerson B, Wiener L, Designing Object-Oriented Software. Englewood Cliffs, New Jersey: Prentice Hall, 1990:3–36.

8. Multi-modal data fusion to combine anatomical and physiological information in the head and heart

DAVID J. HAWKES, DEREK L.G. HILL and
EMMA C.M.L. BRACEY

Summary

This chapter describes our recent experiences in multi-modal image combination and fusion at Guy's Hospital in London. We are investigating opportunities for synergism that might derive from the combination of images from different modalities.

A prequisite for image combination is the accurate registration of data between modalities. Applications in the head are described which use external skin markers to register 3D MRI and SPECT images with an accuracy of about 4 mm. Using user identified point-like landmarks we can register MR and CT images of the head for skull base surgery with an accuracy of between 1 and 2 mm.

Preliminary work using object centred representations of an anatomical structure has shown that we can register reconstructions of the vascular tree, derived from DSA images, with the brain surface, derived from MR images, with an accuracy of about 1.5 mm. We demonstrate the combination of gated MR and SPECT images of the heart based on establishing the long axis of the left ventricle in each modality.

Introduction

Motivation

In the last 3 decades there have been major advances in our ability to examine the structure and function of the human body using a wide range of imaging sensors. Medical imaging primarily provides spatial information on the location of anatomical structures, their size and shape, and whether any pathological structures exist. This wealth of information can be duplicatory (and therefore redundant), confirmatory (necessary at certain critical stages of patient management), complementary (providing separate but useful information), synergistic (the combination of information provides useful extra information) or, occasionally, conflicting (although conflict will always demand explanation).

Johan H.C. Reiber & Ernst E. van der Wall (eds.), Cardiovascular Nuclear Medicine and MRI, 113–130.
© 1992 *Kluwer Academic Publishers*.

Our group is engaged in work to address issues arising from the clinical use of multiple imaging modalities. We pose the following questions:

1. Are we extracting all relevant clinical information potentially available from the combination of these multiple modalities?
2. Would this extra information change patient management (by improving diagnosis and therapy planning or by removing the necessity for other more expensive investigations)?   Our particular interest is in the opportunities for synergism that might be provided by using image processing techniques to combine or 'fuse' data from multiple imaging modalities. We take the term 'data fusion' to mean the process which combines relevant information from two or more separate sources to produce new information.

As all imaging modalities primarily provide spatial information, key prerequisites for data fusion are the establishment of a common coordinate frame, i.e. image registration, and determining the accuracy with which we can achieve this.

In this paper we present our experiences in establishing image registration in a number of clinical applications. We will also describe our methods for computing and presenting the extra information available following registration. An appropriate term that has been coined for these processes is 'synergistic imaging'.

Image registration

Conventionally, image data are acquired with a coordinate system relative to the imaging device. Good radiographic practice usually results in images in which the patient is positioned carefully in relation to the imaging device. External anatomical landmarks, laser positioning devices, etc., are routinely used to 'set-up' the patient for imaging. Images are usually acquired with a positional reproducibility of between 5 and 20 mm and at an orientation within 5 to 10 degrees depending on the modality, the region of the body and the clinical application.

Images can be registered to a common coordinate system after identifying features, visible in each image, which are equivalent, or have known correspondence. These features might be external markers or frames attached to the patient, or features such as points, lines, surfaces or volumes which correspond to specific anatomical structures.

In surgical or radiotherapy treatment planning it may also be necessary to establish the geometric relationship between the patient and the surgical or therapy equipment.

Registration using external markers attached to the head

Markers attached to the skull provide an excellent basis for a coordinate system for registration of images of the head. The most invasive yet until recently most accurate means of establishing registration between images of the head is to use markers attached to the base ring of a stereotaxic frame which is bolted or pinned directly to the skull. Several groups have shown that in stereotaxic neurosurgery registration to an accuracy of about 1 mm can be achieved when combining images obtained by magnetic resonance (MRI), x-ray computed tomography (CT), positron emission tomography (PET) and digital subtraction angiography (DSA), for example [1–4]. Accuracy better than 1 mm is unlikely to be useful due to the finite resolution of the imaging devices, the natural movement of the brain during the cardiac and respiratory cycles and the distortion of brain tissue that occurs during stereotaxic procedures [5]. Thomas et al. have reported the use of a relocatable frame which is attached to a dental impression to register MR, CT, and PET images [6]. We have also experimented with such a device and our experiences are outlined below.

External markers attached to the skin and visible in each modality provide a convenient, non-invasive method for registering images of the head. In our implementation described below, the markers are fixed in position for the duration of acquisition of all images to be registered. The markers are difficult to relocate. Elsen and Viergever claim to have overcome this problem by designing 'V' shaped markers which point to marks drawn on the skin with indelible ink [7]. They have applied this technique to the registration of images of electric dipole activity derived from the EEG with MR images of the head.

Anatomical landmarks and features

The use of external landmarks necessarily requires changes to the acquisition routine and therefore the decision to register data must be taken prior to image acquisition. These limitations have precluded the widespread use of multi-modal or synergistic imaging. Images of the head, however, provide a large number of natural landmarks which may be used for registration. Pelizzari et al. have shown how images of the skin surface or brain surface derived from MRI and PET transmission data can be used for registration [8]. They have developed an algorithm which automatically registers points derived from one surface with the other surface. This technique has been widely used and has been found to be robust when sufficiently well defined overlapping skin surface data is available from the two modalities. Below we outline an improvement which allows explicit coding of uncertainty in surface location and the use of different surfaces which have a well defined anatomical relationship. Evans et al. [9] have demonstrated registration of PET and MRI images using user identified landmarks to establish the rotation and translation transformations between two image data sets. They propose that by identifying more than the three landmarks strictly necessary to derive the transformations of rotation and translation, they can improve the accuracy of registration of PET and MRI data.

Lemoine et al. have developed a potentially effective system for registration of DSA, CT and MRI images based on the identification of the midline fissure, the surface of the brain and corpus callosum on MRI, the vessels around the corpus callosum visible on DSA and the inner surface of the skull and mid-line fissure on CT [2]. Their system is used for planning neurosurgery.

These techniques rely on identification of structures which form a part of the object being imaged. We propose that an 'anatomical object centred' representation will provide the most effective framework for data representation not only for developing software to achieve registration but also for data fusion, display and interaction. In an object centred representation a co-ordinate system and geometric description is defined for a particular feature, anatomical structure or object of interest. This approach is particularly important outside the head where external landmarks do not have fixed relationships to internal structures and internal landmarks are difficult to define. In this paper we outline and show preliminary results of such schemes, firstly, for registering 3D information on blood vessels derived from DSA images and the surface of the brain derived from MR images and, secondly, for registering MR and SPECT (single photon emission tomographic) images of the heart.

Assessment of registration accuracy

The validity and hence clinical utility of the combined or fused data sets are critically dependent on the accuracy of registration. The required registration accuracy will depend on the inherent spatial resolutions of the individual imaging modalities and on the specific clinical applications for which the registered data sets are required. Previous work in this area has tended to neglect thorough assessment of registration accuracy. Although our work is not complete in this area we will present results achieved to date.

Registration to anatomical atlases

In many parts of the body, but in particular in the brain, anatomical atlases can assist in the interpretation of medical image data and in therapy planning. In the brain there is remarkable consistency of size and shape of anatomical structures between individuals provided that the image of the brain is scaled and orientated relative to deep internal structures. Tailarach has proposed a co-ordinate system based on the AC-PC line with proportional squaring to the most anterior, posterior, inferior, superior and two most lateral dimensions of the brain [10]. This significantly reduces inter-individual variations.

Keyserlingk in his statistical voxel model has shown that deep basal structures can be located with an accuracy of 5 mm after this alignment and scaling [11].

We have implemented a simple scheme, described below, in which MRI data from a volunteer is labelled approximately according to tissue type and aligned and scaled to external skin markers.

Multi-modal or synergistic imaging at UMDS

In this paper we will outline several techniques for achieving registration that we have devised and evaluated for accuracy. To date multi-modal registration work has been mainly confined to the head due to the greater ease of establishing a common coordinate system relative to the skull. Our applications of multi-modal synergistic imaging have been confined to two main clinical areas:

1. The use of anatomical information derived from high resolution data (usually MRI, CT or x-ray), to aid in the interpretation of lower resolution functional or physiological nuclear medicine images; and
2. The accurate registration of high resolution images to aid in surgical planning.

Image transformation

Image registration requires the derivation of a transformation between the coordinate frames of each set of images. In most of our work at UMDS we assume that geometric distortion in each modality is negligible or has been corrected and that the pixel dimensions of each modality are known before registration. Only rigid body translation and rotation transformations are therefore required. The co-ordinates of at least three non-collinear points are required to register 3D images.

In general no skewing or warping of either data set is performed. We calculate the transformation which minimizes the root mean square displacement error of each marker point. We use the algorithm presented by Arun et al. which decouples the rotation and translation components [12].

Display strategies

We display our registered images as slices of the registered 3D data sets. Either images are displayed side by side with a linked cursor indicating corresponding locations, or a color overlay technique is used, or a single fused grey scale image is generated. In the color overlay method alternate pixels are assigned, as in a chequer board pattern, to each modality. For one modality, usually the anatomical image (MR, CT or X-ray), the pixel is displayed grey with an intensity related to the pixel value. For the other modality, usually nuclear medicine, the image pixel value is assigned a saturated color on a 'rainbow' color scale. By sacrificing half the potential spatial resolution of the display and half the potential dynamic range, this technique allows the viewer to perceive, in principle, 128×128 colors on a display only physically capable of displaying 256 separate colors.

A single combined grey scale display of bone derived from CT and soft tissue derived from MR is used to display registered MR and CT data of the head.

3D Registration of SPECT images of the brain to MR images or an MR derived atlas

Method

We have devised two methods in which we use MRI data to assist in the delineation of anatomical structures in SPECT images of the brain. In the fir : method we register 3D MRI and SPECT images of the head of the same pa ient acquired consecutively with markers visible in each modality. In the second method we have constructed a segmented and labelled 3D MRI data set from a normal volunteer. This data set is acquired with markers in the same position on the skin surface. More technical detail is provided in [13,14].

Registration of the 3D image data sets was accomplished by means of four external markers which were attached to the skin surface above the mastoid processes of the temporal bones and the zygomatic processes of the frontal bone. The markers were designed to be visible in both modalities and they were left in place on the patient's skin for the duration of both scans. The position of the vertex of the skull was also used when aligning image data to the atlas.

Results

Two examples of registered MRI and SPECT images are shown on Figs. 1 and 2. The transaxial MR scans were acquired on a Philips Medical Systems Gyroscan S15. The pulse sequences and slice thicknesses were determined by the routine clinical protocol. The SPECT images were acquired on an IGE Starcam AC400 Tomographic Gamma Camera using 64 30 second acquisitions and a 360 degree camera rotation. The patients were injected with hexamethylpropyleneamine oxime (HMPAO) labelled with 750 MBq of Tc-99m 20 minutes prior to image acquisition. Figure 1a shows a study of a patient after interstitial radiotherapy showing the correspondence between oedematous changes in the MR image and reduced blood flow in the

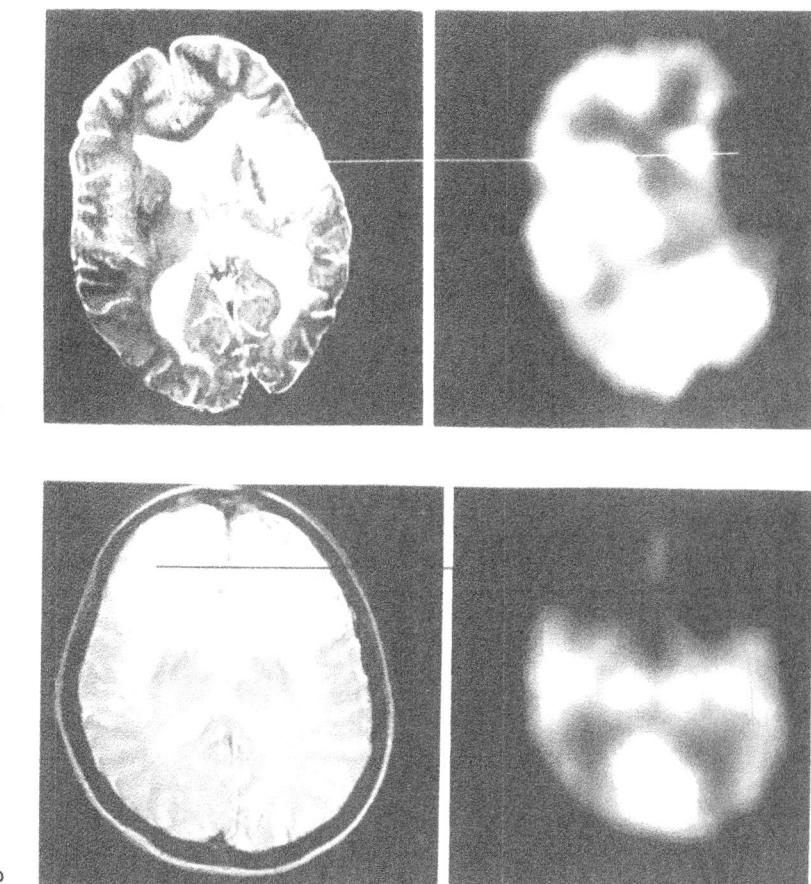

Figure 1. Registered transaxial slices through the brain showing an MR image on the left and corresponding Tc-99m HMPAO SPECT image on the right. A 'linked cursor' connects corresponding points in the two studies. (a) Shows correspondence between the oedematous region after interstitial radiotherapy seen in the MR image and the region of reduced blood flow in the nuclear image. (b) Shows correspondence between MR image and nuclear medicine image of an infarcted region.

HMPAO study. Figure 1b shows aligned transaxial images of a patient with established infarct. The clinical images are displayed with a linked cursor indicating corresponding points in the two images. Our clinical colleagues have found this display the most informative and intuitive and therefore most useful. Occasionally the alternate pixel display has proved useful. An example is shown in Fig. 2a. This display was derived from the images shown on Fig. 1b. Hue is related to isotope activity, with blue through to red corresponding to the lowest through to the highest isotope activities. In this image a narrow rim of lower activity is seen posterior to the infarct site which was not immediately apparent in the image displayed in Fig. 1b.

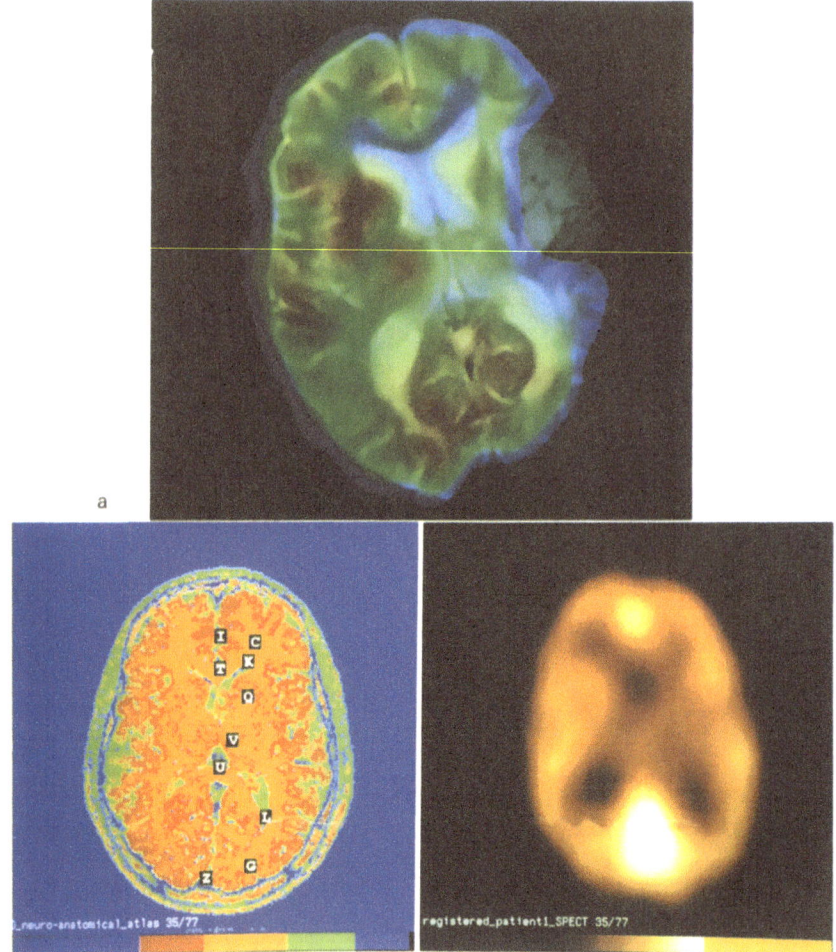

Figure 2. (Colour plate.) (a) Colour overlay display of images in Fig. 1b showing rim of reduced isotope uptake posterior to the infarct. Red corresponds to the highest isotope uptake and blue corresponds to the lowest uptake. (b) One transaxial slice of the atlas data, derived by labelling a high resolution MR data set, aligned with a normal Tc-99m HMPAO scan [14]. (c) Shows the combined gated MR and Tc-99m SestaMIBI image of a horizontal long axis slice through the apex of the heart. The isotope activity is colour coded as in Fig. 2a. Alignment was achieved by defining the long axis of the left ventricle in each modality.

For each study the individual RMS displacement between corresponding markers in the aligned data sets was calculated. The mean RMS displacement for the three studies described above was 4.1 mm. Experiments with a phantom constructed from Lego Technic have shown that internal structures can be located with an accuracy of better than 4 mm when four markers, corresponding in position to the skin surface, were used for registration. Separate work on the measurement of the geometric distortion produced by our MR scanner has shown that distortion is less than 2 mm within the field of view of the head coil [15].

Figure 2b shows an example of the atlas data aligned with a normal transaxial HMPAO scan. For the anatomical atlas 126 transaxial 256 × 256 pixel 2 mm thick contiguous MR slices were collected (TR 350 msec, TE 30 msec). In order to assess the accuracy of location of neuro-anatomical structures using the atlas we acquired seven MR scans with markers in place on patients undergoing routine brain imaging. We assessed the accuracy of registration of several anatomical structures including the optic chiasma and the anterior and posterior horns of the lateral ventricles. As expected the tips of the lateral ventricles showed the greatest discrepancy (12 mm standard deviation) while the optic chiasma had a discrepancy of only 4.6 mm. These results showed that the location accuracy for internal structures compares well with the inherent resolution of SPECT (approximately 10 mm) despite using only linear scaling, rotation and translation to establish registration to external skin markers on a single individual's MR scan.

High precision registration of MRI and CT images of the head for neurosurgery and skull base surgery

We have identified applications in neuro-surgery and skull base surgery in which accurate registration of MR and CT images of the head could be of considerable benefit in surgical planning. We have developed two alternative methods to achieve image registration. The first method uses an adaptation of a localizing frame attached to a dental impression first proposed by Thomas et al., while the second method relies on the identification of a number of corresponding anatomical point-like structures in both data sets [6].

Method 1: registration using the frame attached to a dental impression

The localizing frame is shown in Fig. 3. The frame is fixed to the patient's teeth by means of a silicone rubber dental impression. The frame consists of two perspex plates, each of which contain two Z-shaped line markers orientated at 90° to each other. The markers are tubes of rectangular cross section (4 mm × 2 mm) which are filled with contrast material with a concentration of 30 mg/ml of iodine. This fluid produces sufficient image contrast to be visible both in CT and MR images without causing artefact. The intersection of the image plane with the marker lines visible in each set of images is used to create a set of points for registration. The method of registration is similar to that used with stereotactic frames except that for patient comfort we use only two localizing plates, one on each side of the head [1–4]. Two Z markers are required in each plate, orientated at 90° to each other, in order to resolve the ambiguity of cranio-caudal tilt. The markers will also be visible in unsubtracted digital angiographic images. The registration accuracy achieved

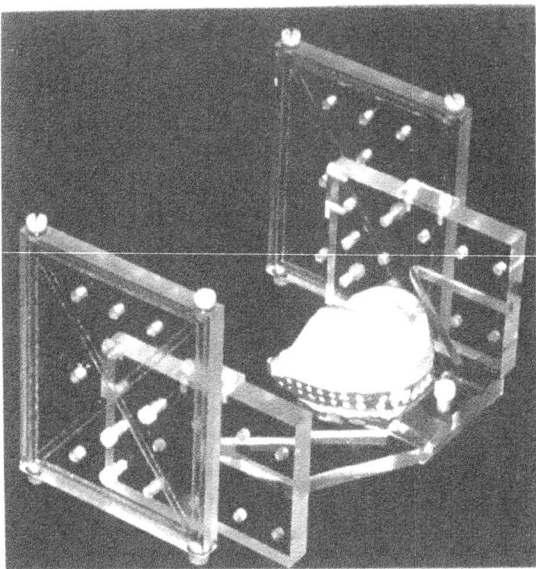

Figure 3. The dental impression attached to two plates. each containing 2 'Z' shaped markers oriented at right angles.

with this frame was assessed by performing an MR scan on a volunteer with the dental impression in position, removing the volunteer from the scanner, repositioning the dental impression and re-scanning.

Results

Two observers identified six anatomical landmarks in both MR images after alignment using the frame and obtained RMS displacements of identified points of 1.9 and 1.15 mm respectively. Figure 4 shows two slices from separate MR scans which had been aligned using the images of the markers attached to the tooth frame. Only one patient has been studied so far using the frame and further work is necessary to evaluate its utility in clinical practice.

Method 2: identification of internal fiducial markers

It became apparent in our assessment of errors in the use of the frame attached to the dental impression that we could identify structures in the base of the skull and temporal bones with a high level of precision in both MR and CT. We have, therefore, used a number of features to register MR and CT images of 6 patients. Images from two will be presented here. The first had an acoustic neuroma on the right side which was surgically removed using a translabyrinthine approach. The second patient had a glomus tumour.

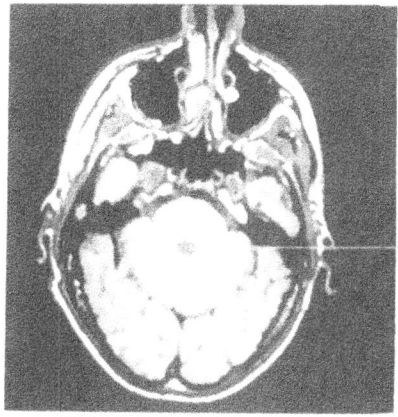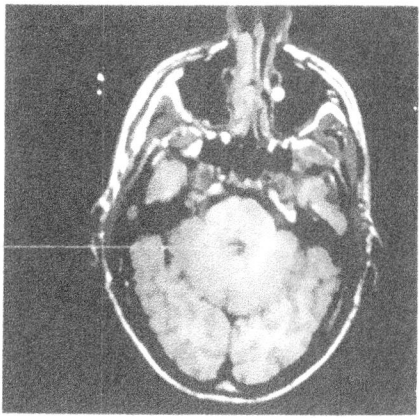

Figure 4. Two corresponding slices from MR scans, acquired on separate occasions and aligned with the aid of the markers on the frame.

The following point-like structures were used to register the two data sets in the first study:

1. The tip of the alar cartilage (visible in both modalities).
2. The most inferior junction of the anterior wall of the sphenoid sinus with the sphenoid inter-sinus septum (visible in both modalities).
3. The modiolus of the left and right cochlea (visible in both modalities).
4. The termination of the nasolacrimal duct in the right maxillary sinus (visible in both modalities).
5. The confluence of the superior sagittal sinus and the transverse sinus (visible using MR) and the internal occipital proturberance (visible using CT).

Further details of this study are provided in [16]. Three non-colinear marker co-ordinates are sufficient to achieve registration. We use between 6 and 12 and this leads to some averaging of registration errors. Our registration algorithm calculates the registration error for all marker points in the registered data sets, together with the root mean square (RMS) error for all points [17]. We use the latter measure to assess registration accuracy.

Results

The inter- and intra-observer error (three observers) in locating the landmarks listed above, for the first patient, were less than the voxel dimensions of the scan data. This patient had CT scans of 1.5 mm slice thickness, and MR scans of 2 mm slice thickness. In the second case, a patient with a glomus tumour, the MR and CT slice thicknesses were both 3 mm. All slices were contiguous. RMS discrepancies of marker location of 1.4 mm for the first patient and 1.8 mm for the second patient were achieved.

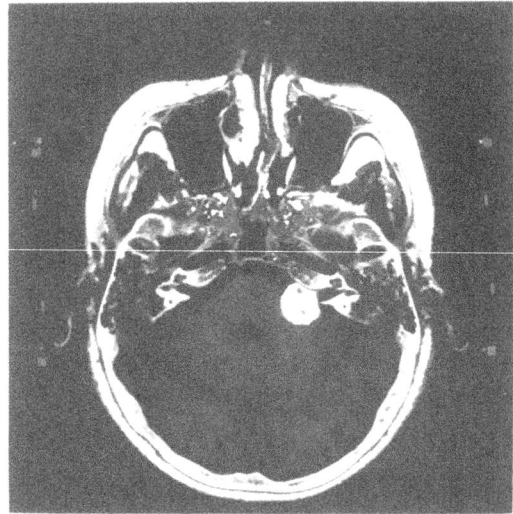

a

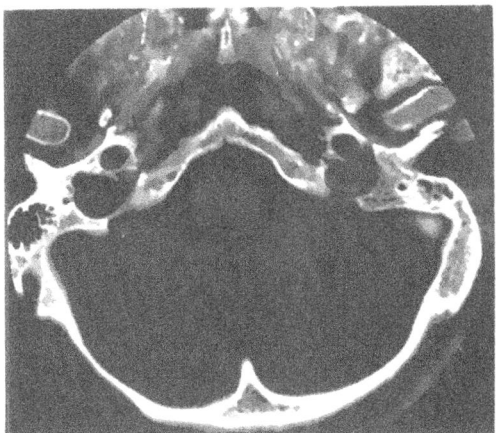

b

Figure 5. Combined transaxial MR and CT scans of the head. The CT value is displayed if it corresponds to bone; otherwise the MR grey value, suitably scaled, is displayed. (a) Patient with acoustic neuroma [16]. (b) Patient with glomus tumour.

Figure 5 shows an example aligned transaxial slice from each study. Figure 5a shows the patient with the acoustic neuroma, Fig. 5b shows the patient with the glomus tumour. In these images the CT number is displayed if the CT number corresponds to bone, otherwise the MR intensity is displayed suitably scaled.

This technique provides a method of incorporating MR data into stereotaxic CT coordinates without the added complication of the patient having to wear a stereotaxic frame for both the MR and CT scans.

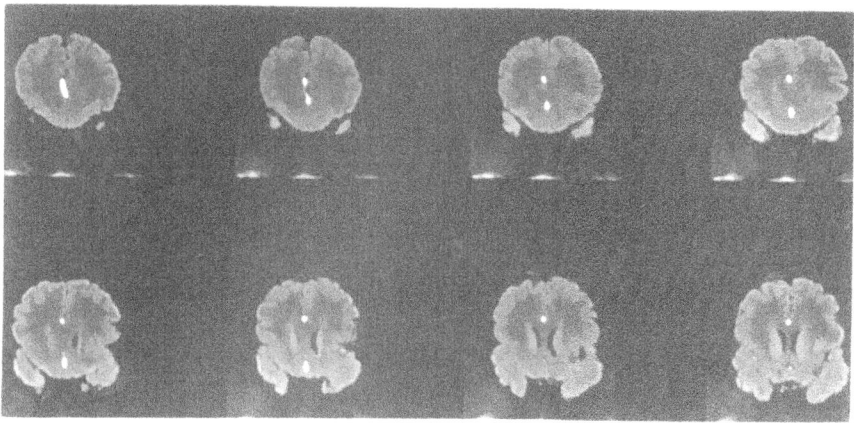

Figure 6. Example coronal slices of a cadaver brain showing the pericallosal artery (white dots of exaggerated radius) after alignment using our 'key-lock' algorithm [19].

Object centred representation to achieve registration

Registration of the cortical surface of the brain, derived from MR images, with 3D vascular data derived from DSA

In an object centred approach entities derived from images from two or more modalities are identified as belonging to specific anatomical structures or their sub-parts. Prior information determining the correspondence or adjacency of these structures is used to build a representation of the object and hence achieve image registration. As described above, this approach has been pioneered by Pelizzari et al. using the location of the skin surface in MRI and PET to achieve registration via their 'head and hat' algorithm [8]. We are investigating two applications of an object centred approach.

In the first we derive the 3D configuration of the cerebral arterial system from bi-plane x-ray views and match this information to the surface of the brain derived from MRI in the manner of fitting a key into a lock [18]. We term this algorithm the 'key-lock' algorithm. We generate, from our knowledge of neuro-anatomy, a voxel representation of the likelihood that a blood vessel exists at a certain location and from the likelihood function generate a cost function used in an optimisation algorithm. More detail is provided in [19].

Preliminary results using data derived from a cadaver brain has shown that a registration accuracy of 1.5 mm should be possible when aligning segments of the pericallosal artery and middle cerebral artery with the surface of the brain. Figure 6 shows examples of coronal MR slices of the cadaver brain with the aligned 3D reconstruction of the pericallosal artery derived from x-ray images superimposed in white (X-ray images were acquired on a Siemens Digitron DSA system and reconstructed using SARA [20]).

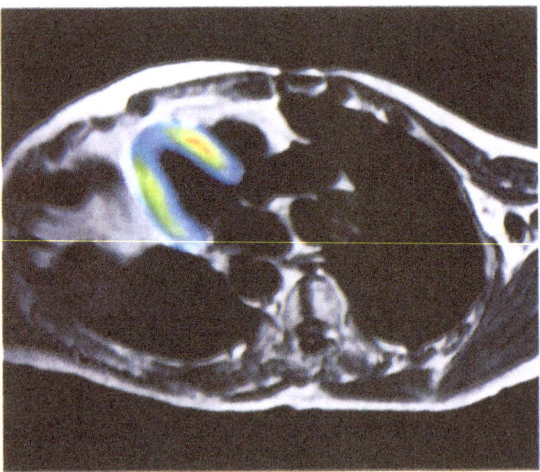

Figure 7. Shows the combined gated MR and Tc-99m SestaMIBI image of a horizontal long axis slice through the apex of the heart. The isotope activity is colour coded as in Fig. 2a. Alignment was achieved by defining the long axis of the left ventricle in each modality.

Combination of SPECT myocardial perfusion data with ECG gated MR images

In a second application we are attempting to combine data derived from gated MR images with SPECT perfusion images of the myocardium. External markers attached to the skin do not have a fixed geometric relationship to cardiac structures and point-like anatomical structures are difficult to define, particularly in SPECT data. We therefore achieve registration by establishing in each modality the long axis of the left ventricle, which is defined as the straight line from apex to mid-point of the valve planes. Horizontal axis, vertical long axis and short axis views are generated relative to this axis. Resulting images in the two modalities only require translation and rotation in the imaging plane to achieve registration, which is relatively straightforward to do interactively.

Figure 7 shows a gated MR image of the horizontal long axis view of the LV of a patient with an established infarct (TR SE of 800 msec, TE of 20 msec and a gated time delay of 312 msec). Superimposed in color on this image is the aligned SPECT image of the uptake of Technetium 99m-Sesta MIBI (Cardiolite - Du Pont) on the same patient (500 MBq of Tc-99m was injected and the patient was scanned 2 hours post injection, with 60 40 sec views taken over 180°). Such an image might allow more accurate determination of a relationship between cardiac wall motion abnormalities, myocardial thinning and perfusion defects. We estimate that the registration accuracy in this application is about 5 mm in plane and within one slice thickness (7 mm) axially.

Discussion

In summary our experiences in image registration would indicate that skin markers are sufficiently accurate (approximately 4 mm) for registering SPECT and MR images of the head provided that the markers are fixed in position for the duration of both scans. Our current markers are limited to use with thin contiguous MR (or CT) slices. For slice thicknesses greater than 5 mm with inter-slice gaps of 2 mm or more we are evaluating the use of larger spherical markers. Alternatively Elsen and Viergever propose the use of 'V' shaped markers stuck to the skin [7].

For combining MR and PET data, the 'head and hat' algorithm of Pelizzari et al. provides an effective solution [8]. The technique requires that sufficient overlapping skin surfaces is sampled in each modality and that strong surface features such as the bridge of the nose are included in each image. The final registration must be carefully assessed to ensure that a local minima in optimisation space has not been returned as the final solution by the algorithm. Techniques for surface segmentation and the representation of uncertainty in surface location would improve the algorithm.

For combining MR and CT images of the skull base there are a large number of anatomical features visible in each modality and these provide sufficient natural markers to achieve registration. In the upper part of the brain and in the absence of skull base features a relocatable frame attached to a dental impression may provide a suitable means of registration when use of a stereotaxic frame pinned to the skull is inappropriate. The use of the relocatable frame requires further assessment.

Alternatively we are developing techniques based on identification of corresponding or adjacent surfaces to achieve registration. We propose that these techniques will use algorithms very similar to our 'key lock' algorithm for registering 3D blood vessel data derived from DSA with brain surface data derived from MRI. Important factors in this work are the appropriate representation of surfaces, the representation of uncertainty in surface location and the representation of the most likely position of adjacent structures. In each application an appropriate optimisation strategy must be devised in order to achieve registration. There is significant work still to be done in this area before these techniques enter routine clinical practice.

In the long term such object centred approaches will become the favored method of combining data from multiple modalities. Our aim is that it should be possible to take the decision to combine images after acquisition and therefore registration should require no (or at least very little) interference with normal radiographic procedures. In the future, the processes of registration and data fusion should be as automated as possible.

Outside the head, where the natural landmarks and rigidity provided by the skull are absent, an object centred approach is generally the only solution. We have presented a single example of such an approach to combine MR and SPECT images of the myocardium.

The widespread implementation of PACS (Picture Archive and Communication Systems) is still hampered by the very large volumes of data generated by routine medical imaging. Object centred representations might provide useful compact intermediate representations of medical data between the conventional voxel or pixel representations and the written report.

Most of the work presented in this paper concerns image registration. Establishing a common coordinate frame for registration opens the possibility of combining information from the two modalities, i.e. data fusion. We have demonstrated a simple example of this in our combination of MR and CT data in the skull base, but there are a large number of possibilities which require further investigation. For example, computation of blood flow (from a nuclear medicine study) with volume estimates from a second modality (such as MR or CT) might be used to calculate blood flow per unit volume.

An important extension of the image registration work is to establish the transformation between the patient's frame of reference, at surgery or radiotherapy, and that of the combined data. Such registration has been available for several years with the use of stereotaxic frames but could now be extended to conventional surgery and radiotherapy. Pelizzari has reported an extension of the use of the 'Head and Hat' algorithm to the use of skin surface coordinates derived from a 3D pointer [21]. A similar technique has been proposed by the Aachen group [22]. These techniques will enable the surgeon or therapist to relate information in the combined image data directly to the patient.

Displays which give the illusion of shaded 3D surfaces in the registered data sets are likely to prove beneficial in surgical planning. However, the use of display intensity to give the visual illusion of shading of an illuminated surface in 3D removes one of the parameters available for visualizing multimodal data. Effective display of 3D multi-modal data requires further research. The additional cues of transparency with stereo or movement parallax will almost certainly be required.

This paper provides an overview of our multi-modal programme at UMDS, Guy's Hospital. As we have demonstrated examples of these techniques to our clinical colleagues we have found that the number of possible clinical applications of multi-modal data fusion has increased dramatically. We now have projects studying the brain, skull base, spine, wrist and heart, with other applications proposed in facial surgery, the kidney, liver, neck and pelvis.

Continued progress in computer science leading to effective image segmentation, object identification, data representation, 3D visualization, interaction and simulation, together with workstations of sufficient power and parallelism to perform these tasks, will provide the necessary technology for these techniques to enter clinical practice.

Introduction of these techniques into clinical medicine requires extensive validation of the accuracy of registration and demonstration that there is clinical benefit in using the extra information. This work may stimulate further research into protocols for the effective use of technology for diagnosis and therapy planning in specific clinical areas, thus ensuring the most efficient use of finite health care resources.

The last two decades have seen a revolution in medical image acquisition technology. Future developments will concentrate on the extraction and presentation of clinically relevant information from medical images. We predict that development of techniques to combine data from multiple imaging modalities will become the dominant activity in medical imaging research in the next few years.

Acknowledgements

By its nature the multi-modal work described in this paper requires the active participation and cooperation of a large number of people working in different disciplines. We are particularly grateful for the help and advice provided by the radiography staff at Guy's Hospital, in particular Phillippa Graves and Julie Shields; Mr. Mike Gleeson, Consultant ENT Surgeon; Dr. Tim Cox, Consultant Radiologist; Dr. Alan Colchester, Consultant Neurologist; Dr. John Chambers of the Department of Cardiology; Dr. André Melizzia of the Department of Psychiatry; John Crossman, Charlie Bird, Eldon Lehmann and Charlie Hardingham, Medical Students; the computing assistance of Clifford Ruff and Glynn Robinson; and the technical assistance of Peter Liepins.

We are grateful to the Leverhulme Trust, the AIM Exploratory Action project MMOMS and the Special Trustees of Guy's Hospital for financial support of this work.

References

1. Peters TM, Clark JA, Olivier A, Marchand EP, Mawko G, Dieumegarde M, Muresan LV, Ethier R. Integrated stereotaxic imaging with computed tomography, magnetic resonance imaging and digital subtraction angiography. Radiology 1986;161:821–6.
2. Lemoine D, Barillot C, Gibaud B, Pasqualini E. An Anatomical-based 3D registration system of multimodality and atlas data in neurosurgery. Colchester AC, Hawkes DJ, editors. Information processing in medical imaging. Berlin: Springer, 1991. In press.
3. Zhang J, Levesque MF, Wilson CL, Harper RM, Engel J, Lufkin R, Behnke EJ. Multimodality imaging of brain structures for stereotactic surgery. Radiology 1990;175:435–41.
4. Vandermeulen D, Suetens P, Gybels J, Oosterlinck A, Marchal G. A prototype medical workstation for computer assisted stereotactic neurosurgery. In: Lemke HU, Rhodes ML, Jaffee CC, Felix R, editors. Computer assisted radiology. Berlin: Springer, 1990:386–9.
5. Thomas DGT. Personal Communication. 1991; Unpub.
6. Thomas DG, Gill SF, Wilson CB, Darling JC, Parkins CS. Use of a relocatable stereotactic frame to integrate positron emission tomography and computed tomography images: applications in human malignant brain tumours. Proceedings of the 10th World Society of Stereotactic and Functional Neurosurgery 1990. S.l.: S.N., 1990:388–92.

7. Van den Elsen PA, Viergever MA. Marker guided registration of electromagnetic dipole data with tomographic images. In: Colchester AC, Hawkes DJ, editors. Information processing in medical imaging. Berlin: Springer, 1991. In press.

8. Pelizzari CA, Chen GT, Spelbring DR, Weichselbaum RR, Chen CT. Accurate three-dimensional registration of CT, PET, and/or MR images of the brain. J Comput Assist Tomogr 1989;13:20–6.

9. Evans A, Marret S, Collins L, Peters T. Anatomical-functional correlative analysis of the human brain using three dimensional imaging systems. Proc SPIE 1989; 1092:264–74.

10. Talairach J, Tournoux P. Co-planar stereotactic atlas of the human brain. Stuttgart: Thieme, 1988.

11. Von Keyserlingk DG, Niemann K, Wasel J. A quantitative approach to spatial variation of human cerebral sulci. Acta Anat (Basel) 1988;131:127–31.

12. Arun KS, Huang TS, Blostein SD. Least-squares fitting of 2 3D point sets. IEEE Trans Pattern Anzal Machine Intelligence 1987;9:698–700.

13. Hawkes DJ, Hill DL, Lehmann ED, Robinson GP, Maisey MN, Colchester AC. Preliminary work on the interpretation of SPECT images with the aid of registered MRI images and an MR derived 3D neuro-anatomical atlas. In: Hoehne KH, Pizer SM, Fuchs H, editors. 3D imaging in medicine: algorithms, systems, applications. Berlin: Springer, 1990:241–52.

14. Lehmann ED, Hawkes DJ, Hill DL, Bird CF, Robinson GP, Colchester ACF, Maisey MN. Computer aided interpretation of SPECT images of the brain using an MRI derived 3D neuro-anatomical atlas. Med Inf (London). In press.

15. Price D. Magnetic resonance imaging brain morphometry: an investigation into its accuracy. (Dissertation). Guildford, Surrey, UK: Univ. of Surrey, 1990.

16. Hill DL, Hawkes DJ, Crossman JE, Gleeson MJ, Cox TCS, Bracey EEC ML, Strong AJ, Graves P. Registration of MR and CT images for skull base surgery using point-like anatomical features. Br J Radiol. In press.

17. Hawkes DJ, Hill DL, Lehmann ED, Robinson GP, Maisey MN, Colchester AC. Preliminary work on the interpretation of SPECT images with the aid of registered MR images and an MR derived neuro-anatomical atlas. In: Hoehne KH, Fuchs H, Pizer SM, editors. 3D Imaging in Medicine: Algorithms, systems, applications. Berlin: Springer, 1990:241–52.

18. Hawkes DJ, Mol CB, Colchester AC. The accurate 3D reconstruction of the geometric configuration of vascular trees from X-ray recordings. In: Guzzardi R, editor. Physics and engineering of medical imaging. Dordrecht: Nijhoff, 1987:250–6.

19. Hill DL, Hawkes DJ. The use of anatomical knowledge to register 3D blood vessel data derived from DSA with MR images. Proc SPIE. In press.

20. Hardingham CR, Hawkes DJ. SARA: A system for angiographic reconstruction and analysis – technical report, radiological sciences, UMDS, University of London, 1991. Unpub.

21. Pelizzari CA, Tan KK, Levin DN, Chen GT, Balter J. Interactive 3D patient – image registration. In: Colchester AC, Hawkes DJ, editors. Information processing in medical imaging. Berlin: Springer 1991. In press.

22. Adams L, Gilsbach JM, Krybus W, Meyer-Ebrecht D, Mosges R, Schlondorff G. CAS – A navigation support for surgery. In: Hoehne KH, Fuchs H, Pizer SM, editors. 3D Imaging in Medicine: algorithms, systems, applications. Berlin: Springer, 1990:411–23.

9. Information preserving compression of medical images

MAX A. VIERGEVER and PAUL ROOS

Summary

A state-of-the-art report on information preserving (or lossless, or error-free, or reversible) compression of medical images is presented. Reversible compression consists of two steps, decorrelation and coding. Methods for intraframe decorrelation of 2D images can be divided into three classes, viz. transform, predictive, and multiresolution decorrelation. A method from the latter class, hierarchical interpolation (HINT), provides for optimum decorrelation. In addition, HINT is free of parameters, easy to implement, and insensitive to channel errors. For temporal and spatial sequences of 2D images, 2D HINT applied to each frame individually generally decorrelates as well as interframe methods which take the temporal or spatial correlation of the sequence into account. The decorrelation performance of 2D HINT is best preserved in the coding step by adaptive arithmetic coding, for which the computation time is quite high, however. A more efficient method, yielding hardly worse bit rates at much higher speed, is model-based Huffman coding. The compression rates which may be expected from 2D HINT followed by model-based Huffman coding depend strongly on image modality, spatial resolution, and quantization level. For 8–bit nuclear medicine images, the coding bit rates found were in the range of 2.5–5 bits per pixel.

1. Introduction

The field of image data compression may rejoice in a vivid interest from the medical imaging community. This interest has been aroused by the growing impact of digital image formation methods in radiology (CT, DSA, MRI, MRA, computed radiography) and nuclear medicine (planar scintigraphy, SPECT, PET). Film-based methods are slowly but surely losing ground in both image formation and image archiving. In fact, a filmless nuclear medicine department has already proven viable [1]. Yet, the growing extent of digital images does not in itself imply a need for data compression, in view of the advancements in optical archiving and transmission which have at least kept pace with image formation technology. The attention to digital image

Johan H.C. Reiber & Ernst E. van der Wall (eds.), Cardiovascular Nuclear Medicine and MRI, 131–149.
© 1992 *Kluwer Academic Publishers.*

compression can, therefore, only be explained by an even stronger increasing demand for efficiency in data storage and communication, a feature which is not uncommon in rapidly developing technological areas.

The aim of image data compression methods is to represent images efficiently, i.e. at low bit rates. This would allow data storage at relatively low cost and data transmission at relatively high speed, both of which are essential in the design of picture archiving and communication systems. In addition to reducing the costs of disk space, efficient storage increases the on-line availability of patient data, which is particularly useful in a fully digital radiological or nuclear medicine image system. Furthermore, in some acquisition systems, notably those involving temporal image sequences such as digital angiography, the flow of image data is so large that compression is required for adequate disk access [2].

Image compression comes in two flavours: (i) irreversible, or lossy, or noisy, or information reducing compression, and (ii) reversible, or lossless, or error-free, or information preserving compression. Compression methods belong to the second class only if the original data can be exactly reconstructed from the compressed representation. Reversible compression may be mandatory for two reasons:

- *legal regulations*. In many countries it is required to keep records of all original patient data for a number of years; it is not allowed to dispense with any – even seemingly useless – information contained in the images.
- *postprocessing*. Irreversible compression methods are capable of representing images at considerably reduced storage costs with hardly perceivable degradation. However, the losses thus introduced may be greatly enhanced by postprocessing operations (as e.g. contour detection) applied to the images.

An additional advantage of lossless compression methods is that a comparison of their performance can be made solely on the basis of their efficiency, as contrasted with lossy compression methods which require a subjective evaluation to indicate whether or not the coding losses are acceptable.

The only drawback of error-free image compression methods is that they do not perform so well as concerns their primary task: representing the images at low bit rates. As we shall show, typical compression ratios for nuclear medicine images are of the order of 2–3. Lossy compression methods are still quite satisfactory in preserving image quality with ratios that are five times as high.

The purpose of the present chapter is to give a state-of-the-art report of reversible data compression in medical imaging with special attention to nuclear medicine images. We want to emphasize that restricting the subject of this paper to error-free compression does not imply that we advise against information reduction. On the contrary, we are of the opinion that putting a ban upon information reduction is inconsistent with the absence of regulations on the accuracy of digital image formation. This permits, if not invites, incorporating lossy compression in the data acquisition step. For a survey of irreversible compression methods, we refer to [3–8].

Information preserving methods can achieve image compression by exploiting the usually high degree of correlation between neighbouring pixels. In the majority of the methods the pixel values are first decorrelated, after which the resulting data are encoded using a variable length coder as, e.g., Huffman coding or arithmetic coding. An exception is the well-known Lempel-Ziv method in which the decorrelation and the variable length coding are combined. We shall return to Lempel-Ziv coding at the end of this chapter, but concentrate on methods which deal with decorrelation and coding separately.

The organization of the chapter is as follows. In section 2, the decorrelation of two-dimensional (2D) images is discussed. Section 3 addresses the decorrelation of time sequences of 2D images, and Section 4 the decorrelation of 3D images. In Section 5 the coding step is considered. Finally, in Section 6 the conclusions are summarized.

2. Intraframe decorrelation of 2D images

This section discusses the decorrelation of 2D image data. Only single frames of 2D data are considered, no allowance is made for correlation with other frames if the image is part of a spatial or temporal image sequence. Therefore, the term intraframe decorrelation is used, as contrasted with interframe decorrelation which does take into account the correlation between consecutive frames in a sequence.

The aim of the decorrelation step is to remove the statistical redundancy in the image. As an illustration, consider Fig. 1a, which shows the histogram of the grey values of a 512×512 coronary angiogram. After decorrelation, the histogram takes the form of Fig. 1b: strongly peaked, centred around the value 0. The peakedness of the histogram is exploited by the variable length coder by assigning short code words to frequently occurring amplitudes, longer code words to less frequent amplitudes.

Before discussing methods for image decorrelation, we first introduce the terms information and entropy. Suppose we have an image with K grey levels $\{f_i ; i = 1,2, \ldots ,K\}$ and probability p_i of grey value f_i. Then the information contained in the image is defined as

$$I = - \sum_{i=1}^{K} \text{Log}_2 p_i \tag{1}$$

The first order entropy is defined as the average information

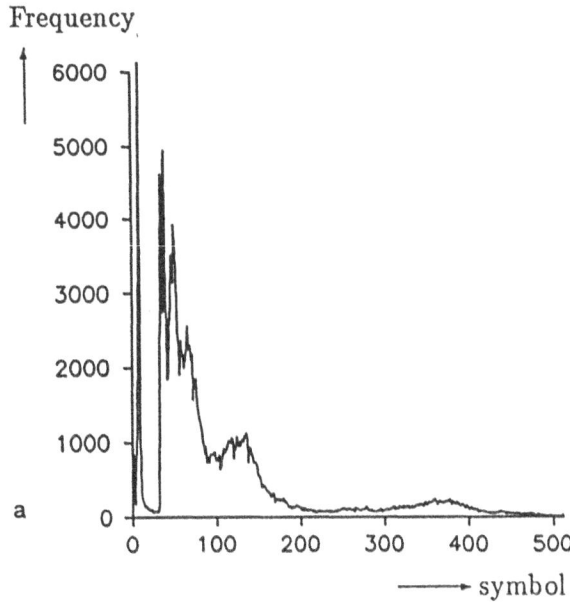

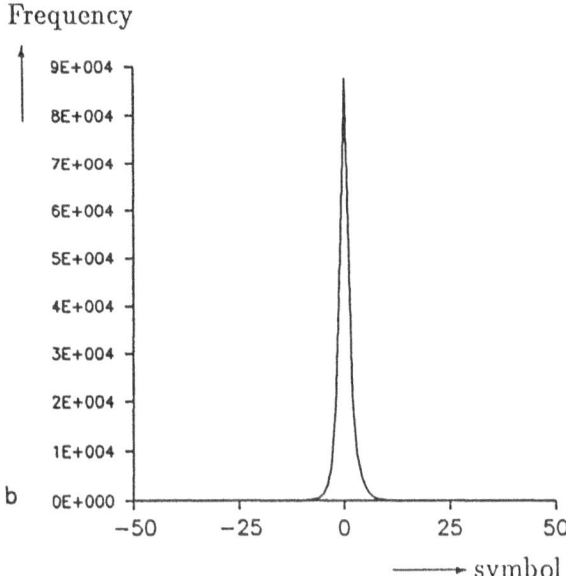

Figure 1. Grey value histogram of a 512 × 512 coronary angiogram, quantized at 9 bits/pixel. (a) original image; (b) decorrelated image. The decorrelation method used was 2D DPCM with φ = 0.95 (see Section 2.2.).

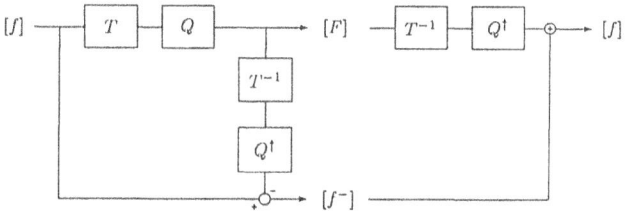

Figure 2. Schematic representing reversible transform decorrelation. T is the discrete image transform, Q the scaling and rounding operator (quantizer), Q^+ an approximation to the inverse of the scaling part of Q, usually provided by a look-up table; f is the original image, F the transformed image, and f^- the differential image (or error image). The decorrelated 'image' consists of F and f^-.

$$H = - \sum_{i=1}^{K} p_i \, Log_2 \, p_i \tag{2}$$

It can be shown [9] that, for independent data samples, H is the lower bound on the average length of the code words obtained by using a variable length coder. This optimum is achieved if the code length distribution is inversely proportional to the logarithm of the histogram amplitudes. The efficiency of the considered decorrelation methods will be judged primarily by the entropy of the decorrelated image.

Intraframe decorrelation methods can be divided into three classes:
– transform decorrelation methods (2.1.);
– predictive decorrelation methods (2.2.);
– multiresolution decorrelation methods (2.3.).
After having discussed the various methods, we shall compare the decorrelation performance of the best three methods in subsection 2.4.

2.1. *Transform decorrelation methods*

Figure 2 presents the functional scheme of reversible transform decorrelation, valid for any digital image transform producing noninteger-valued transformed images. Transforms applied in image compression are notably the Karhunen-Loève (KL) transform, the (real) discrete Fourier transform (DFT, RDFT), the discrete Hartley transform (DHT), the discrete cosine transform (DCT), and the Walsh-Hadamard transform (WHT); see [6] for a brief description of the methods. In practice, the transform is not applied to the entire image, but the image is divided into smaller blocks so as to save CPU time. Customary block sizes are 4×4, 8×8 or 16×16 pixels.

The image transform (T in Fig. 2) produces noninteger-valued coefficients which have to be quantized (i.e., scaled and rounded) before encoding. This quantization introduces errors in the reconstruction process. These errors

Entropy (bits/pixel)

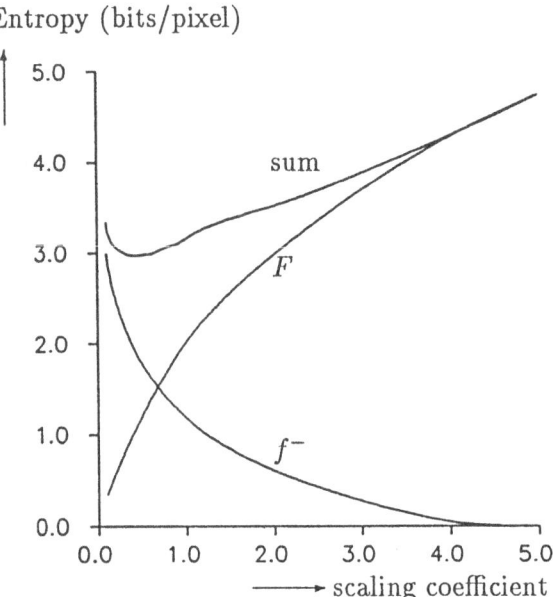

Figure 3. Average entropy of a series of 15 512 × 512 angiographic images with a quantization level of 9 bits/pixel, decorrelated using the DCT, as a function of the scaling coefficient. The DCT block size was 8 × 8. F is the DCT transformed image (cf. Fig. 1), f^- is the differential image, 'sum' is the sum of F and f^-.

can be made arbitrarily small by increasing the quantization accuracy. However, well before reaching an almost reversible situation, the compression efficiency will have dropped severely, most likely even below one. The solution to this problem is sketched in Fig. 2. The reconstruction error (f^-) is transmitted together with the transformed image F, thus ensuring reversibility. The entropy of the transformed image increases with increasing quantization accuracy, while the entropy of the error decreases.

Fig. 3 shows the average entropy of a series of 512^2, 9–bits coronary angiograms, transformed using the DCT, as a function of the quantization accuracy; q = 1 corresponds to equal normalization of F and f^-. The block-size of the DCT was 8 × 8. The optimal value of q is achieved when the sum entropy is minimal; for the images considered here, q = 0.4.

The result portrayed in Fig. 3 is representative of the performance of noninteger-valued transform methods. The resulting sum entropy of 2.97 for q = 0.4 is higher than that of methods to be discussed in the sequel. Furthermore, the optimal scaling coefficient is not known a priori, so in general, by using a preset value of q, the result will be worse. Finally, the coding step is nontrivial here because two images with relatively low entropy have to be dealt with. For instance, Huffman coding is inadequate for this purpose owing to its lower bound of 1 bit/pixel. While other coding methods have this problem to a lesser degree, the final compression result (i.e., after the coding step) may be expected to deviate more from the decorrelation entropy than in the case of a single decorrelated image of higher entropy.

It is possible to avoid the quantization step in Fig. 2, and hence the need for storing a differential image f⁻, by using an integer-valued discrete image transform. Such an option is impractical for the (R)DFT, DHT, DCT, and certainly for the KL transform. Only the WHT allows for a feasible integer-valued version, as outlined in [10]. In [2] the integer WHT is modified to provide optimal reversible compression.

The integer WHT does not have two of the three drawbacks of real image transforms, viz. the presence of a scaling parameter and the necessity to code a differential image in addition to the transformed image. The decorrelating power of the integer WHT is quite poor, however, despite the improvement mentioned above. In consequence, transform decorrelation is inadequate for error-free image compression.

2.2. *Predictive decorrelation methods*

The second class of decorrelation methods has data prediction as its central concept. The idea is well illustrated by considering a sequence of integers which has to be stored. Rather than storing the values as such, the value of every element of the sequence (except for the very first) is predicted by a weighted sum of its predecessors. In the simplest version, the value of the previous element is used as the prediction. The differences between the estimates and the actual values are stored, with the exception of the first element which is stored as such. The resulting histogram is similar to that of Fig. 1b. As an alternative, the prediction of the element values can be based on statistical properties of the sequence rather than on the previous element values.

The method outlined in the preceding paragraph is called one-dimensional differential pulse code modulation (1D DPCM). While this method can be applied to decorrelate an image by scanning it row by row (or column by column), a 2D version of the method is more suitable. The prediction in 2D DPCM can be written as

$$\hat{f}(i,j) = \sum_{p,q \in W} a(p,q)f(i-p, j-q) \tag{3}$$

with $a(p,q) \in R$, and W is the prediction window which defines the previously coded elements that are used in the estimation. Since the coefficients $a(p,q)$ are generally real-valued (i.e., noninteger), $\hat{f}(i,j)$ must be rounded to produce an integer-valued differential image $u = f - \hat{f}$, (Fig. 4).

If the image is assumed to be a homogeneous random field with zero mean and an exponentially decaying autocovariance function, the variance

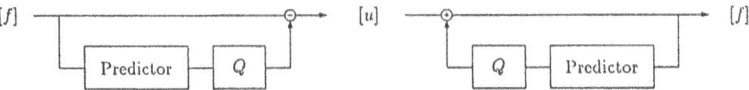

Figure 4. Scheme for reversible DPCM. Left: decorrelation, right: reconstruction. f is the original image, u the differential image which is stored. R is a rounding operator, the customary option for which is nearest integer.

of the differential image u is minimum for a predictor of the form (see e.g., [4] for a derivation).

$$\hat{f}(i, j) = -\phi^2\hat{f}(i - 1, j - 1) + \phi\hat{f}(i - j, j) + \phi\hat{f}(i - j - 1) \qquad (4)$$

where ϕ is the correlation coefficient of the image; its value is usually around 0.95. The predictor can be denoted symbolically by

$$\begin{matrix} -\phi^2 & \phi \\ \phi & . \end{matrix} \qquad (5)$$

A small variation is to use the energy-conserving prediction scheme (Roos et al. 1988)

$$\begin{matrix} 1 & -\tau^2 & \tau \\ \tau(2 - \tau) & \tau & . \end{matrix} \qquad (6)$$

in which the sum of the coefficients equals one.

The correlation coefficient ϕ will generally not satisfy the assumption of being constant. The local variations in image statistics may be taken into account in the prediction coefficients, as proposed in [12]. It has been found [11] that this is inefficient for images with a high signal-to-noise ratio, but may yield improved decorrelation for noisy images. The computational expenses of adaptive DPCM are, however, significantly higher than those of straightforward DPCM, which makes adaptive DPCM unattractive.

2.3. Multiresolution decorrelation methods

Multiresolution techniques, also called hierarchical techniques, decorrelate an image at several hierarchically connected scale levels. Three multiresolution decorrelation methods, the Laplacean pyramid, subband coding, and the S-transform are briefly discussed. A fourth method, hierarchical interpolation, is reviewed in more detail.

The Laplacean pyramid [13] is a hierarchical data structure based on splitting the frequencies of the original image into a member of bands (Fig.

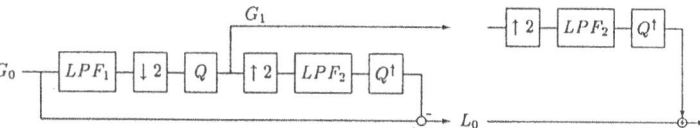

Figure 5. Construction of the lowest level L_o of the Laplacean pyramid (left part of the figure) and reconstruction of the original image (right part). LPF$_1$ and LPF$_2$ are low-pass filters, Q is a scaling and rounding operator, Q$^+$ is an approximation to the inverse scaling operator, $\downarrow 2$ and $\uparrow 2$ represent downsampling and upsampling by a factor of 2, G_0 is the original image, G_1 is the first low-pass filtered version of G_0.

5). The scheme bears a close resemblance to that of transform coding, cf. Fig. 2. The levels L_0, L_1, L_2, ... of the Laplacean pyramid serve as differential images. In addition to this feature, which has proven a disadvantage (Fig. 3), the Laplacean pyramid suffers from an increase in data samples. The number of elements of the data structure is 4/3 times that of the original image. Accordingly, the Laplacean pyramid is unsuited for reversible image decorrelation.

Subband coding is based on the same frequency band splitting concept as the Laplacean pyramid. We do not outline the method here; the interested reader is referred to [14]. The performance of subband coding was found to be even poorer than that of the Laplacean pyramid.

The S-transform (or, in full, sequential transform) is a multiresolution extension of the Walsh-Hadamard transform [15]. The method has drawn attention because of its attractive simplicity (e.g., [16]). Its decorrelating properties are less attractive, however; the performance is in the same range as that of the two previous methods. To give a numerical example, the decorrelation result for the series of 9–bit angiographic images mentioned in section 2.1 was an average first order entropy of 3.32 bits per pixel for the Laplacean pyramid, 3.36 for subband coding, and 3.25 for the S-transform, all with optimal block size and/or scaling coefficient.

Hierarchical interpolation (HINT, proposed in [17] and further elaborated in [11] has a multilevel decorrelation scheme as shown in Fig. 6. First, a subsampled (i.e., low-resolution) version of the original image, consisting of the 4–dot elements, is stored, for example using DPCM. In the second step the 3–dot pixels are estimated from the four surrounding 4–dot pixels by linear or median interpolation. The estimates are rounded to the nearest integer to ensure reversibility and subtracted from the actual pixel value; the differences are variable length coded and stored. Then the 2–dot pixels can be estimated from the 3– and 4–dots elements, etcetera. Notice that the interpolation is in fact a prediction, analogous to DPCM.

The reconstruction is straightforward. The 4–dot elements are first decoded. Upon interpolating these pixels and adding the (decoded) corresponding differential elements, the 3–dot pixels are recovered. Continuation of this procedure gives the 2–dot, 1–dot, and open circle elements.

In practice, an 8×8 block size is used for HINT rather than the 4×4

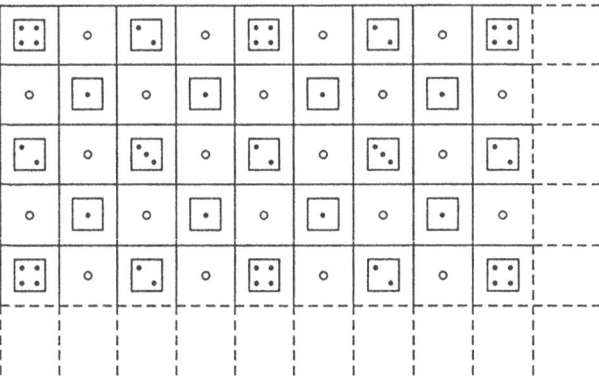

Figure 6. Pixel classification scheme for 2D HINT (block size 4 × 4). See the text for further explanation.

block structure of Fig. 6. The decorrelation efficiency is quite insensitive to the block size, however. The choice of interpolation method does not influence the resulting entropy appreciably either. Consequently, HINT is a parameter-free method.

2.4. *Decorrelation results*

This subsection presents the results of the best three decorrelation methods, viz. DPCM with the predictor of eq. 5, normalized DPCM (nDPCM) with the predictor of eq. 6, and HINT. The methods have been evaluated on a number of medical images stemming from various modalities, see Table 1.

The main conclusion which can be drawn from Table 1 is that HINT has the best decorrelation performance. Since HINT is in addition free of parameters, easy to implement, and insensitive to channel errors, it is the most appropriate method for intraframe 2D image decorrelation. A second conclusion is that normalized DPCM with a predictor as given by eq. 6 is generally better than unnormalized DPCM (eq. 5). This implies that the assumption underlying the derivation of eq. 5. viz. that the image is a zero-mean homogeneous random field with an exponentially decaying autocorrelation function, is not justified. An interesting observation is the variation in the optimum values of the correlation coefficient ϕ and the normalized correlation coefficient τ; ϕ is around 0.5 for the nuclear medicine images considered here and significantly higher for the other modalities, while τ has a very high value for the angiogram, the only high signal-to-noise ratio image, and low values for all other images. This parameter dependence of DPCM and (n)DPCM nicely illustrates the attractiveness of a parameter-free method like HINT.

Table 1. Comparison of the decorrelation performance of HINT, DPCM, and nDPCM on medical images acquired from various modalities

Image type	CT Head Transverse	MR Head Sagittal	Coronary Angiogram	Liver Scintigram	Bone Scintigram	Lung Scintigram
Dimension	256×256	256×256	512×512	128×128	256×256	256×256
Quantization level (bits)	12	12	9	8	8	8
Entropy before decorrelation (bits/pixel)	7.64	6.76	7.55	3.66	3.96	2.94
Entropy after HINT decorrelation (bits/pixel)	6.73	5.68	2.66	3.01	3.18	2.58
Entropy after DPCM decorrelation	7.12	5.91	2.76	3.15	3.33	2.65
optimal ϕ	0.91	0.70	0.95	0.49	0.49	0.49
Entropy after nDPCM decorrelation	6.78	5.75	2.73	3.15	3.26	2.69
optimal τ	0.04	0.10	0.85	0.05	0.04	0.02

3. Interframe decorrelation of 2D image sequences

It seems likely that time series of 2D images can be compressed more efficiently than the individual frames by utilizing the temporal correlation in addition to the spatial correlation. Temporal decorrelation methods are either based on extrapolation (like DPCM in spatial decorrelation) or on interpolation (like HINT). Furthermore, temporal decorrelation methods may or may not try to register possible motion artefacts.

An extensive discussion of all interframe decorrelation methods is beyond the scope of this chapter. A recent comparative study of such methods [18, 19], showed that (i) motion estimation is not advantageous for image compression, (ii) interpolation-based methods are superior to extrapolation-based methods, (iii) interframe compression yields entropies that are generally not lower than intraframe HINT, while the computational expenses are higher. The latter conclusion can be explained by the fact that the temporal decorrelation destroys the spatial correlation of the individual frames.

If the speed of the decorrelation step is essential, two other methods

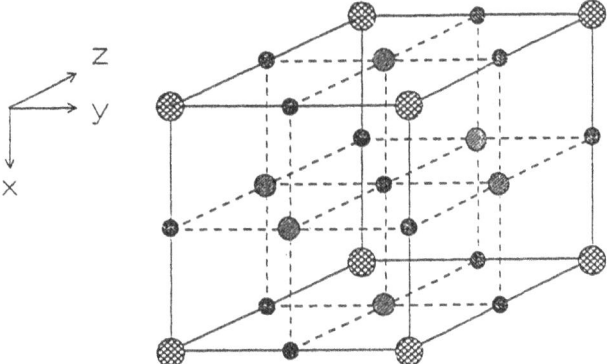

Figure 7. Voxel classification scheme for 3D HINT (block size $2 \times 2 \times 2$). The first step in 3D HINT is downsampling, in this example by a factor of 2^3 (large spheres). By 2D interpolation of the large sphere voxels, estimates for the elements indicated by the mid-size spheres are obtained, which are subtracted from the actual values. Next, 3D interpolation of the mid-size and large sphere voxel values gives estimates for the small sphere elements, which again are subtracted from the actual values. In practice, a $4 \times 4 \times 4$ block size is used.

come into consideration. Unregistered (that is, non motion-compensated) interpolation gives slightly worse results than 2D HINT at reduced (approximately 2/3) computational cost, unregistered extrapolation gives significantly worse – but for many purposes still acceptable – results at significantly lower (approximately 1/5) cost than 2D HINT.

While these figures may seem attractive, it should be noted that the computation time of the decorrelation step is generally much smaller than that of the coding step. A crude estimate is that the coding step requires five times as much CPU time. Consequently, the factor of 5 gain of unregistered extrapolation over 2D HINT results in only a marginal improvement in speed for the complete procedure of decorrelation and coding.

4. Decorrelation of 3D images

3D image compression is still a largely unexploited area of investigation. In the literature, considerable improvements of 3D over 2D image compression have been predicted [20], but so far have not been confirmed for either lossy or lossless coding. We have examined the possible gain of 3D hierarchical interpolation over its 2D pendant, by a variance analysis of the (linear) interpolation estimators used in 2D and 3D HINT. The interpolation steps in 3D HINT are outlined in Fig. 7.

The result of the variance analysis is that only a minor improvement can be expected of 3D decorrelation [21]. Indeed, preliminary experiments on multi-slice 3D image data sets showed that 3D decorrelation performs slightly better than 2D decorrelation applied to the individual slices [22]. A more extensive study, however, revealed that this observation is not supported for all multi-slice images. In fact, for SPECT images we found that more often than not 3D HINT proved inferior to 2D HINT, see Table 2.

The reason why 3D decorrelation is not consistently better than 2D decorrelation is that the interslice correlation in a multi-slice medical data set generally is much lower than the intraslice correlations. This is mainly due to the large distance between the slices in standard imaging protocols for CT, MRI, SPECT, and PET. Cubic or near-cubic 3D data acquisition will not become common practice in medical imaging in the near future, however, with the possible exception of MRI. The only way to enhance the performance of 3D decorrelation methods then is to adapt the decorrelation strategy to the image statistics. In keeping with the results referred to in subsection 2.2, this might give some improvement for noisy images at the expense of more CPU time, but will deteriorate the decorrelation of high signal-to-noise images. In consequence, we advocate decorrelation of multi-slice 3D data sets by applying 2D HINT to the individual slices.

5. Image coding

The decorrelation step of reversible image compression produces a decorrelated image which needs to be coded for storage or transmission. The coding step should ideally yield a bit rate close to the entropy of the decorrelated image. We have examined a number of reversible coding methods, all of which are based on one of the standards – Lempel-Ziv, Huffman, or arithmetic coding.

Lempel-Ziv coding [23] maps substrings of input symbols into fixed length output codes. It detects high usage patterns and symbol repetition rather than symbol frequency distribution. Consequently, Lempel-Ziv coding is particulary suited for low entropy signals which have a high probability of containing high usage patterns; reversibly decorrelated medical images are not within this class, except perhaps for nuclear medicine images. The pattern detection ability entails that Lempel-Ziv coding has decorrelating properties. Nonetheless, the method is generally unsuitable for direct application to the original, uncorrelated images because the data correlation is utilized only in one dimension, viz. the coding order of the symbols. The exceptions to this first rule are images having a low correlation as, again, some nuclear medicine images.

In summary, Lempel-Ziv coding is neither a promising method for reversible coding of HINT decorrelated images, nor for straightforward compression of 2D medical images. For nuclear medicine images, however, Lempel-Ziv coding may be suitable in view of the low information content and the low spatial correlation. This statement is endorsed by the numerical experiments reported in Table 3.

Huffman coding [24] is a variable length coder in which the length of a

Table 2. Comparison of 2D and 3D decorrelation using Hierarchical Interpolation on multi-slice images acquired from various modalities

Image type	CT Head	CT Spine	MR Head	MR Head	SPECT Brain	SPECT Heart	SPECT Bone
Dimension	256 × 256 × 120	256 × 256 × 128	128 × 128 × 32	256 × 256 × 64	64 × 64 × 25	64 × 64 × 20	64 × 64 × 23
Quantization level (bits)	12	12	12	12	8	8	8
Original entropy before decorrelation (bits/pixel)	7.43	9.40	10.70	8.77	4.46	5.42	3.61
Entropy after decorrelation by 2D HINT (bits/pixel)	6.53	8.32	9.79	8.19	2.82	2.87	2.54
Id, 3D HINT	6.24	8.23	9.59	8.08	3.09	3.30	2.49

Table 3. Comparison of reversible coding performances of model-based Huffman coding, adaptive arithmetic coding, and Lempel-Ziv coding

Image type	CT Head Transverse	MR Head Sagittal	Coronary Angiogram	Liver Scintigram	Bone Scintigram	Lung Scintigram	Heart SPECT
Original entropy (bits/pixel)	7.64	6.76	7.55	3.66	3.96	2.94	5.64
HINT entropy	6.73	5.68	2.66	3.01	3.18	2.58	4.46
Adaptive arithmetic coding entropy (a)	6.96	5.77	2.67	3.25	3.25	2.64	5.45
(b)	6.89	5.74	2.72	3.07	3.21	2.60	4.73
Model-based Huffman entropy (a)	7.01	5.81	2.72	3.27	3.27	2.67	5.48
(b)	6.93	5.79	2.88	3.10	3.23	2.63	4.77
Lempel-Ziv entropy (HINT images)	8.62	7.05	2.98	3.36	3.19	2.62	5.99
Lempel-Ziv entropy (original images)				3.37	3.35	2.51	6.74

All methods have been applied to images decorrelated using 2D HINT. Lempel-Ziv coding has also been applied to the original data. The results a/b for Huffman and arithmetic coding refer to the coder being applied to (a) each level of the HINT pyramid separately, and (b) the entire HINT image. The images used are those of Table 1 and the SPECT heart image of Table 2.

code word is based on the probability of the symbol (i.e., decorrelated image value). The method is optimal given the – severe – constraint that an integral number of bits be assigned to each symbol. The bit rate has a lower bound of 1 bit/pixel.

The symbol probability can either be measured from the histogram of the data, estimated beforehand, or determined by an adaptive procedure. The first option may require a significant number of bits/pixel to store the code tables, especially for large images, the second option may be highly inaccurate, and the third option is slow.

We have developed a probability model which combines the positive elements of these options. Based on a histogram calculation, an initial probability model is constructed which is minimally adapted during the coding. The procedure also includes a runlength coding preprocessing step to identify a repetition of zero-valued symbols in the decorrelated image. For further details we refer to [25]. The results of this model-based Huffman coding are shown in Table 3.

Arithmetic coding [26, 27] represents the decorrelated image values as a whole by one real-valued number between 0 and 1. Each symbol is allotted a subinterval of $[0,1)$ with a size proportional to its probability. The first symbol thus comprises a subinterval of $[0,1)$, the second symbol a subinterval of this subinterval, etc. Each symbol coded narrows the interval until the final interval is obtained which represents the symbol set uniquely; any number within this interval may be used for storage or transmission.

The performance of arithmetic coding depends, just as Huffman coding, on the probability model. The combined model outlined above may be used (and indeed has been used); it yields minute improvements in bit rate over its Huffman analogue at much higher computational cost. In Table 3, arithmetic coding with an adaptive probability model has been included, since this option gives optimum decorrelation results. Because of its huge computational load, it should be viewed as a reference only.

If we judge the results of Table 3 using the bit rate as sole criterion, adaptive arithmetic coding is generally the best coding technique for HINT decorrelated images. Model-based Huffman coding is slightly worse for all data sets. On the average, the best results are obtained by considering the entire HINT pyramid as the message to be coded, rather than the individual levels of the pyramid.

Lempel-Ziv coding of the HINT data is not an attractive option for the radiological images, nor for the SPECT image; it does quite well for the other nuclear medicine images, however. Similar results are obtained when Lempel-Ziv is applied to the original data (shown here only for the 8–bit images using UNIX compress).

Table 3 does not show the computational speed of the methods. Huffman coding is the fastest method, Lempel-Ziv coding takes about 1.5 times as long, while arithmetic coding is on the average 5 times slower than Huffman. Since model-based Huffman coding approximates the optimum bit rate closely for all images, it is the most suitable method for reversible coding of HINT decorrelated images.

6. Summary of conclusions

The conclusions drawn in this chapter may be summarized as follows:

2D intraframe decorrelation

- Transform decorrelation methods are unsuited for reversible compression.
- DPCM is a good decorrelator, but has a great disadvantage in its dependency on a parameter.
- HINT has the best decorrelation performance, is free of parameters, and is in addition insensitive to channel errors and easy to implement. Consequently, HINT is the optimum method for lossless image decorrelation.

Interframe decorrelation of image sequences

Interframe decorrelation of temporal image sequences gives no improvement over intraframe decorrelation of the individual images.

3D decorrelation

3D decorrelation of multi-slice images is not consistently superior to 2D decorrelation of the individual slices. For SPECT images, 3D decorrelation is generally worse.

Coding

The most suitable reversible coding method for HINT decorrelated images is model-based Huffman coding. This method is fast and approximates the optimum bit rate closely in all cases.

In summary, 2D HINT followed by model-based Huffman coding is an appropriate compression strategy for all types of medical images. The compression ratios depend strongly on image modality, spatial resolution, and quantization level. For the 8–bits nuclear medicine images considered in this paper, the bit rates vary between 2.6 and 4.8 bits/pixel, which amounts to compression ratios of 1.7–3.0.

Acknowledgements

This research was supported in part by the Dutch ministry of Economic Affairs through a SPIN grant, and by the industrial companies Hewlett-Packard, Agfa Gevaert, Philips Medical Systems, KEMA, and Tektronix.

References

1. Anema PC, de Graaf CN, Wilmink JB, et al. One year clinical experience with a fully digitized nuclear medicine department: organizational and economical aspects. In: Jost RG, editor. Medical Imaging V: PACS design and evaluation. Bellingham: SPIE Press. In press.
2. Peters JH, Roos P, van Dijke MC, Viergever MA. Loss-less image compression in digital angiography. In: de Graaf CN, Viergever MA, editors. Information processing in medical imaging. New York: Plenum Press, 1988:335-46.
3. Netravali AN, Limb JO. Picture coding: review. Proc IEEE 1980;68:366-406.
4. Jain AK. Image data compression: a review. Proc. IEEE 1981;69:349-89.
5. Rosenfeld A, Kak AC. Digital picture processing. 2nd ed. New York: Academic Press, 1982.
6. Netravali AN, Haskell BG. Digital pictures: representation and compression. New York: Plenum Press, 1988.
7. Jain AK. Fundamentals of digital image processing. Englewood Cliffs, NJ: Prentice-Hall, 1989.
8. Rabani M, Jones PW. Digital image compression techniques. Bellingham: SPIE Press, 1991.
9. Shannon CE, Weaver W. The mathematical theory of communication. Urbana: University of Illinois Press, 1949.
10. Ahmed N, Rao KR. Orthogonal transforms for digital signal processing. Berlin: Springer-Verlag, 1975.
11. Roos P, Viergever MA, van Dijke MCA, Peters JH. Reversible intraframe compression of medical images. IEEE Trans Med Imag 1988;7:328-36.
12. Heiss R, Zschunke W. An adaptive DPCM intraframe prediction method without switching. In: Proceedings of the Picture Coding Symposium. Tokyo: S.N.;1986:202-3.
13. Burt PJ, Adelson EH. The Laplacian pyramid as a compact image code. IEEE Trans Commun 1983;31:532-40.
14. Woods JW, O'Neil SD. Subband coding of images. IEEE Trans Acoust Speech Signal Processing 1986;34:1278-88.
15. Lux P. Novel set of closed orthogonal functions for picture coding. AEU Arch Elektron Ubertragungstech 1977;31:267-74.
16. Ranganath S, Blume H. Hierarchical image decomposition and filtering using the S-transform. In: Schneider RH, Dwyer SJ, editors. Medical Imaging II: image data management and display. Bellingham: SPIE Press, 1988.
17. Endoh T, Yamazaki Y. Progressive coding scheme for multi level images. In: Proceedings of the Picture Coding Symposium. Tokyo: S.N.;1986:21-2.
18. Roos P, Viergever MA. Interframe vs intraframe compression of image sequences. In: Viergever MA, editor. Science and engineering of medical imaging. Bellingham: SPIE Press, 1989:145-9.
19. Roos P, Viergever MA. Reversible interframe compression of medical images: a comparison of decorrelation methods. IEEE Trans Med Imag. In press.
20. Todd-Pokropek A. Image data compression: a survey. In: Viergever MA, Todd-Pokropek A, editors. Mathematics and computer science in medical imaging. Berlin: Springer-Verlag, 1988:167-95.
21. Roos P, Viergever MA. Reversible 3D compression of medical images. In press.

22. Roos P, Viergever MA. Reversible 3D compression of CT data using HINT. In: Ortendahl DA, Liacer J, editors. Information processing in medical imaging. New York: Wiley-Liss, 1991:505–13.
23. Ziv J, Lempel A. Universal algorithm for sequential data compression. IEEE Trans Inf Theor 1977;23:337–43.
24. Huffman DA. A method for the construction of minimum redundancy codes. Proc IRE 1952;40:1098–1101.
25. Roos P, Appelman FJ, Viergever MA. Reversible coding of medical images. In press.
26. Langdon GG. An introduction to arithmetic coding. IBM J Res Dev 1984;28:135–49.
27. Witten IH, Neal RM, Cleary JG. Arithmetic coding for data-compression. Commun ACM 1987;30:520–40.

PART III

SPECT: Advances in cardiovascular imaging

10. Quantitative computer assessment of regional contractility from ECG-gated planar Tc-99m SestaMIBI images

FRANS J.Th. WACKERS and PIOTR MANIAWSKI

Summary

Tc-99m SestaMIBI images are of relatively high count density. This makes it practical to acquire ECG-synchronized planar images for simultaneous evaluation of myocardial perfusion and contraction. However, interpretation of these studies by visual inspection of endless loop cine, as commonly is done for equilibrium radionuclide angiocardiographic (ERNA) studies, is not straightforward. Because of cross-talk of walls and thickening of the facing wall, endocardial motion is difficult to assess. In normal hearts cavity obliteration frequently occurs, which does not agree with perceived motion of ERNA. On the other hand, epicardial motion is frequently minimal even in normal subjects.

Accordingly, we developed a new non-geometric method to evaluate and quantify simultaneously myocardial perfusion and function. This image was generated by subtracting 15 frames from the end-systolic frame, normalizing the 15 functional images to the end-systolic image and by summing all functional images, and by comparison to a normal data base. Quantitative Regional Function Index (QRFI) was derived from these profiles. The method was validated by computer simulation, comparison to regional ejection fraction and semiquantitative wall motion score on ERNA. Computer simulation demonstrated QRFI measurement to be relatively independent of the presence of a perfusion defect, but to agree well with simulated contraction. Good agreement was found between QRFI and assessment of regional left ventricular function in patients. In conclusion, this new count-based technique allows reliable simultaneous quantitative assessment of regional myocardial perfusion and function.

Introduction

Tc-99m SestaMIBI is a new myocardial perfusion imaging agent that is now widely employed for clinical imaging. Favourable dosimetry makes it possible to administer up to 30mCi per study. Consequently, typical Tc-99m Sesta-

Johan H.C. Reiber & Ernst E. van der Wall (eds.), Cardiovascular Nuclear Medicine and MRI, 153–162.
© 1992 *Kluwer Academic Publishers.*

MIBI images are characterized by relatively high count density in comparison to that usually with Thallium-201 [1,2].

Since the beginning of imaging with Tl-201, it was realized that static myocardial perfusion images, acquired by either planar of SPECT technique, display a blurred projection of the distribution of the radiopharmaceutical within the contracting heart. Therefore, electrocardiographic synchronization, or 'gating' as used for equilibrium gated blood pool imaging was proposed as a means to remove the blur of the beating heart and improve detection of small perfusion defects. This approach was considered the more attractive since cine display of the contracting perfusion image could provide simultaneous diagnostic information with regard to regional perfusion and regional contractile function.

ECG-gated Tc-99m SestaMIBI imaging

The usefulness of ECG-gated Tl-201 images has been investigated in the past, but this approach virtually was abandoned as being too impractical because of its long acquisition times [3]. The above mentioned high count density in Tc-99m SestaMIBI images make it feasible to explore the usefulness of this approach anew. Standard computer software as employed for equilibrium radionuclide angiocardiography, can be used for ECG-gating of perfusion images. After administration of 20–30 mCi of Tc-99m SestaMIBI, usually 16 frames are acquired per RR-cycle for planar imaging, and 8 frames per RR-cycle for SPECT imaging.

Analysis of regional wall motion on planar images: endocardium or epicardium?

Cine display of ECG-gated planar SestaMIBI images shows the contracting heart. However, on close inspection it becomes clear that interpretation of these motion pictures is not straightforward. Contracting myocardial perfusion images show information different from dynamic display of equilibrium radionuclide angiocardiography. Analysis of regional wall motion on equilibrium gated blood pool studies involves analysis of endocardial movement. On gated SestaMIBI studies both the motion of the endocardial and epicardial border can be analyzed. However, the 'endocardial' border on planar Tc-99m SestaMIBI images is not a fixed border, but a continuously changing border during the cardiac cycle. Due to thickening of overlying facing myocardium the apparent endocardial border may shift up on the gray scale confluence with the opposite wall (Fig. 1). This may give an exaggerated impression of motion and visually an overestimation of the degree of contraction.

In a preliminary evaluation we compared visual analysis of motion of the

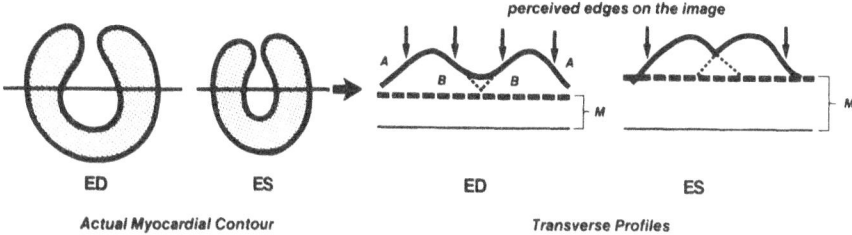

Figure 1. Explanation of overestimation of regional wall motion by analyzing the 'endocardial' border on ECG-gated Tc-99m SestaMIBI images. The myocardium has an epicardial outer (a), edge and an 'endocardial' inner (b), edge gradient. During systole, A moves over a constant background and thus the perceived edge is unchanged. (This is a similar to the endocardial edge on equilibrium radionuclide angiocardiography). During systole, the B edges move toward each other and confluence. In addition, there is increased foreground activity by contracting overlying myocardium (M). Thus, the 'endocardial' edges appear to have greater motion. The 'cavity' may even obliterate during systole. The perceived edges are dependent upon the setting of the gray scale.

endocardial and of the epicardial border on gated SestaMIBI studies with that of the endocardial border on equilibrium radionuclide angiocardiography (Figs. 2 and 3) [4]. Analysis of the *endocardial* border alone (thus comparable to analysis of a gated bloodpool study) showed substantial underestimation of regional wall motion abnormalities. On the other hand assessment of regional *epicardial* motion on the ECG-gated SestaMIBI studies showed significant agreement in 80 % of segments (Table 1). Therefore, it appeared that *visual* analysis of regional wall motion on planar SestaMIBI studies is best performed from the *epicardial* border. However, as is obvious from echocardiography, magnetic resonance imaging, or open chest animal studies, epicardial motion is usually less and more subtle than endocardial motion.

Although the epicardial border may be the most appropriate border to analyze, reliable detection of changes in contraction may be difficult, because of the small excursion of this border. In particular when visual inspection is employed, the accuracy and reproducibility of interpretation may be suboptimal.

Moreover, this one-dimensional analysis of left ventricular borders does not take advantage of the three-dimensional count information that potentially can be derived from these dynamic perfusion studies.

Count-Based functional image of regional contraction

The changes that can be observed on dynamic display of ECG-gated Sesta MIBI studies, are changes in count density during the cardiac cycle that reflect inward endocardial motion and myocardial thickening. Traditionally

ED   ES

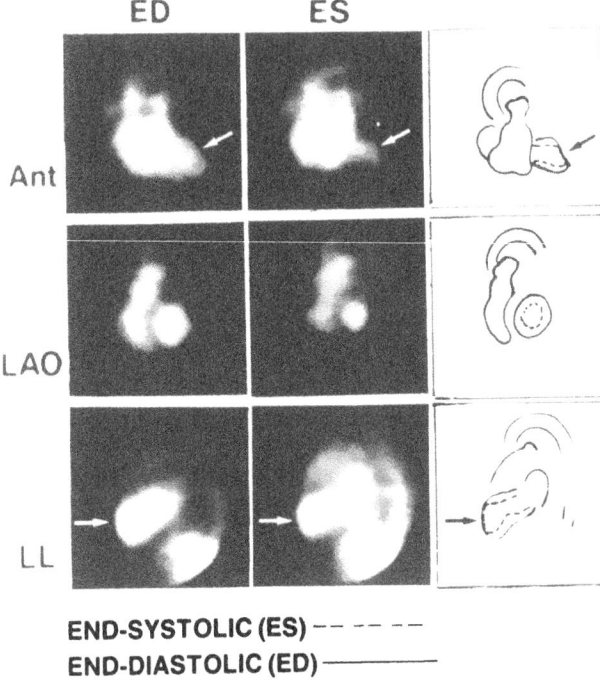

Ant

LAO

LL

END-SYSTOLIC (ES) — — — — —
END-DIASTOLIC (ED) —————

Figure 2. Analysis of regional wall motion on equilibrium radionuclide angiocardiography in a patient with an anterior infarction. Regional wall motion is analyzed by inspection of the motion of the endocardial border in three views: anterior (ANT), left anterior oblique (LAO) and left lateral (LL). On the anterior view there is akinesis of the anterolateral segment (arrow). On the LAO view motion appears to be normal since the abnormal segment is seen 'enface'. On the LL view the anterior segment is akinetic.

such difference can be displayed in a 'difference' image, i.e. an end-systolic frame minus the end-diastolic frame. However, such an image is relatively poor in counts (Fig. 4). In particular when the motion is abnormal, changes may be minimal and indistinguishable from random noise. We developed a new algorithm for creating a functional image with improved count statistics and incorporating count changes throughout the entire cardiac cycle [5]. This functional image of regional myocardial contraction is generated as follows: the end-systolic frame is identified and each of the remaining 15 frames is subtracted from this end-systolic image resulting in 15 initial functional images. Subsequently, each image is normalized on a pixel-by-pixel basis to the end-systolic image. Finally, all 15 functional images are summed to a final functional image (Fig. 4).

These functional images can be derived from the left anterior oblique view and the left lateral view. Because of overlap of the right ventricle, they are not readily generated from the anterior view. This methodology was developed and validated for planar ECG-gated perfusion studies. However, the same algorithm should also be applicable to ECG-gated SPECT images.

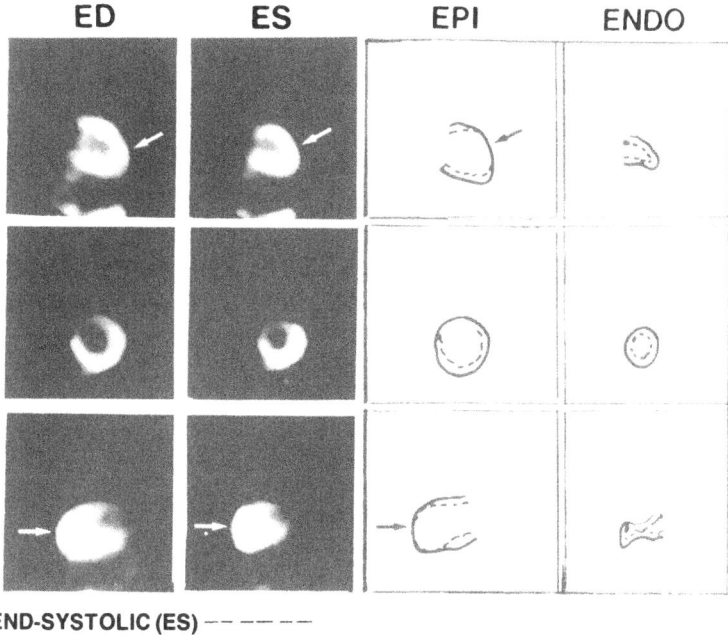

ED ES EPI ENDO

END-SYSTOLIC (ES) — — — — —
END-DIASTOLIC (ED) —————

Figure 3. Analysis of regional wall motion from ECG-gated Tc-99m SestaMIBI images in the same patient as in Fig. 2. The patient received thrombolytic therapy for acute anterior wall infarction. The perfusion images show near normal perfusion of the anterior wall, indicating successful reperfusion. Regional wall motion can be analyzed from the epicardial (EPI) and endocardial (ENDO) border. The excursion of the epicardial border agrees well with endocardial motion in Fig. 2. However, the endocardial motion incorrectly gives the impression of near normal motion. The potential mechanism for this is explained in Fig. 1. This patient had successful reperfusion of the anterior wall. However, because of 'stunning', myocardial contraction was still abnormal.

Table 1. Segment by segment comparison of regional wall motion on equilibrium radionuclide angiocardiography (ERNA) and ECG-gated Tc-99m SestaMIBI imaging. (209 segments in 19 patients)

| | | G-MIBI | | | |
| | | Endocardium | | Epicardium | |
		NL	ABN	NL	ABN
ERNA	NL	94	4	73	25
	ABN	63	48	17	94
McNemar Test		$p < 0.001$		$p = NS$	
agreement			68%		80%

Abbr.: NL = normal; ABN = abnormal.

SINGLE FRAME

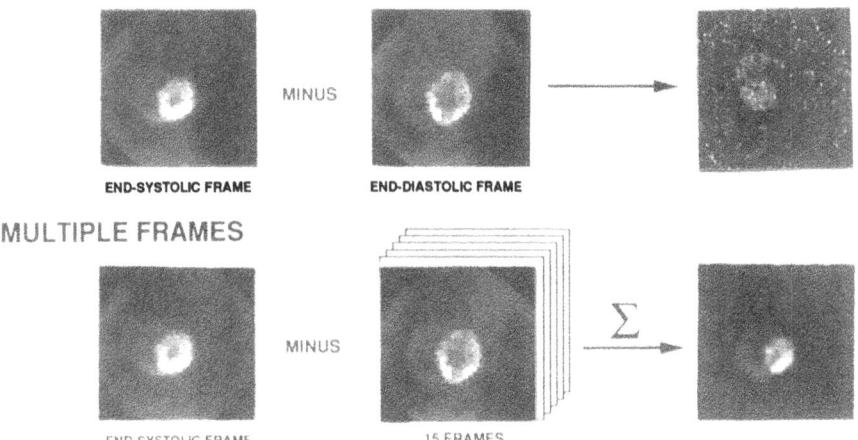

Figure 4. Generation of a functional image of myocardial contraction. *Top*: Although a functional image can be created by simple subtraction of the end-diastolic frame from the end-systolic, the resulting image is relatively poor in counts and has a poor signal-to-noise ratio. *Bottom*: iterative substraction of all remaining 15 frames in the RR-cycle from the end-systolic image, followed by normalization to the end-systolic image and summation results in a functional image with adequate count density and improved signal-to-noise ratio.

Quantification of functional images

A normal functional image displays an ellipse with more or less homogenous distribution of counts since endocardial motion and thickening is uniform. On an abnormal functional image the abnormally contracting area is displayed as a segmental area with relatively less counts (Fig. 5). It should be emphasized that because of image normalization, only *relative* contraction abnormalities can be identified on functional images. Therefore, global left ventricle dysfunction cannot be recognized or even measured. Although these functional images can be analyzed by visual inspection, because of the relatively high count density, quantification of regional contraction is feasible. For quantification we employed circumferential count profiles. The functional image is divided into 36 segments of 10° each, radiating from the centre. The maximal counts in each segment is displayed as a circumferential profile. The profile is normalized to the segment with highest counts which is assigned the value of 100 %. The patient's profile is displayed simultaneously with a curve displaying the lower-limit-of-normal regional motion. This curve is derived from functional images obtained in subjects with a low (< 3 %) likelihood of having coronary artery disease. Segments with abnormal function can be identified as a portion of the circumference profile below the lower-limit-of-normal curve. The area below the lower-limit-of-normal curve is integrated and expressed as a percentage of the entire area below the curve (Fig. 5). This integral is the Quantitative Regional Function Index (QRFI). When

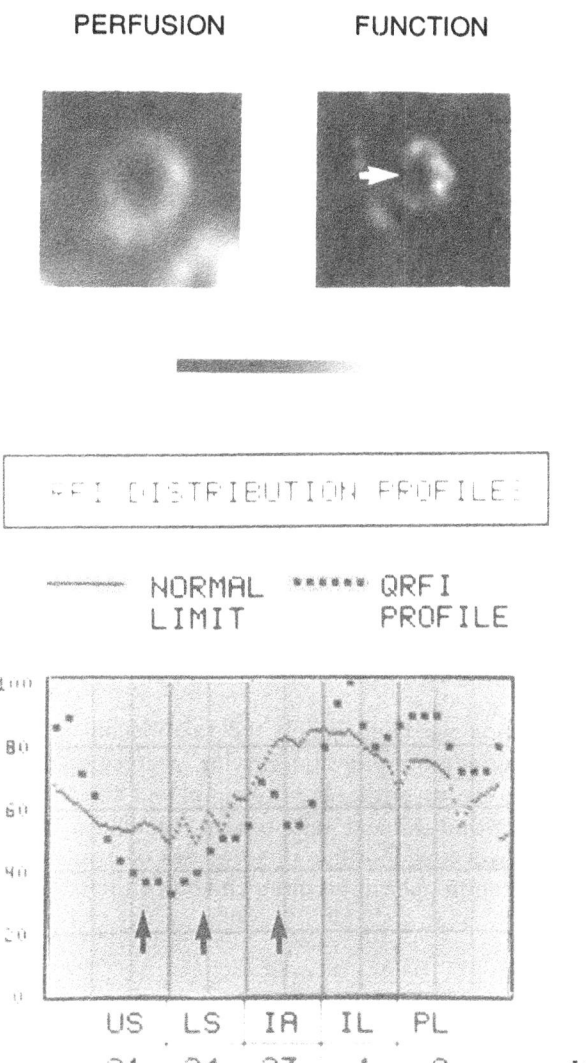

Figure 5. Example of quantification of a Functional Regional Contraction Image. *Top*: The Tc-99m SestaMIBI perfusion image (LAO view) is shown at the left (perfusion). The derived functional image (function) is shown at the right. The perfusion image shows slightly decreased uptake in the septum. The functional image shows an abnormal area (arrow) at the septum and inferoapical segment. A normal functional image displays an ellipse (see Fig. 4). *Bottom*: The functional image is quantified as a circumferential count profile (see text). The portion of the Quantitative Regional Function Index (QRFI) profile below the normal limit curve (arrow) indicates abnormal contraction. This is expressed quantitatively as an integral. QRFI is abnormal in the upper septum (US), lower septum (LS), inferoapical (IA) region and inferolateral (IL) region. The posterolateral (PL) segment is normal. QRFI in each segment as shown. Total QRFI in this image is 69.

contraction is normal, QRFI is zero. The higher the value for QRFI, the more abnormal regional functional abnormality.

Validation of quantitative regional function index

This new quantitative functional index was validated in several ways.
1. Comparison to visual analysis of regional wall motion on equilibrium radionuclide angiocardiography in the same patient. Regional wall motion was scored subjectively as 'normal', 'mildly hypokinetic', 'severely hypokinetic', and 'akinetic'. We found a good agreement between the semiquantitative regional wall motion score and QRFI. By statistical analysis each category was significantly different from each other.
2. Comparison to regional left ventricular ejection fraction on equilibrium radionuclide angiocardiography. A good relationship existed between regional left ventricle ejection fraction and QRFI in the same region. However, since LVEF is a continuous variable in normally contracting regions and QRFI is zero, a logarithmic curve fitted these data best.

QRFI, varying contraction abnormality and varying defect severity

By computer simulation we investigated the relationship between varying degrees of contraction abnormality and varying degrees of defect intensity and measured QRFI. Over a wide range of simulated abnormal contraction abnormality QRFI showed a linear relationship. Similarly, QRFI measurements were reliable over a wide range of severities of myocardial perfusion defect. Thus, QRFI can be measured independent of these variables.

Comments

We demonstrated that it is feasible to quantify regional myocardial contraction using a newly developed count-based algorithm from ECG-gated Tc-99m SestaMIBI images. At the present time, our experience with QRFI is restricted to planar images. However, this algorithm should be readily applicable to ECG-gated tomographic images, provided that sufficient count density is obtained. Because of cross-talk and overlap of myocardial segments during contraction, we believe that count-based quantification of regional motion is a necessity for interpretation of planar images. On ECG-gated tomographic images the overlap should be less of a problem. However, partial volume effect and movement of myocardial segments in and out of the reconstructed plane should be considered as a potential confounding factor. Importantly, the problem with the 'shifting endocardial border', as observed on planar images, is not present on SPECT images.

We have successfully applied the presently described method in patients who received thrombolytic therapy for acute myocardial infarction [6]. In these patients recovery of regional left ventricular function after successful thrombolysis could be demonstrated by serial measurements of QRFI. In patients with successful thrombolysis myocardial perfusion defects became smaller and QRFI improved significantly over time. On the other hand, in patients who failed thrombolysis and had occluded infarct arteries, myocardial perfusion defects remained unchanged and no improvement of regional function as measured by QRFI was noted.

An expected future application of this method is in rest-exercise myocardial perfusion studies with Tc-99m SestaMIBI. It is anticipated that in patients without prior myocardial infarction, and exercise-induced myocardial ischemia, measurement of QRFI potentially provides information with respect to myocardial viability and therefore, defect reversibility. For example, the initial perfusion defect reflects myocardial blood flow at peak exercise. However, since imaging is performed 30 minutes or longer after exercise, myocardial ischemia should no longer be present and regional wall motion (QRFI) should be normal. In such a patient images obtained after an injection at rest would show defect reversibility. Therefore, a single (ECG-gated) image obtained directly after exercise could suffice to predict defect reversibility by analyzing perfusion and function. This approach is at the present time under investigation by a number of investigators.

In summary, ECG-gated Technetium-99m labelled myocardial perfusion images can provide simultaneous, quantitative information on myocardial perfusion and regional myocardial contraction. Our initial clinical experience suggests that this combined and integrated analysis may be invaluable in patients with acute and chronic ischemic heart disease.

References

1. Wackers FJ, Berman DS, Maddahi J, et al. Technetium-99m hexakis 2–methoxyisobutyl isonitrile: human biodistribution, dosimetry, safety, and preliminary comparison to thallium-201 for myocardial perfusion imaging. J Nucl Med 1989;30:301–11.
2. Kiat H, Maddahi J, Roy LT, et al. Comparison of technetium-99m-methoxy isobutyl isonitrile with thallium-201 for evaluation of coronary artery disease by planar and tomographic methods. Am Heart J 1989;117:1–11.
3. Hamilton GW, Narahara KA, Trobaugh GB, Ritchie JL, Williams DL. Thallium-201 myocardial imaging: characterization of the ECG-synchronized images. J Nucl Med 1978;19:1103–10.
4. Wackers FJ, Mattera JA, Bowman L, Zaret BL. Gated Tc-99m-isonitrile myocardial perfusion imaging: disparity between endo-, and epicardial wall motion (abstract). Circulation 1987;76 Suppl 4:302.
5. Maniawski PJ, Allam AH, Wackers FJ, Zaret BL. A new non-geometric technique for

simultaneous evaluation of regional function and myocardial perfusion from gated planar isonitrile images (abstract). Circulation 1989;80 Suppl 2:544.

6. Allam AH, Maniawski PJ, Verani MS, Gibbons RJ, Zaret BL, Wackers FJ. Simultaneous assessment of recovery of regional ventricular function and perfusion after thrombolysis using serial gated Tc-99m-isonitrile imaging (abstract). Circulation 1989;80 Suppl 2:620.

11. Myocardial perfusion imaging by single photon emission computed tomography (SPECT)

JAMSHID MADDAHI*, KENNETH VAN TRAIN,
ERNEST GARCIA, HOSEN KIAT, JOHN FRIEDMAN
and DANIEL S. BERMAN

Summary

Single Photon Emission Computed Tomography (SPECT) is superior to the planar imaging method because it provides a higher image contrast resolution and allows separation of overlapping myocardial regions. Several computerized methods are now available and are being developed for quantitative analysis of SPECT myocardial perfusion by Tl-201 or the new Tc-99m labeled myocardial perfusion agents. In patient studies, all short axis and apical portions of vertical long axis Tl-201 SPECT images are quantified by dividing each myocardial slice into 60 equal sectors and displaying the maximal count per sector as a linear profile. The best threshold for defining normal limits was developed in a pilot group of 45 patients. After comparing patients' profiles with normal limits, abnormal and normal portions of the patients' profiles are plotted on a 2–dimensional polar map which is divided into specific coronary artery territories based on a scheme developed in a group of patients with disease of different coronary arteries. ROC analysis for defect size showed that the optimal thresholds for a definite perfusion defect were 12 % for the LAD and LCX and 8 % for the RCA territories. These criteria were prospectively applied to an additional 138 patients which yielded respective sensitivity, specificity and normalcy rates for overall detection of CAD of 96 %, 56 % and 86 % with high sensitivity and specificity for identification of CAD in individual coronary arteries. The accuracy of this quantitative SPECT technique was further assessed in a multicenter trial consisting of 318 patients whose SPECT images were obtained by various cameras, computers and operators. The results indicated that the quantitative SPECT method, utilizing standard normal limits developed at Cedars-Sinai Medical Center, can be applied at other institutions with similar accuracies. In 66 patients with prior myocardial infarction, new quantitative criteria were developed by ROC analysis that took into consideration contiguity of defects with the infarct zone. The new defect thresholds (40 % for LCX, 20 % for RCA and 12 % for LAD) were 86 % accurate for detection of patients with

*Supported in part by a grant 1RO1–HL41628 from the National Institute of Health, Bethesda, Maryland.

Johan H.C. Reiber & Ernst E. van der Wall (eds.), Cardiovascular Nuclear Medicine and MRI, 163–180.
© 1992 *Kluwer Academic Publishers*.

multivessel coronary disease after myocardial infarction. SPECT is superior to the planar imaging method in detecting patients without prior myocardial infarction, and those with moderate or single vessel coronary disease.

SPECT is increasingly being used in conjunction with Tc-99m labeled myocardial perfusion agents. The results of qualitative analysis of SPECT Tc-99m SestaMIBI studies in a multicenter study have been similar to those of Tl-201 SPECT for detection of perfusion defects and evaluation of the patterns of defect reversibility. Using an approach similar to that used for quantitation of Tl-201 SPECT studies, a quantitative method has recently been developed for the interpretation of exercise-rest Tc-99m SestaMIBI images. Furthermore, methods are being developed for the analysis of same day rest-stress protocols and for the absolute quantification of myocardial perfusion by performing attenuation and scatter correction on Tc-99m Sesta-MIBI myocardial perfusion images. Myocardial perfusion SPECT images are being quantified with respect to the extent of myocardial perfusion deficit which holds promise for assessing percent infarcted and jeopardized myocardium as important prognostic indicators in coronary artery disease.

Introduction

Planar Tl-201 myocardial perfusion scintigraphy has been widely used for the detection and evaluation of coronary artery disease. With the planar imaging method, however, normally and abnormally perfused myocardial regions frequently overlap one another limiting the ability of the method to detect, localize and size myocardial perfusion defects. To overcome these limitations, the technique of Single Photon Emission Computed Tomography (SPECT) has been developed. With SPECT, multiple planar images of the myocardium are obtained over 180 or 360 degrees and the image data are reconstructed to provide multiple slices of the myocardium at desired planes. This increased angular sampling results in a higher image contrast resolution and allows separation of overlapping myocardial regions. Over the past decade, SPECT myocardial perfusion imaging with Tl-201 has undergone several technical developments and its clinical application in patients with coronary artery disease has been extensively evaluated. Recently, SPECT application has expanded to its use in conjunction with the new Tc-99m labeled myocardial perfusion agents. This manuscript will review the current state and future directions of SPECT imaging of myocardial perfusion with Tl-201 and Tc-99m labeled agents.

SPECT myocardial perfusion imaging with Tl-201

Technical aspects

Imaging protocol

As with planar Tl-201 imaging, SPECT technique is generally used in conjunction with exercise or pharmacological stress testing using coronary vasodilators such as dipyridamole [1–4] or adenosine [5]. The patient is injected with 3–4 mCi of Tl-201 at least 1 min prior to termination of exercise or pharmacologic stress. For imaging, a large field-of-view camera which is especially designed to rotate around the patient is used. The most common protocol includes the use of an all purpose, parallel hole colimator and a 64×64 16–bit matrix. The patient lies on the imaging table in supine position and images are obtained over a semi-circular 180° arc extending from the 45° RAO to the 45° LPO position, imaging 32 projections each for 40 sec. Recently, SPECT imaging in the prone position has been advocated for reducing the inferoseptal attenuation artifact [6]. SPECT imaging does not begin till at least 10 min after injection of Tl-201 in order to diminish the frequency of the 'upward creep' artifact [7]. During this 10–15 min waiting period, a single 5 min anterior view planar image may be acquired to assist evaluation of several image patterns that are better assessed by the planar imaging method; i.e., lung uptake of Tl-201 [8–12], transient ischemic dilation of the left ventricle [13], and the breast attenuation artifact. Due to the length of acquisition and the nature of the equipment, SPECT imaging is technically very demanding and requires more attention to quality control than planar imaging. An important step in quality control for SPECT acquisition is correction for nonuniformity. For this purpose, a 3 million count image is obtained weekly from a uniform cobalt 57 flood source. This image is then used to correct each of the projection images for nonuniformity. Another important step prior to acquisition is the determination of the mechanical center of rotation. The center of rotation is then used to align the detector data with respect to the reconstruction matrix. Failure to correct for the center of rotation causes misregistration of pixels during the reconstruction process which leads to artifactual myocardial perfusion defects. Since patient motion during SPECT imaging is a frequent cause of image artifacts [14], patients should be instructed to lie still during the entire acquisition and projection images should be displayed at the end of acquisition in a cine loop format to evaluate whether patient motion has occurred.

Image processing and quantitation protocol

Several methods for image processing and quantitation are now available [15–18]. In this manuscript, the method developed at Cedars-Sinai Medical Center [17] will be described as a model to discuss various steps involved in

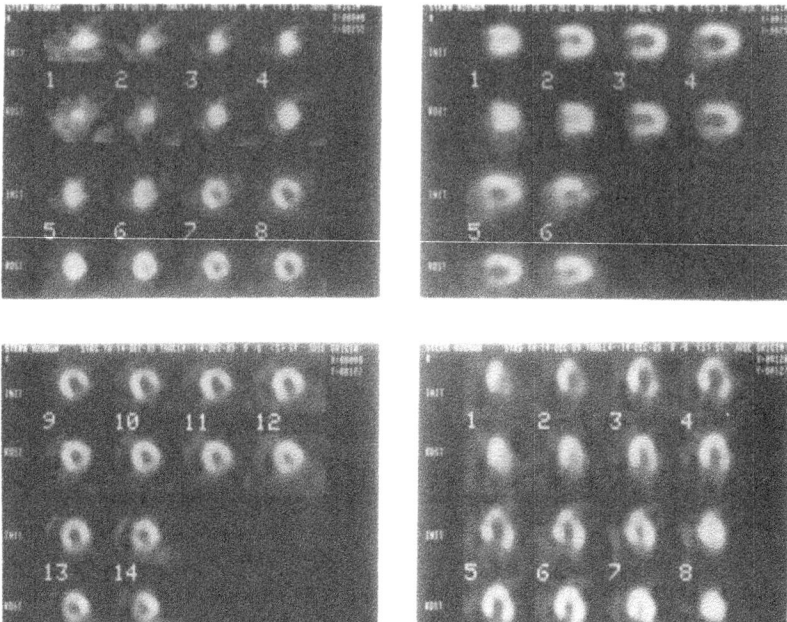

Figure 1. TL-201 myocardial perfusion SPECT images reoriented in the short axis (Tomograms 1 through 14), vertical long axis (Tomograms 1 through 6) and horizontal long axis (Tomograms 1 through 8) planes. In each quadrant, the first and third rows represent the initial post exercise images and the second and fourth rows represent the corresponding redistribution images. A reversible inferolateral wall defect is noted.

image processing and quantitation that are similar between the different methods. Raw image data are smoothed using a 9–point weighted averaging algorithm. The filtered-back projection technique is used to reconstruct images. A Butterworth filter with a cutoff frequency of 0.2 cycles per pixel and order 5 is used for filtering of the images prior to reconstruction. Images are reoriented in planes that are perpendicular and parallel to the long axis of the left ventricle (Fig. 1). All tomograms are reconstructed at 1 pixel per slice, which represents a thickness of approximately 6.2 mm. No attenuation or scatter correction is used. The resulting short axis and vertical long axis myocardial images are then quantified utilizing the circumferential profile technique. With this method, the center of the left ventricular cavity and the radius of search are defined by the operator. From the center, 60 equidistant radii (6° apart) are then generated. Along each radius, the computer searches and selects the maximum count value. The values are then normalized to the highest value found in each slice and are plotted for each angular location on the myocardial periphery, thereby generating a circumferential count profile. For proper comparison of stress and redistribution images with the normal profiles and with one another, an anatomic landmark is defined at the inferior junction of the right and left ventricles on the short axis slices

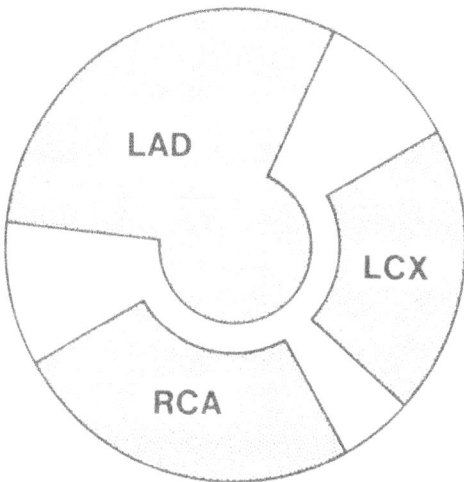

Figure 2. Polar map display of the three coronary artery territories. LAD = the left anterior descending, LCX = the left circumflex and RCA = the right coronary artery.

to which the 102° angle is assigned. On the vertical long axis slices, the most apical point is used for alignment and the 90 angle is assigned to it. The circumferential profiles are then compared to the normal data base to determine whether a perfusion defect is present. The normal data base consists of 35 males and 20 females with a less than 5 % likelihood of coronary artery disease based on Bayesian analysis of their age, sex, symptoms and the results of their exercise electrocardiograms [19–21]. The myocardium was divided into five separate myocardial zones in the short axis and long axis orientation. Gender specific lower limits of normal were then developed for each zone. Since the distribution of normal profile points around the mean is not gaussian in all regions of the myocardium, the range approach rather than standard deviation approach was used to define the lower limit of normal. The range approach is based on the lowest observed value below the mean normal profiles. The patient's circumferential profiles are then compared to the corresponding normal limit profiles. The results of this comparison are displayed in a 'polar map' format in which the entire myocardium is represented as a disc with the center corresponding to the left ventricular apex and the periphery to the atrio- ventricular junction (Fig. 2). In a systematic study, different portions of the polar map were assigned to the distributions of the left anterior descending (LAD), left circumflex (LCX), and posterior descending (PDA) coronary arteries. With this approach, the territory of the LAD is represented by the anterior, anterolateral, anteroseptal and apical regions of the left ventricle. The territory of the posterior descending coronary artery is represented by the inferior and inferoseptal regions of the left ventricle and the territory of the LCX is represented by the posterolateral wall. In order to develop criteria for a definite perfusion defect, receiver operating characteristic (ROC) curve analysis was used to identify the best defect size criterion, for each of the coronary territories, that provided the optimum true positive and false positive tradeoff for detection of disease. These optimum defect size thresholds were: greater than or equal to 12 % for the LAD and LCX territories and greater than or equal to 8 % for the PDA territory (Fig. 2).

Clinical applications of Tl-201 SPECT

Detection of coronary artery disease

As with the other tests applied for the detection of coronary artery disease (CAD), the diagnostic accuracy of the exercise Tl-201 SPECT study is expressed by sensitivity and specificity. These parameters depend on several factors such as qualitative vs quantitative analysis and exercise vs pharmacologic stress testing. In addition, several characteristics of the patient population under study may affect the sensitivity and specificity such as presence or absence of myocardial infarction, threshold for defining significant CAD, referral bias, level of exercise and the severity (percentage stenosis) and extent (number of diseased vessels) of CAD in the referred population. Table I summarizes the results of the Tl-201 SPECT imaging method using qualitative analysis of images. In a total of 706 reported patients [15,18,22,23], the sensitivity is 92 % and specificity is 77 %. The sensitivity and specificity of quantitatively analyzed Tl-201 SPECT images has also been studied by various investigators. In a prospective study of 138 patients, the Cedars-Sinai method of quantitation had a sensitivity of 95 %, specificity of 56 % and normalcy rate of 86 % [17]. Normalcy rate is defined as the true negative rate in a group of patients with a low (< 5 %) likelihood of CAD. In this study, SPECT had a sensitivity of 100 % in patients with prior myocardial infarction compared to 90 % in those without prior myocardial infarction. Similar results were observed when this method was applied at multiple centers to a total of 318 patients [24]; sensitivity, specificity and normalcy rates were 94 %, 43 % and 82 % respectively. Based on the results of 1066 reported patients in five published manuscripts [15,17,18,22,24], the average sensitivity, specificity and normalcy rate of quantitative Tl-201 SPECT method for detection of CAD has been 93 %, 72 % and 83 % respectively (Table 1). It is of note that the specificity of Tl-201 SPECT appeared to be lower in the study of DePasquale and colleagues reported in 1988 [15] compared to the study of Tamaki and colleagues reported in 1984 [22] both using qualitative image analysis. A similar trend is also noted for the quantitative SPECT method with a decrease in specificity from 91 % to 47 % from 1984 [22] to 1989 [24]. The decline of specificity with time is likely to be due, in part, to an increase in referral bias in the more recent studies.

Table 1. Sensitivity and specificity of Tl-201 SPECT for detection of coronary artery disease

Visual analysis

Year	Lead author	Sensitivity (%)	Specificity (%)	Normalcy rate
1984	Tamaki [22]	76/82 (93)	20/22 (91)	–
1988	DePasquale [15]	173/179 (97)	21/31 (68)	–
1989	Fintel [23]	88/96 (92)	*	–
1990	Mahmerian [18]	193/221 (87)	57/75 (76)	
Overall		530/578 (92)	98/128 (77)	

*Results of patients with normal coronary arteries and low likelihood of CAD not reported separately.

Quantitative analysis

Year	Lead author	Sensitivity (%)	Specificity (%)	Normalcy rate
1984	Tamaki [22]	80/82 (98)	20/22 (91)	–
1988	DePasquale [15]	170/179 (95)	23/31 (74)	–
1989	Maddahi [17]	88/92 (96)	10/18 (56)	24/ 28 (86)
21989	Van Train [24]	185/196 (94)	30/46 (43)	62/76 (82)
1990	Mahmerian [18]	192/221 (87)	65/75 (83)	–
Overall		715/770 (93)	138/192 (72)	86/104 (83)

Normalcy rate has been proposed as an alternative to the biased specificity [21]. Although the true unbiased specificity of the SPECT technique has not been determined, it is expected to be higher than the average literature specificity of 70 % but it may not be as high as the average literature normalcy rate of 82 %. It is likely that the true specificity of the SPECT technique is slightly lower than the planar imaging method because of the fact that SPECT imaging is technically more demanding and has many more sources of acquisition and processing artifacts than the planar imaging method. Fintel and colleagues [23] compared the diagnostic performance of planar and SPECT imaging methods in 136 patients using qualitative image analysis. They found that Tl-201 SPECT was superior to planar imaging in males, in patients without prior myocardial infarction, those with single vessel disease, and in patients with 50–69 coronary stenosis.

Detection of disease in individual coronary arteries

The coronary arteries and their branches supply different regions of the left ventricular myocardium. Based on the known anatomic relationships between coronary arteries and various myocardial regions and actual study of patients with single and multivessel CAD who had Tl-201 myocardial perfusion studies, general guidelines have been developed for assignment of various myocardial regions to specific coronary arteries. It is therefore possible to infer disease of a given coronary artery by noting the location of perfusion defect on Tl-201 SPECT myocardial images. The mean literature

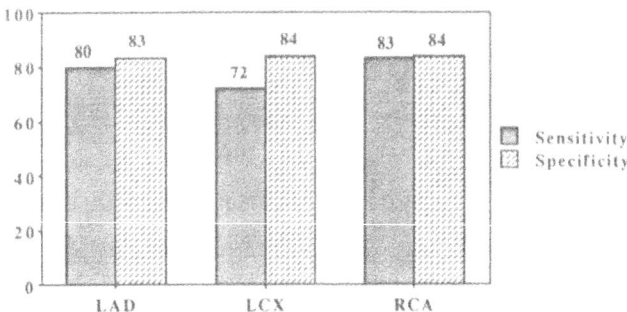

Figure 3. The mean literature sensitivities and specificities of the quantitative TL-201 SPECT for identification of disease in the LAD, LCX and RCA territories.

[15,22,18] sensitivities and specificities of the qualitative Tl-201 SPECT are respectively 72 % and 87 % for LAD, 56 % and 96 % for LCX, and 85 % and 80 % for PDA. The mean literature [15,17,18,22,24] sensitivities and specificities of the quantitative Tl-201 SPECT are respectively 80 % and 83 % for LAD, 72 % and 84 % for LCX, and 83 % and 84 % for PDA (Fig. 3).

The pooled literature results and direct comparison of SPECT and planar quantitative imaging methods in the same patient population [25] have shown that SPECT has a higher sensitivity for detection of disease in the LCX territory. This improved sensitivity may be related to improved defect contrast and decreased defect overlap associated with SPECT imaging. In the study of Maddahi, et al. [17], the specificity of SPECT for localization of disease in patients with prior myocardial infarction was 41 % compared to 81 % in those without prior myocardial infarction. This higher false positive rate in patients with prior myocardial infarction was caused by frequent extension or 'tailing' of the infarct related perfusion defect into the adjacent myocardial territories that were supplied by normal coronary arteries. In a subsequent study of 66 patients [26] with prior myocardial infarction, new quantitative criteria were developed by ROC analysis that took into consideration contiguity of defects with the infarct zone. The new defect thresholds were defined as 40 % for LCX, 20 % for RCA and 12 % for LAD. These new criteria significantly improved specificity for detection of disease in the LCX and RCA territories from 37 % to 87 % and 60 % to 73 % respectively (Fig. 4). Overall, quantitative Tl-201 SPECT was 86 % accurate for detection of multivessel coronary disease patients with prior myocardial infarction.

Sizing of myocardial perfusion defect

Prognosis in CAD has been shown to be related to the extent of necrotic and jeopardized myocardium. SPECT has theoretical advantages over planar imaging for sizing of myocardial perfusion defects because of increased angular sampling of the myocardium which results in reduced regional overlap

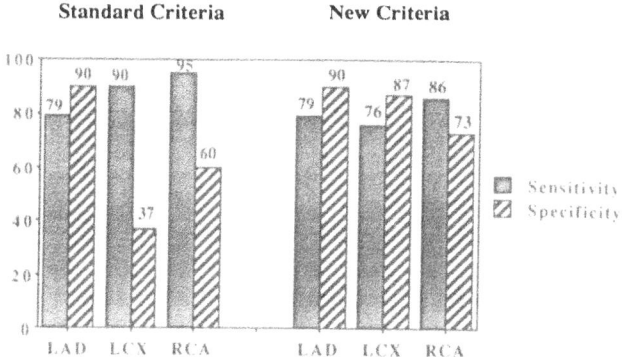

Figure 4. Comparison of standard versus new criteria for localization of coronary disease in patients with prior myocardial infarction. The new criteria significantly improved specificity for detection of disease in the LCX and RCA territories.

and improved contrast of perfusion defects. In an experimental animal study, Prigent et al. [27] compared SPECT Tl-201 myocardial perfusion defect size with post sacrifice pathologic infarct size in 14 dogs with 6–8 hr closed-chest coronary occlusion. Tl-201 SPECT images were quantified by automatically generating circumferential profiles which were then compared with normal limit profiles derived from 6 normal dogs. SPECT and pathologic infarct sizes correlated highly (r = 0.93, SEE = 9.4 %) on 71 individual myocardial slices. In order to determine SPECT infarct size as percent of the total left ventricular myocardium, infarct sizes from each slice were added to one another after each was multiplied by a coefficient that reflected the contribution of that slice to the total left ventricular weight. A close correlation was noted between SPECT and pathology for sizing the total left ventricular myocardial perfusion defect; r = 0.86, SEE = 4.5 %. In a subsequent study [28], different methods were compared for assessing the contribution of each slice to the total left ventricular mass. Prigent et al. [29] also compared SPECT and planar Tl-201 myocardial perfusion imaging for quantifying myocardial infarct size in experimental animals. In this study, SPECT more closely approximated pathological infarct size than the planar imaging method.

SPECT myocardial imaging using Tc-99m myocardial perfusion agents

Tl-201, despite widespread clinical use, does not have ideal imaging characteristics mainly because it has low energy photons and a long half-life. The photon energy of Tl-201 (68–80 keV) is not well suited for standard gamma cameras, which perform best at the 140 keV photon peak of Tc-99m. Furthermore, the 73 hr half-life of Tl-201 limits the injected dose to 3–4 mCi, resulting in relatively low count density of the images. In order to circumvent these physical limitations of Tl-201, two groups of Tc-99m labeled compounds; Tc-99m SestaMIBI [30–34] and Tc-99m-teboroxime [35–40], have been developed and were recently approved for clinical use.

Clinical results using qualitative analysis of Tc-99m SestaMIBI SPECT

This has been extensively evaluated through the North American multicenter clinical trial [41] and studies by several investigators [42–44]. In the multicenter study, 22 centers in the United States and 2 centers in Canada compared Tc-99m SestaMIBI with Tl-201 imaging and coronary angiography. Rest and exercise Tc-99m SestaMIBI SPECT were performed on two separate days using an average of 20 mCi for each study. A total of 278 patients and 6677 myocardial segments were evaluated. The overall image quality of Tc-99m SestaMIBI was superior to that of Tl-201. With respect to identifying stress perfusion defects, the concordance between Tc-99m SestaMIBI and Tl-201 SPECT was 92 %. The two tracers were also compared with respect to identifying different patterns of defect reversibility. This comparison is of particular interest since the mechanism for stress defects reversibility of Tc-99m SestaMIBI is different from that of Tl-201. Tl-201 defect reversibility is the result of differential washout rate of Tl-201 from the normal and viable but hypoperfused myocardial regions. Tc-99m SestaMIBI, however, does not redistribute significantly. Therefore, defect reversibility is assessed by comparing the stress image with that obtained after injection of Tc-99m SestaMIBI in the resting state. Exact agreement for the pattern of defect reversibility was 83 % for patients and 89 % for segments. With respect to detection of CAD, Tc-99m SestaMIBI and Tl-201 sensitivities, specificities and normalcy rates were respectively 89 % and 90 %; 49 % and 41 %; and 81 % and 82 %. These results from the multicenter study suggest that SPECT Tc-99m SestaMIBI has superior image quality and is clinically as effective as Tl-201 SPECT for detection of myocardial perfusion defects, assessment of defect reversibility patterns and evaluation of CAD. It is of note, however, that in this trial Tc-99m SestaMIBI imaging and processing parameters were similar to those used for Tl-201. Due to differences between the two agents, research is underway to optimize acquisition parameters for Tc-99m Sesta-MIBI. This topic is discussed in more detail below. In a recent study [42], Tc-99m SestaMIBI-SPECT was compared to planar imaging method for detection of CAD and assessment of disease in individual coronary arteries. The two methods were not significantly different from one another with respect to overall detection of CAD. However, sensitivity of Tc-99m SestaMIBI SPECT for detection of disease in individual coronary arteries was 89 % which was significantly higher than the 60 % obtained by Tc-99m SestaMIBI planar studies with a similar specificity of 86 %.

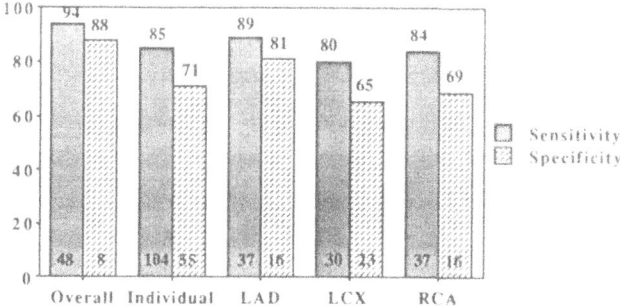

Figure 5. Sensitivities and specificities of Tc-99m SestaMIBI SPECT quantitative analysis for overall detection and identification of disease in individual coronary arteries. The latter is subcategorized to LAD, LCX and RCA territories.

Clinical results using quantitative analysis of Tc-99m SestaMIBI SPECT

As with Tl-201, quantitative analysis is an important adjunct to the interpretation of Tc-99m SestaMIBI myocardial perfusion images. Two computerized methods have been described for quantitative analysis of Tc-99m SestaMIBI. Kahn et al. [44] developed a gender specific normal data base from 12 normal volunteers and evaluated their quantitative method in 36 patients with angiographically documented CAD. The overall sensitivity for detection of CAD was 95 %. The sensitivity and specificity were 74 % and 83 % for LAD, 91 % and 76 % for LCX, and 74 % and 69 % for RCA. Kiat et al. [45] developed a gender specific normal data base from patients with a low likelihood of CAD, using a quantitative method similar to that used for quantitation of Tl-201–SPECT studies. In a collaborative study between the two groups, similar inter-institutional results were observed (Fig. 5) even though different camera / computer systems were used in the two institutions and the normal data base developed at Cedars-Sinai was used to analyze images from both institutions [45].

Quantitation of perfusion defect size

This aspect of Tc-99m SestaMIBI SPECT has been evaluated by several investigators. Verani et al. [46] studied 13 dogs with permanent coronary occlusion and showed a high correlation (r = 0.95) between Tc-99m Sesta-MIBI SPECT and postmortem pathologic defect size as determined by TTC staining. Gibbons et al. [47] developed and validated a quantitative technique in a heart phantom in which the SPECT defect size was defined as the areas enclosed between the count profiles and a 60 % threshold. There was virtually a one to one relation between the SPECT and true defect size (r = 0.99). This method was then applied to patients with evolving myocardial infarction to assess the effect of thrombolytic therapy in reducing the size of myocardium at risk. Bergin et al. [48] showed a high correlation (r = 0.79) between

Tc-99m SestaMIBI SPECT and the risk area in experimental animals. More recently, Prigent et al. [49,50] assessed the possibility of sizing both transmural and nontransmural myocardial perfusion defects by Tc-99m SestaMIBI SPECT using 128×128 image acquisition matrix, a high resolution collimator and 64 projections over 180°. Defect size was defined as the area enclosed between the count profile and a threshold which was optimized in a pilot study. Using this method, there was a high correlation between the Tc-99m SestaMIBI and TTC infarct size for transmural ($r = 0.90$) and nontransmural ($r = 0.89$) perfusion defects.

New developments

In order to fully utilize the superior characteristics of Tc-99m SestaMIBI, there is a need to optimize the technical aspects of SPECT imaging for this agent. Performance may be enhanced through the careful selection of optimal radiopharmaceutical doses, imaging sequences, acquisition parameters, reconstruction filters, perfusion quantification methods and multidimensional methods of displaying myocardial perfusion. These aspects are currently being studied in a collaborative research between the investigators at Emory University and Cedars-Sinai Medical Center [51]. In order to complete the rest and stress studies in the same day, a low dose resting study is followed by a high dose stress study in a few hours [52,53]. The protocols for patient preparation, acquisition parameters and reconstruction are summarized in Tables 2 and 3. These protocols are the result of the extensive phantom studies and preliminary patient results given the existing instrumentation and recommended dose limits. The group has also developed a hybrid method for extracting the three-dimensional myocardial count distribution by radial sampling that is mostly perpendicular to the myocardial wall. This is accomplished by spherical coordinate sampling of the apex and cylindrical coordinate sampling of the rest of the myocardium (Fig. 6). The presence,

Table 2. Patient acquisition protocol for rest-stress Tc-99m SestaMIBI

	Rest	Exercise
Dose	8–9 mCi	22–25 mCi
Injection to imaging interval	1 hr	30 min
Rest to stress study interval	3–4 hours	
Energy window	20 % symmetric	Same
Collimator	High resolution	Same
Orbit	180°, circular	Same
Number of projections	64	Same
Matrix	64 × 64	Same
Time/projection	25 sec	20 sec
Total Time	30 min	25 min
ECG gated	No	Yes
Frames/cycle	1	8
R-to-R window (%)	100	100

Table 3. Reconstruction protocol for rest-stress Tc-99m SestaMIBI same day studies

	Rest	Exercise
Decay correction	yes	yes
Filter (General Electric)	2D Butterworth	Same
Cutoff frequency	0.4 cycles/cm	0.52
Power	10	5
Filter (Siemens)	2D Butterworth	Same
Cutoff frequency	0.5 Nyquist	0.66
Order	5	2.5
Reconstruction Filter	Ramp	Same
Short axis slice thickness	12.88 mm	12.88 mm
Short axis slice increment	6.4 mm	6.4 mm

location and extent of myocardial perfusion defects are quantified by comparing the extracted counts with a normal limit data base. New methods for visualizing the myocardial distribution in multiple dimensions have also been developed. The methods represent the myocardial distribution in two-dimensional polar maps (Fig. 7) and in three-dimensional and four-dimensional displays [51]. The three-dimensional rendering of the myocardial count distribution has the advantage of accurately representing the extent and location

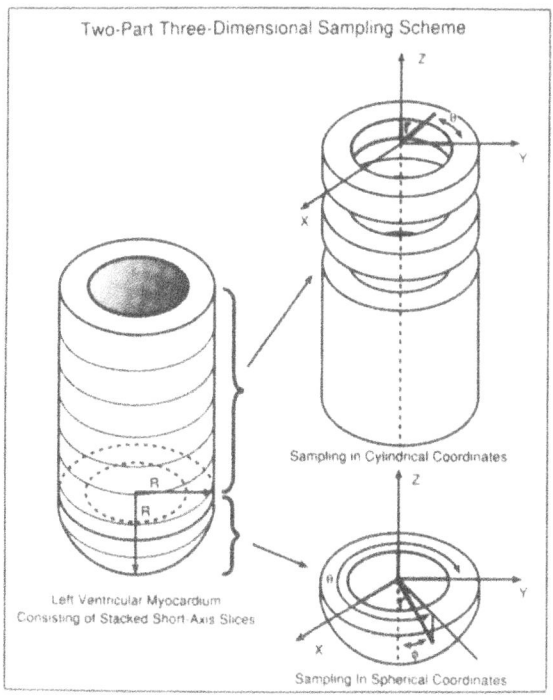

Figure 6. Diagrammatic demonstration of the method used for three dimensional sampling of Tc-99m SestaMIBI SPECT images [reprinted with permission (51)].

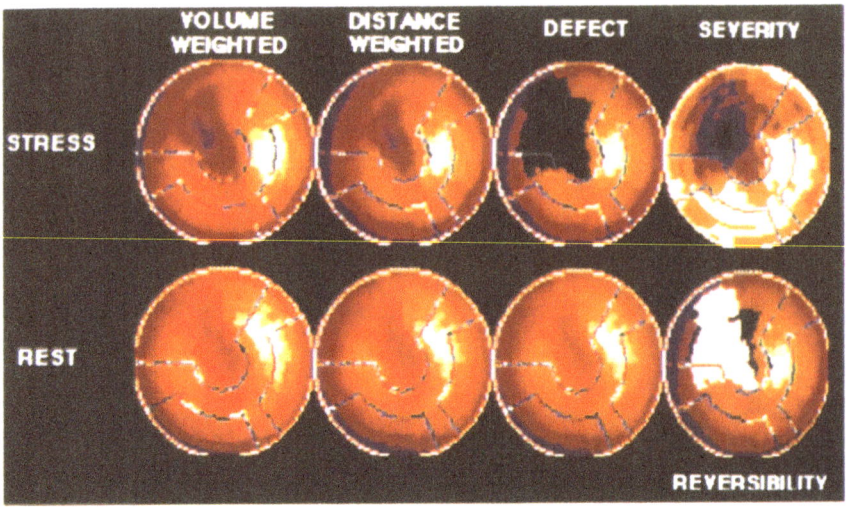

Figure 7. Different polar map displays of stress/rest Tc-99m SestaMIBI SPECT images in a patient with reversible anteroseptal and apical perfusion defects.

of perfusion defects which are distorted on polar maps. Since no one type of polar map can accurately represent the volume of perfusion defects and their distance from the apex, volume-weighted and distance-weighted polar maps have been developed. This new acquisition, processing, reconstruction, and image display methods for Tc-99m SestaMIBI should improve image quality as compared to current Tl-201 imaging and early Tc-99m SestaMIBI studies which utilized Tl-201 protocols. Another area of current investigation is development of algorithms for attenuation and scatter correction with Tc-99m SestaMIBI SPECT images. A major problem with Tl-201 and Tc-99m SestaMIBI studies is variable attenuation caused by varying distance of myocardial regions from the collimator and variable thickness of tissues interposed between the myocardium and the collimator. These attenuation patterns are frequently the source of false positive studies. Through the collaborative effort between the Emory University and Cedars-Sinai Medical Center investigators, various algorithms are being developed and validated in phantoms and experimental animals for correcting the effects of attenuation and scatter [54]. Attenuation correction is accomplished by first obtaining a transmission map of the heart and the surrounding structures. An attenuation correction matrix is then generated from this transmission map which is applied to the raw data before reconstruction, using the first order Chang correction method. This approach may ultimately add 10 min to the acquisition time and another 10 min to the processing time. For scatter correction, myocardial images are simultaneously obtained on two different photopeaks; 106 KeV to yield a scatter image that is then used to correct the 140 KeV 'on peak' study. Incorporation of these corrections may ultimately improve the diagnostic accuracy of Tc-99m SestaMIBI SPECT for detection of coronary artery disease.

SPECT myocardial perfusion imaging by Tc-99m-teboroxime

Tc-99m-teboroxime differs from Tc-99m SestaMIBI because it has a higher peak myocardial extraction fraction (90 % vs 65 %), much faster myocardial clearance (T1/2 of 10–15 min vs 5 hr) and the possibility of perfusion defect redistribution. These differences in physiologic properties of the two agents necessitates utilization of a different imaging protocol with Tc-99m-teboroxime. The total effective imaging time available after injection of teboroxime is approximately 10 min. The feasibility of SPECT teboroxime imaging with single headed rotating cameras has been demonstrated by Bellinger et al., Drane et al., and Carretta et al. but the results have not yet been published. The optimal mode of acquisition is continuous rather than step and shoot. Alternatively, three headed SPECT cameras may be utilized which further reduces the total acquisition time by 30 % [55]. With Tc-99m-teboroxime, both rest and stress myocardial perfusion studies may be completed in less than an hour. In a large multicenter trial [56], 177 patients were studied with Tc-99m-teboroxime using either planar or SPECT imaging methods and the results were compared with cardiac catheterization and/or Tl-201 imaging. The overall sensitivity for detection of coronary artery disease was 84 % and specificity was 91 %. Tc-99m-teboroxime imaging results agreed with Tl-201 interpretation in 91 % of the cases. The ability to do complete rest-stress study in a very short period of time appears to be an advantage of Tc-99m-teboroxime over Tl-201 or Tc-99m SestaMIBI. With the advent of three detector SPECT imaging systems, teboroxime may be particularly well suited to kinetic SPECT imaging, allowing rapid tomographic assessment of initial uptake and washout of the tracer. Preliminary data have suggested that compartmental modelling kinetic data with this tracer could permit the quantification of regional myocardial blood flow [57,58]. The feasibility of very rapid stress delayed imaging with a single injection of this tracer is currently being investigated.

Acknowledgements

The authors are grateful to Mercedes Bocanegra for typing of the manuscript and Lee Griswald for preparation of the figures.

References

1. Gould KL. Noninvasive assessment of coronary stenoses by myocardial perfusion imaging during pharmacologic coronary vasodilation. I. Physiologic basis and experimental validation. Am J Cardiol 1978;41:267–78.
2. Gould KL, Westcott RJ, Albro PC, Hamilton GW. Noninvasive assessment of coronary stenosis by myocardial imaging during pharmacologic coronary vasodilation. II. Clinical methodology and feasibility. Am J Cardiol 1978;41:279–87.
3. Leppo JA. Dypiridamole-thallium imaging: the lazy man's stress test. J Nucl Med 1989;30:281–7.

4. Ranhosky A, Kempthorne-Rawson J. The safety of intravenous dipyridamole thallium myocardial perfusion imaging. Intravenous dipyridamole thallium imaging study group. Circular 1990; 81: 1205–9. Comment in: Circulation 1990;81:1425–7.

5. Verani MS, Mahmarian JJ, Hixson JB, Boyce TM, Staudacher RA. Diagnosis of coronary artery disease by controlled coronary vasodilation with adenosine and thallium-201 scintigraphy in patients unable to exercise. Circulation 1990; 82: 80–7. Comment in: Circulation 1990;82:308–9.

6. Segall GM, Davis MJ. Prone versus supine thallium myocardial SPECT: a method to decrease artifactual inferior wall defects. J Nucl Med 1989; 30: 548–55. Comment in: J Nucl Med 1989;30:1738–9.

7. Friedman J, Van Train K, Maddahi J, et al. 'Upward creep' of the heart: a frequent source of false positive reversible defects during thallium-201 stress-redistribution SPECT. J Nucl Med 1989;30:1718–22.

8. Boucher CA, Zir LM, Beller GA, et al. Increased lung uptake of Thallium-201 during exercise myocardial imaging: clinical, hemodynamic and angiographic implications in patients with coronary artery disease. Am J Cardiol 1980;46:189–96.

9. Gibson RS, Watson DD, Carabello BA, Holt ND, Beller GA. Clinical implications of increased lung uptake of thallium-201 during exercise scintigraphy 2 weeks after myocardial infarction. Am J Cardiol 1982;49:1586–93.

10. Bingham JB, McKusick KA, Strauss HW, Boucher CA, Pohost GM. Influence of coronary artery disease on pulmonary uptake of thallium-201. Am J Cardiol 1980;46:821–6.

11. Kushner FG, Okada RD, Kirschenbaum HD, Boucher CA, Strauss HW, Pohost GM. Lung thallium-201 uptake after stress testing in patients with coronary artery disease. Circulation 1981;63:341–7.

12. Levy R, Rozanski A, Berman DS, et al. Analysis of the degree of pulmonary thallium washout after exercise in patient with coronary artery disease. J Am Coll Cardiol 1983;2:719–28.

13. Weiss AT, Berman DS, Lew AS, et al. Transient ischemic dilation of the left ventricle on stress thallium scintigraphy: a marker of severe and extensive coronary artery disease. J Am Coll Cardiol 1987;9:752–9.

14. Friedman J, Berman D, Van Train K, et al. Patient motion in thallium-201 myocardial SPECT imaging. An easily identified frequent source of artifactual defect. Clin Nucl Med 1988;13 (5):321–4.

15. De Pasquale EE, Nody AC, DePuey EG, et al. Quantitative rotational thallium-201 tomography for identifying and localizing coronary artery disease. Circulation 1988;77 (2):316–27.

16. Garcia EV, Van Train K, Maddahi J, et al. Quantification of rotational thallium-201 myocardial tomography. J Nucl Med 1985;26:17–21.

17. Maddahi J, Van Train K, Prigent F, et al. Quantitative single photon emission computed thallium-201 tomography for detection and localization of coronary artery disease: optimization and prospective validation of a new technique. J Am Coll Cardiol 1989; 14: 1689–99. Comment in: J Am Coll Cardiol 1989;14:1700–1.

18. Mahmarian JJ, Boyce TM, Goldberg RK, Cocanougher MK, Roberts R, Verami MS. Quantitative exercise thallium-201 single photon emission computed tomography for the enhanced diagnosis of ischemic heart disease. J Am Coll Cardiol 1990;15:318–29. Comment in: J Am Coll Cardiol 1990;15:330–3.

19. Diamond GA, Forrester JS. Analysis of probability as an aid in the clinical diagnosis of coronary artery disease. N Engl J Med 1979;300:1350–8.

20. Diamond GA, Forrester JS, Hirsch M, et al. Application of conditional probability analysis to the clinical diagnosis of coronary artery disease. J Clin Invest 1980;65:1210–21.

21. Rozanski A, Diamond GA, Forrester JS, Berman DS, Morris D, Swan HJ. Alternative referent standards of cardiac normality. Implications for diagnostic testing. Ann Intern Med 1984;101:164–71.

22. Tamaki N, Yonekura Y, Mukai T, et al. Stress thallium-201 transaxial emission computed

tomography: quantitative versus qualitative analysis for evaluation of coronary artery disease. J Am Coll Cardiol 1984; 4(6): 1213–21.

23. Fintel DJ, Links JM, Brinker JA, Frank TL, Parker M, Becker LC. Improved diagnostic performance of exercise thallium-201 single photon emission computed tomography over planar imaging in the diagnosis of coronary artery disease: a receiver operating characteristic analysis. J Am Coll Cardiol 1989;13:600–12.

24. Van Train KF, Maddahi J, Berman DS, et al. Quantitative analysis of tomographic stress thallium-201 myocardial scintigrams: a multicenter trial. J Nucl Med 1990;31:1168–79.

25. Maddahi J, Van Train K, Wong C, et al. Comparison of thallium-201 single photon emission computed tomography (SPECT) and planar imaging for evaluation of coronary artery disease. J Nucl Med 1986;27:999. (Abstract)

26. Chouraqui P, Maddahi J, Ostrzega E, et al. Quantitative exercise thallium-201 rotational tomography for evaluation of patients with prior myocardial infarction. Am J Cardiol 1990;66:151–7.

27. Prigent F, Maddahi J, Garcia EV, Satoh Y, Van Train K, Berman DS. Quantification of myocardial infarct size by thallium-201 single photon emission computed tomography: experimental validation in the dog. Circulation 1986;74(4):852–61.

28. Prigent F, Maddahi J, Garcia EV, Resser K, Lew AS, Berman DS. Comparative methods for quantifying myocardial infarct size by thallium-201 SPECT. J Nucl Med 1987;28:325–33

29. Prigent F, Maddahi J, Van Train K, Berman D. Comparison of rotational tomography and planar imaging for quantification of experimental infarct size. Am Heart J. In press.

30. Williams SJ, Mousa SA, Morgan RA,Carroll TR, Maheu LJ. Pharmacology of Tc-99m s: agents with favorable characteristics for heart imaging. J Nucl Med 1986;27:877–8. (Abstract)

31. Sia ST, Holman BL, McKusick K, et al. The utilization of Tc-99m-TBI as a myocardial perfusion agent in exercise studies: comparison with Tl-201 thallous chloride and examination of its biodistribution in humans. Eur J Nucl Med 1986;12:333–6.

32. McKusick K, Holman BL, Jones AG, et al. Comparison of 3 Tc-99m s for detection ischemic heart disease in humans. J Nucl Med 1986;27:878. (Abstract)

33. Wackers FJ, Berman DS, Maddahi J, et al. Technetium-99m hexakis 2–methoxy-isobutyl : human biodistribution, dosimetry, safety, and preliminary comparison to thallium-201 myocardial perfusion imaging. J Nucl Med 1989;30:301–11.

34. Picard M, Dupras G, Taillefer R, Arsenault A, Boucher P. Myocardial perfusion agents: compared biodistribution of 201–thallium, Tc-99m tertiary butyl (TBI) and Tc-99m-methoxy isobutyl (MIBI). J Nucl Med 1987;28:654–5. (Abstract)

35. Narra RK, Nunn AD, Kuczynski BL, Feld T, Wedeking P, Eckelman WC. A neutral technetium-99m complex for myocardial imaging. J Nucl Med 1989;30:1830–7.

36. Leppo JA, Meerdink DJ. Comparative myocardial extraction of two technetium labeled BATO derigative (SQ30217, SQ(32014) and thallium. J Nucl Med 1990;31:67–74.

37. Maublant JC, Moins N, Gachon P. Uptake and release of two new Tc-99m labeled myocardial blood flow imaging agents in cultured cardiac cells. Eur J Nucl Med 1989;15:180–2.

38. Stewart RE, Hutchins GD, Brown D, et al. Myocardial retention and clearance of the flow tracer Tc-99m SQ30217 in canine heart. J Nucl Med 1989;30:860–1. (Abstract)

39. Narra RK, Feld T, Wedeking P, Matyas J, Nunn AD, Coleman RE. SQ30217, a technetium-99m labeled myocardial imaging agent which shows no interspecies difference in uptake. Nuklearmedizin 1987;23 (suppl):489–91.

40. Seldin DW, Johnson LL, Blood DK, et al. Myocardial perfusion imaging with technetium-99m SQ30217: comparison with thallium-201 and coronary anatomy. J Nucl Med 1989;30:312–9.

41. Maddahi J, Kiat H, Van Train KF, et al. Myocardial perfusion imaging with technetium-99m SestaMIBI SPECT in the evaluation of coronary artery disease. Am J Cardiol 1990;66 (13):55E-63E.

42. Kiat H, Maddahi J, Roy LT et al. Comparison of technetium 99m methoxy isobutyl with

thallium 201 for evaluation of coronary disease by planar and tomographic methods. Am Heart J 1989;117:1-11.

43. Iskandrian AS, Heo J, Kong B, Lyons E, Marsch S. Use of technetium-99m (RP-30A) in assessing left ventricular perfusion and function at rest and during exercise in coronary artery disease, and comparison with coronary arteriography and exercise thallium-201 SPECT imaging. Am J Cardiol 1989;64:270-5.

44. Kahn JK, McGhie I, Akers MS, et al. Quantitative rotational tomography with 201Tl and 99mTc 2-methoxy-isobutyl-. A direct comparison in normal individuals and patients with coronary artery disease. Circulation 1989;79:1282-93.

45. Kiat H, Van Train KF, Maddahi J, et al. Development and prospective application of quantitative 2-day stress-rest Tc-99m methoxy isobutyl SPECT for the diagnosis of coronary artery disease. Am Heart J 1990;120:1255-66.

46. Verani MS, Jeroudi MO, Mahmarian JJ, et al. Quantification of myocardial infarction during coronary occlusion and myocardial salvage after reperfusion using cardiac imaging with technetium-99m hexakis 2-methoxy isobutyl isonitrile. J Am Coll Cardiol 1988;12:1573-81.

47. Gibbons RJ, Verani MS, Behrenbeck T, et al. Feasibility of tomographic 99mTc-hexakis-2-methoxy-2-methylpropyl- imaging for the assessment of myocardial area at risk and the effect of treatment in acute myocardial infarction. Circulation 1989;80:1277-86.

48. Bergin JD, Sinusas AJ, Smith WH, et al. Quantitative imaging for risk area determination following transient coronary occlusion. J Nucl Med 1990;31:784. (Abstract)

49. Prigent F, Maddahi J, Nichols K, et al. Quantification of myocardial infarct size by gated Tc-99m MIBI tomography (SPECT): experimental validation in the dog. J Nucl Med 1990;31:832-3. (Abstract)

50. Prigent F, Maddahi J, Nichols K, et al. Effect of matrix size and gating on myocardial infarction sizing with Tc-99m SestaMIBI SPECT. Circulation 1990;82 (4 Suppl 3):III-204. (Abstract)

51. Garcia EV, Cooke CD, Van Train KF, et al. Technical aspects of myocardial SPECT imaging with technetium-99m SestaMIBI. Am J Cardiol 1990;66:23E-31E.

52. Taillefer R, Laflamme L, Dupras G, Picard M, Phaneuf C, Leveille J. Myocardial perfusion imaging with 99mTc-methoxy-isobutyl- (MIBI): comparison of short and long term intervals between rest and stress injections. Preliminary results. Eur J Nucl Med 1988;13:515-22.

53. Taillefer R, Gagnon A, Laflamme L, Gregoire J, Leveille J, Phaneuf DC. Same day injections of Tc-99m methoxy isobutyl hexamibi for myocardial tomographic imaging: comparison between rest-stress and stress-rest injection sequences. Eur J Nucl Med 1989;15:113-7.

54. Maddahi J, Prigent F, Garcia E, Nichols K, Galt J, Cook J, Berman D. Validation of newly developed attenuation and scatter correction methods for quantitating myocardial perfusion by Tc-99m SestaMIBI SPECT. Circulation 1990;82 (4 Suppl 3):III-651. (Abstract)

55. Kim AS, Akers MS, Faber TL, Corbett JR. Dynamic myocardial perfusion imaging with Tc-99m teboroxime in patients: comparison with thallium-201 and arteriography. Circulation 1990;82 (4 Suppl 3):III-321. (Abstract)

56. Zielonka JS, Bellinger R, Coleman RE, et al. Multicenter clinical trial of 99m-Tc teboroxime (SQ30,217, Cardiotec) as a myocardial perfusion agent. J Nucl Med 1989;30:1745. (Abstract)

57. Stewart RE, Schwaiger M, Hutchins GD, et al. Myocardial clearance kinetics of technetium-99m SQ30217: a marker of regional myocardial blood flow. J Nucl Med 1990;31:1183-90.

58. Drane WE, Decker M, Stickland P, Tineo A, Zmuda S. Measurement of regional myocardial perfusion using Tc-99m teboroxime (Cardiotec) and dynamic SPECT. J Nucl Med 1989;30:1744. (Abstract)

12. Acquisition and processing of tomographic radionuclide ventriculograms

TRACY L. FABER and JAMES R. CORBETT

Summary

Acquisition and quantification methods for tomographic radionuclide ventriculograms (TRVG) are discussed. The approach takes advantage of the three-dimensional data to measure left ventricular (LV) volumes and endocardial motion. The methods were validated using tomograms from normal volunteers; LV volumes and motion from the SPECT studies were compared to values computed from magnetic resonance (MR) images of the same persons. The clinical usefulness of the methods was evaluated by analyzing the TRVGs of 21 patients with known infarcts. Regional motion was compared to the computed normal values to determine areas of abnormally contracting tissue, and the results were compared to known infarct location. Ejection fractions computed from the TRVGs were compared to values calculated from planar radionuclide ventriculograms (RVG) for these 21 patients. The average error in motion measurements when TRVG and MR values were compared was -5 mm. The correlation between planar and TRVG ejection fractions was 0.94. Automatic analysis found 19 of the 21 abnormalities; the locations of all detected abnormalities and the known infarcted tissue corresponded correctly.

Introduction

Gated tomographic radionuclide ventriculograms (TRVG) are the 3–D analogues to standard planar radionuclide ventriculograms (RVG). The advantage of TRVG over planar studies is the ability to completely sample the cardiac blood pool in three dimensions, and to slice the resulting volume in any plane while maintaining complete separation of the chambers.

Tomographic acquisition of RVGs was first proposed by Moore et al. in the early 80s [1]. Since then, various studies have shown TRVG to have better sensitivity than RVG for detecting regional wall motion abnormalities in general and to allow better analysis of inferior wall motion abnormalities in particular [2,3], to permit accurate calculations of global left ventricular (LV) volumes and ejection fractions (EF) [2–4], and to allow quantitative

Johan H.C. Reiber & Ernst E. van der Wall (eds.), Cardiovascular Nuclear Medicine and MRI, 181–191.
© 1992 *Kluwer Academic Publishers.*

assessment of wall motion comparable to that from contrast ventriculography [2,5].

However, gated tomographic studies contain large amounts of image data that are difficult to analyze and integrate. Gated tomographic reconstructions are typically composed of 64 × 64 × 32 or 128 × 128 × 64 3–D images at 8–16 frames through the cardiac cycle. For TRVG to become a useful clinical tool, automatic quantification methods need to be developed that will process and condense the entire 3–D image data set into meaningful and well-presented information. The first step in calculating global or regional LV parameters is the separation of the blood pool from the background. Then an appropriate model must be applied to quantify LV motion for all points on the 3–D boundary.

We have previously described a boundary detector that we will present only superficially in this manuscript [6]. We describe a 3–D motion model that is not dependent on any coordinate system. A set of normal studies is processed with these methods, and motion values are compared to those computed using the same model applied to hand-traced magnetic resonance (MR) studies of the same patients. Finally, the normal motion values are used to predict wall motion abnormalities in 21 patients with known LV myocardial infarcts.

Methods

The surface detector is based on a model of the LV generated from normal patients. Image intensity gradients are used to revise initial likelihoods of each voxel's being on the LV surface. The model is used to modify these likelihoods and determine the most likely smooth, connected, 'LV-shaped' surface for each frame of the gated study. The output is a set of 288 points for each frame; the points are distributed about the LV as shown in Fig. 1. Since the boundary detector has been described in [6], it will be discussed further only to describe its effects on motion quantification.

The surface points were triangulated to create a polygonal solid model of the LV. The volume could be computed at each frame, and the end-diastolic (ED) and end-systolic (ES) volumes and EF could be calculated. Using the ED and ES frames, motion was calculated using a system based on a 3–D extension of the model known as the 'centerline' method [7]. A set of points midway between those at ED and ES were created; these were connected into a 'center surface'. For each point on this central surface, a normal to that point was constructed. The distance between the ED and ES surfaces along the central surface normal was considered to be the motion of the endocardium at that point. This is diagrammed in Fig. 2.

LV endocardial surfaces were displayed using 3–D graphics. Motion values were color-coded onto the surface, using the color or gray scale of the user's choice, so that the location and extent of any abnormality could be

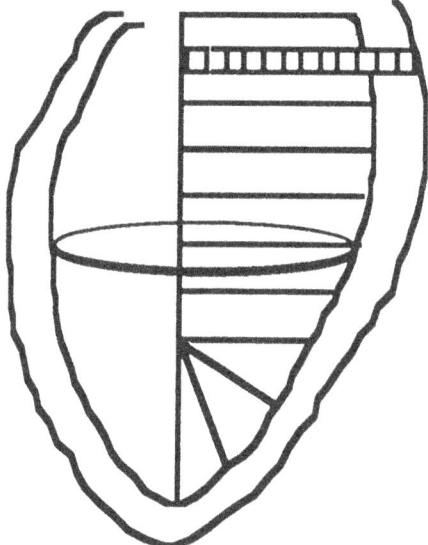

Figure 1. Coordinate system used to detect endocardial surface. The basal 3/4 of the LV is detected using a cylindrical coordinate system; the apical 1/4 is detected using a spherical coordinate system. There are points detected at 24 angles about the LV long axis for each of twelve contours, which are parallel only within the cylindrical coordinate system. For each angle at each contour, consecutive pixels from the coordinate system origin out to ~7 cm are investigated for their likelihood of being surface points.

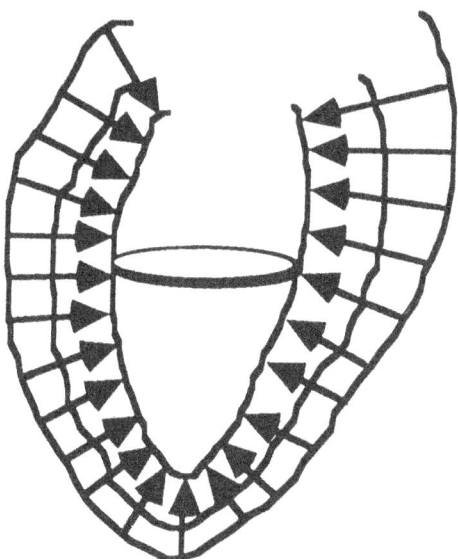

Figure 2. Motion is considered to be perpendicular to a surface halfway between end diastole and end systole.

easily visualized. The surfaces could be interactively rotated, even while displayed in a cine 'beating' mode, and viewed from any perspective.

TRVGs were acquired using a 3–headed rotating gamma camera equipped with a low energy general purpose collimator (PRISM, Ohio Imaging, Picker Inc, Highland Heights, OH). One hundred and twenty gated projections were acquired over 360° using the closest elliptical orbit. Temporal discrimination was achieved by using the electrocardiogram (ECG) to create 16 equally spaced time frames over the cardiac cycle. Each projection was acquired for a preset time of 25 sec into a 64×64 matrix with a pixel size of 5 mm $\times$ 5 mm. Total imaging time was ~ 17 min. Projections were reconstructed into transverse image sets using filtered backprojection with a Butterworth filter of cutoff $= 0.43$ and order $= 4$. Neither scatter nor attenuation correction was performed. Only those projections from 45° right anterior oblique to 45° left posterior oblique, 180° total, were reconstructed. Short axis sections were created as input into the surface detection software. Total time required for reconstruction and reformatting was ~ 10 min.

MR images were acquired using a .35Tesla MR device (Toshiba America, MRI, Inc., South San Francisco, CA). LV short axis images were obtained using spin-echo acquisitions with a repetition time equal to cardiac cycle length and an echo time of 30 msec. Using a repeated multislice or rotation technique [8], images were acquired in each slice at 100 msec intervals throughout the cardiac cycle, from end diastole, through systole, and into early diastole. Five time frames and ten slices were acquired; pixel sizes were 1.70 mm $\times$ 1.70 mm, and slice thickness was 10.0 mm.

Planar RVGs were acquired using a standard field of view gamma camera equipped with a low energy general purpose collimator (Picker DynaMo). Gated equilibrium septal projections were obtained at a temporal resolution of 16 frames per cardiac cycle; all studies were performed at a spatial resolution of 64×64. Standard software was used to interactively outline the LV boundaries at ED and ES, and a count-based method was used to compute the ejection fractions.

Four normal volunteers with a low pretest likelihood of coronary artery disease were studied using both TRVG and MR. The TRVGs were processed with automatic boundary detection and motion quantification software. MR boundaries were traced interactively, but motion was calculated using the same method as for TRVG. Motion values were grouped into nine geometrically defined LV regions, including the apex, and mid-ventricular and basal anterior, lateral, inferior, and septal regions. The mean and standard deviation of the difference in motion computed from TRVG and MR were determined for each LV region. The lower limit of normal motion for each region was considered to be the mean-2 $\times$ standard deviation of motion computed from the normal TRVGs.

Twenty one patients were studied 8 $\pm$ 5 days following an acute myocardial infarction. TRVGs were acquired and processed as described above; RVGs were also acquired from these patients. Motion quantification was

Table 1.

Region	TRVG Motion x̄ (mm)	s (mm)	Lower Limit of Normal	MRI Motion x̄ (mm)	s (mm)	Motion Error (mm)
apical	6.4	2.0	2.4	5.9	2.0	0.5
lateral	9.1	2.0	5.1	10.7	2.1	−1.6
basal lateral	9.2	3.4	2.4	11.2	3.9	−2.0
inferior	7.5	1.7	4.1	7.5	2.0	−0.1
basal inferior	7.4	3.5	0.4	11.7	4.4	−4.3
septal	5.0	1.2	2.6	8.3	2.3	−3.2
basal septal	7.4	3.5	0.4	7.1	3.0	0.3
anterior	7.4	1.4	4.6	7.6	1.7	−0.1
basal anterior	9.9	2.6	4.7	7.8	3.0	2.1

performed, and EFs were computed for each study. The motion of each LV surface point was compared to the 'normal' value for the region containing that point. The area and location of any contiguous group of abnormally moving points was output in a printed report. The existence and location of the known infarcts were compared to the abnormalities detected by the automatic software. In addition, EFs computed from the TRVGs were compared to those calculated from the RVGs.

Results

Normal motion values determined from TRVG using the automatic software ranged from an average of 9.9 mm in the basal anterior region to 5.0 mm in the mid-ventricular septal region. Standard deviations ranged from 4.4 mm in the basal inferior region to 1.2 mm in the septal region. See Table 1 for a list of normal values.

MR motion calculations agreed well with TRVG values. Disagreements were largest in the basal regions. However, in the apical and mid-ventricular regions, the average difference between TRVG and MR motion was less than 0.5 mm. Table 1 displays the the error in motion for all LV regions.

Good correlations between planar and tomographic EF were obtained. The regression equation was $y = 1.05x - 2.2\%$; the correlation was 0.94. The standard error of the estimate was 4.8%. Figure 3 shows the data with the regression line.

Analysis of TRVG revealed motion abnormalities in 19 of the 21 infarct patient studies; the abnormalities were in the region of infarction as indicated by ECG. Figure 4 shows ED and ES slices from the TRVG of a normal volunteer. Motion is coded onto the LV surface using shades of gray as displayed in Fig. 5. This color-coding scheme ranges from black, which indicates motion ≤ -2 mm (dyskinetic) to white, which indicates motion ≥ 6 mm. In this case, the LV is entirely white, indicating normal motion. Figure 6 shows ED and ES slices from the TRVG of a patient with a anterior

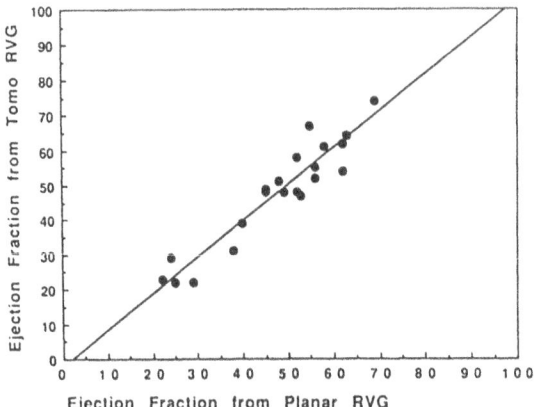

Figure 3. Comparison between ejection fractions computed using tomographic vs planar radionuclide ventriculograms. The correlation coefficient is 0.95; the regression equation is y = 1.01x −9.0 %

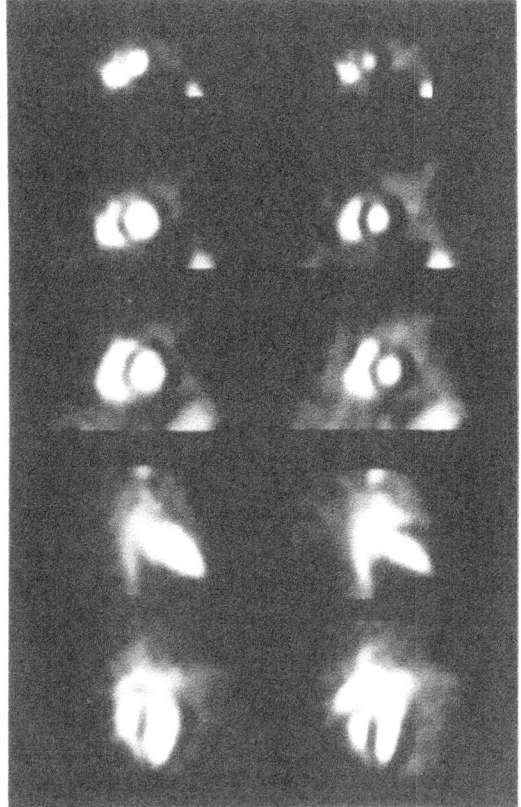

Figure 4. Tomographic radionuclide ventriculogram acquired from a normal volunteer. End-diastolic slices are on the left; end-systolic slices are on the right. From top to bottom, the sections are apical short axis, mid-ventricular short axis, basal short axis, vertical long axis, and horizontal long axis.

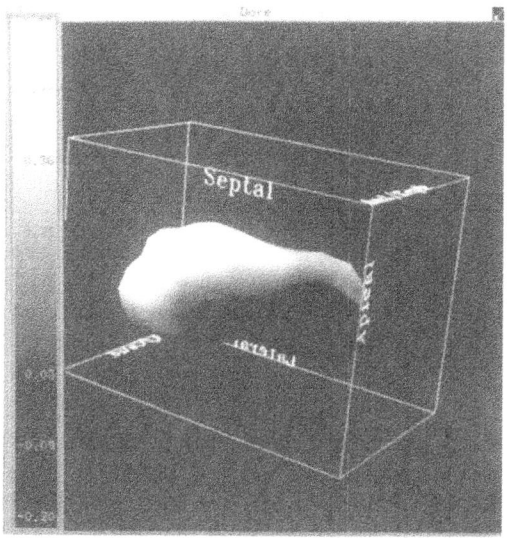

Figure 5. End-diastolic view of the endocardial surface detected from TRVG in Fig. 4; the view is approximately anterior. This surface is coded for endocardial motion; the overall white color of the surface indicates normal motion.

infarct. Note the obvious aneurysm in the apical regions of the horizontal long axis and short axis slices. Figure 7 shows the LV endocardial surface of this patient color-coded for motion. The dark gray and black area in the apical and septal regions corresponds to the aneurysm; the lighter shade of gray in the anterior and septal regions indicates hypokinesis.

Discussion

Normal motion values are close to those numbers reported in echocardiographic studies [9]. MR and TRVG values agree best in apical and midventricular regions, and differ mainly in basal regions. EF measurements from TRVG correlate well with those computed from planar studies. The correlation coefficient we have computed is similar to those reported by previous investigators [2–4]. Finally, wall motion diagnosis found nearly all of the existing abnormalities in actual patient studies; furthermore, all abnormalities were found in the proper locations.

Previous studies have compared quantitated wall motion in a single vertical long axis slice from TRVG to that in contrast ventriculograms [2,5]. One of these [2] used second derivatives of intensity to define the LV; the other [5] used interactive tracing. We have attempted to quantify wall motion in the entire 3–D LV, and have used the second derivative in conjunction with a model that ensures 3–D smoothness and connectivity. Of course, the accur-

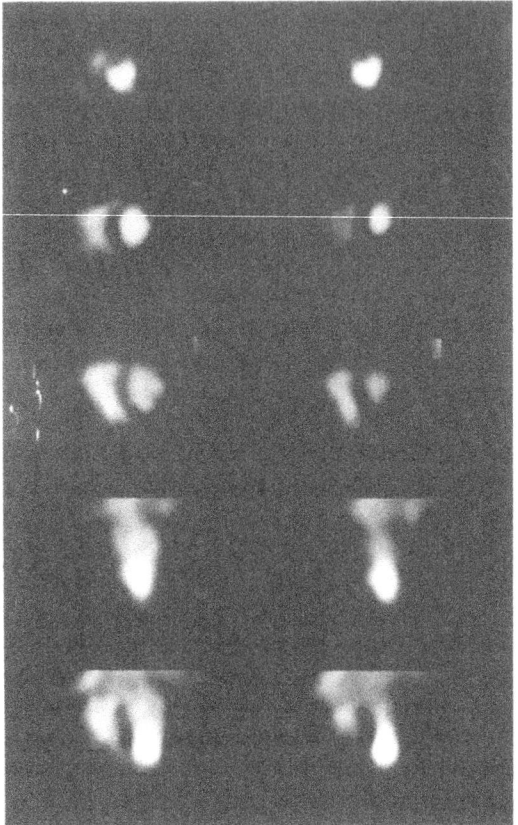

Figure 6. TRVG acquired from a patient with an anterior infarct. End-diastolic slices are on the left; end-systolic slices are on the right. From top to bottom are shown apical, mid-ventricular and basal short axis, vertical long axis, and horizontal long axis slices.

acy of motion quantification depends upon the accuracy of edge detection. The boundary detector that we use assumes that the actual LV border is located at a zero-crossing of the second derivative of image intensity. Unfortunately, even in a noiseless system, the image intensity and its derivatives are affected by both the system point spread function (PSF) and partial volume effects caused by sampling. The degradation in boundary location caused by both of these depends on the shapes of the blood pool components. Primarily, the effects of the PSF and sampling will cause the LV blood pool boundaries to be detected outside the true edges in regions where the LV blood pool has a small diameter and inside the true edges in regions where it is separated from other cardiac chambers by thin structures. The result will be an underestimation of motion, particularly in the septal and valve plane regions. The negative TRVG motion errors seen in comparison with

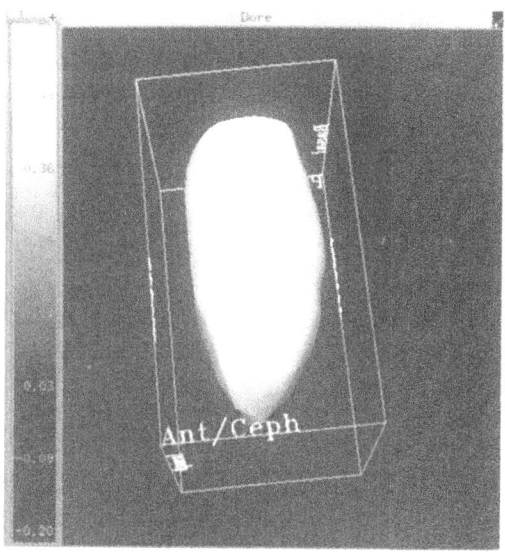

Figure 7. End-systolic view of the endocardial surface detected from the TRVG in Fig. 6. The endocardium is displayed with an approximately septal view. The dark gray and black r ions seen in the septal and apical region indicate an aneurysm; lighter gray areas indicate surrou ding hypokinetic tissue.

MR in the septal and basal regions illustrate this problem. In addition, the low intensity derivatives of thin structures, such as the valve planes and septum, may lead to edge detection errors when high intensity gradient boundaries nearby are erroneously detected. Once again, this will occur mostly in basal and septal regions, and explains the positive motion error seen in the basal septal region.

Current high resolution collimators and image restoration software will decrease PSF effects and lessen the likelihood of the occurrence of both errors. Also, multiple detector tomographs, with increased system sensitivity, allow smaller pixel sizes and/or higher collected counts and should decrease partial volume effects and/or noise.

Previous studies employed models of motion which assumed contraction toward a single LV point, either the center of the slice [2] or the 69 % point along the LV long axis [5]. The advantages to this approach include the automatic correction for LV translation and the normalization of motion for LV size with the computation of values such as % shortening. The disadvantages are the difficulty in correctly determining the long axis and the movement of the LV center point due to wall motion abnormalities rather than translation. Also, limiting analysis to a single slice not only ignores much of the data but also requires an assumption that contraction occurs within that slice.

Because our boundary detector requires the user to identify the LV aortic valve plane, both the length of the resulting LV long axis and the centroid of the LV are subject to observer error. Thus, motion calculations based on these variables would be subject to the same problems. By using only local shape for our model of motion, only the basal portion of the LV, where the valve plane must be identified, will be affected by user interaction. Although our implementation of the 'centerline' method does not correct for translation and may cause overestimation of motion abnormalities, corrections for apparent translation caused by motion abnormalities can cause their underestimation.

However, other revisions in our approach to motion quantification should improve its performance. Currently, the angular sampling detects approximately every other voxel on the endocardial surface; analysis of more surface points would improve identification of small abnormalities. Our grouping of motion into rather arbitrary regions for averaging and analyzing should be refined. Since motion varies over the LV surface, an experimentally determined grouping that minimizes variance over each region could improve analysis. These regions should also be defined so that they do not overlap more than one coronary artery supply. Finally, more normal studies should be processed to improve the statistical information.

Conclusion

We have described and validated a method for endocardial motion quantification and visualization from tomographic radionuclide ventriculograms. The clinical use of these methods has been demonstrated in a preliminary manner.

The clinical studies indicate that our technique may be a useful tool for evaluating endocardial wall motion and the diagnosis of abnormalities. The addition of more normal studies, with the improvements described above, should decrease the variance of motion within regions and improve our ability to discriminate between normal and abnormal studies. Although motion measurements are quite accurate, we expect them to improve as SPECT hardware and software improves, making these methods even more reliable.

References

1. Moore ML, Murphy PH, Burdine JA. ECG-gated emission computed tomography of the cardiac blood pool. Radiology 1980;134:233–5.
2. Gill JB, Moore RH, Tamaki N, et al. Multi-gated blood-pool tomography: a new method for the assessment of left ventricular function. J Nucl Med 1986;27:1916–24.
3. Corbett JR, Jansen DE, Lewis SE, et al. Tomographic gated blood pool radionuclide ventriculography: Analysis of wall motion and left ventricular volumes in patients with coronary artery disease. J Am Coll Cardiol 1985;6:349–58.
4. Stadius ML, Williams DL, Harp G. Left ventricular volume determination using single-photon emission computed tomography. Am Cardiol 1985;55:1185–91.

5. Barat J-L, Brendel AJ, Colle J-P, et al. Quantitative analysis of left-ventricular function using gated single photon emission tomography. J Nucl Med 1984;25:1167–74.

6. Faber TL, Stokely EM, Corbett JR. Surface detection in dynamic tomographic myocardial perfusion images by relaxation labeling. SPIE Visual Communications and Image Processing. 1988;Vol 1001:297–300.

7. Sheehan FH, Bolson EL, Dodge HT, Mathey DG, Schofer J, Woo HK. Advantages and applications of the centerline method for characterizing regional ventricular function. Circulation 1986;74:293–305.

8. Crooks LE, Barker B, Chang H, et al. Strategies for magnetic resonance imaging of the heart. Radiology 1984;153:459–65.

9. Feigenbaum H. Echocardiography. 3rd ed. Philadelphia: Lea and Febiger, 1986:550.

PART IV

Cardiovascular clinical applications

13. New perfusion agents in clinical cardiology

SIMON H. BRAAT, PIERRE RIGO and HEIN J.J. WELLENS

Summary

For more than a decade thallium 201 (Tl-201) has been used for measurement of myocardial perfusion and viability although its physical characteristics, i.e. a photon energy of 68–80 keV and a half-life of 73 hr, are far from ideal. For a couple of years two groups of tracers, isonitriles and boronic acid adducts of technetium dioximes (BATO) compounds, both labeled to technetium-99m (Tc-99m), have been available. The uptake of these agents in the myocardium is proportional to regional blood flow and because of the Tc-99m label, with a photon energy of 140 keV and a half-life of 6 hr, they have better physical characteristics. The isonitrile with the best properties for myocardial imaging is Tc-99m SestaMIBI (Cardiolite). It has transient hepatic uptake and little or no myocardial redistribution making it to an ideal single photon emission computed tomography tracer. The commercially developed agent of the BATO group is Tc-99m teboroxime (Cardiotec). Its extraction fraction by the myocardium is higher than that of Tl-201 and of Tc-99m SestaMIBI but its washout is very rapid and flow-related.

Because of the lack of redistribution or of rapid washout, two separate injections are always necessary with these new tracers to be able to distinguish ischemia from scar tissue. It is advisable to start with the resting study and to give the second injection after exercise when a one-day protocol is done. In clinical trials Tc-99m SestaMIBI and Tc-99m teboroxime have been shown to be at least as good as Tl-201 in detecting coronary artery disease with planar imaging. Whereas Tl-201 redistribution can cause logistic problems if no camera is available in the coronary care unit, Tc-99m SestaMIBI does not redistribute and has the potential of overcoming these problems.

In several studies Tc-99m SestaMIBI has proven to be reliable in localizing and detecting myocardial infarction in the coronary care unit and it is also able to assess the myocardial area at risk and the effect of treatment with thrombolytic therapy. Tc-99m SestaMIBI also has been shown to be of value in the catheterization laboratory in visualizing the size of the myocardium perfused by the different coronary arteries and in detecting the area at risk during short episodes of ischemia.

Johan H.C. Reiber & Ernst E. van der Wall (eds.), Cardiovascular Nuclear Medicine and MRI, 195–206.
© 1992 *Kluwer Academic Publishers.*

Introduction

Thallium 201 (Tl-201) has been used for more than 15 years for measurement of myocardial perfusion and viability. Its physical characteristics, i.e. a photon energy of 68–80 keV and a half-life of 73 hr, make it suboptimal for scintillation camera imaging while radiation dosimetry limits the dose to be administered. To circumvent these limitations investigators have attempted, immediately after the introduction of Tl-201, to develop a myocardial perfusion agent labeled with technetium-99m (Tc-99m). This tracer (photon energy of 140 keV and a half-life of 6 hr) exhibits much better physical characteristics for scintillation imaging than Tl-201. Success was met in 1982 when a group at the Peter Bent Brigham Hospital reported the development of Tc-99m isonitriles [1]. These agents demonstrated uptake in the myocardium proportional to regional blood flow. Recently, another group of Tc-99m labeled tracers, called boronic acid adducts of technetium dioximes (BATO) compounds, were demonstrated to have high myocardial extraction with subsequent myocardial concentration also proportional to regional perfusion [2]. Many Tc-99m labeled isonitriles compounds have been developed, but only three compounds have been applied clinically. Tc-99m t-butyl-isonitrile (TBI) was suboptimal for myocardial imaging due to its prominent hepatic and pulmonary uptake. The persistent liver uptake could obscure defects in the inferior wall of the left ventricle. The activity of TBI in the lungs acted as a reservoir of the tracer and with the subsequent washout a significant amount would be delivered to the myocardium and altered the resulting perfusion pattern from that corresponding to the initial injection and uptake of TBI (3–6).

The disadvantage of another isopropyl Tc-99m carboxy-isopropyl- isonitrile (CPI) was the progressive hepatic accumulation over time, while the myocardial uptake was excellent with rapid washout from the myocardium [7]. The isonitrile with the most favorable biological properties for myocardial imaging till now is Tc-99m methoxy-isobutyl-isonitrile, also known as RP30, Cardiolite or Tc-99m SestaMIBI [8]. Tc-99m SestaMIBI shows only minimal lung uptake and transient hepatic uptake [9]. The combination of transient early hepatic uptake and minimal myocardial redistribution makes it an ideal tracer for single photon emission computed tomography [10].

The BATO compounds, which form another class of Tc-99m myocardial perfusion agents, are neutral lipophilic complexes of boronic acid. The commercially developed agent of this group is Tc-99m teboroxime or Cardiotec [11,12].

Physiological characteristics of Tc-99m isonitriles

Tc-99m SestaMIBI, which is a lipophilic cationic Tc-99m complex, has the most favorable myocardial to background ratio of any of the nitriles. The uptake and clearance kinetics of this new myocardial agent have been investigated in a number of experimental animal models. Tc-99m SestaMIBI uptake in the myocardium occurs in proportion to myocardial blood flow [8,13–16]. This uptake is similar to that of Tl-201. In animal models a good correlation was found between microsphere-determined myocardial blood flow and Tc-99m SestaMIBI distribution in the myocardium at rates up to 2.0 ml/min/g [8,17].

Like other diffusible indicators, Tc-99m SestaMIBI underestimates myocardial blood flow at higher flow rates. In low flow regions the myocardial uptake of Tc-99m SestaMIBI was higher compared to the microsphere-determined regional blood flow. This is explained by an increased extraction of the agent at low flows. The increased extraction has also been observed with Tl-201. Increased extraction was seen when flow was reduced to 10–40 % of control [13]. When the flow was even more reduced to 0–10 % of control this increased extraction was not longer evident [16]. It can be concluded from these studies that myocardial uptake of Tc-99m SestaMIBI is proportional to regional flow in the physiologic flow range with enhanced extraction of the tracer in low flow regions where some tissue is still viable. Also Tc-99m teboroxime shows an uptake in the myocardium which is proportional to blood flow at rates up to 1,5 ml/min/g [18]. This study also showed that the initial extraction of Tc-99m teboroxime is higher compared to Tl-201 and that the cellular washout is fairly rapid and flow-related. Leppo and Meerdink [19] showed in the blood perfused isolated rabbit heart that the first-pass myocardial extraction for Tc-99m SestaMIBI was less than that of Tl-201, and that Tl-201 had a higher transcapillary exchange rate than Tc-99m SestaMIBI. However, Tc-99m SestaMIBI showed a significantly higher parenchymal cell permeability and a higher volume of distribution than Tl-201. The overall effect of these differences in permeability results in little difference in the myocardial uptake of the two agents when imaged in vivo.

From another study by Meerdink and Leppo [20], it appeared that the uptake mechanisms of Tc-99m SestaMIBI are less dependent on active transport processes compared to Tl-201. When the cellular membrane is intact and cellular viability persists, intracellular extraction of Tc-99m SestaMIBI can proceed. Myocardial clearance of Tc-99m SestaMIBI is negligible. This lack of redistribution probably can be explained by low blood levels of Tc-99m SestaMIBI and long myocardial cellular retention so that little amount of tracer is available for reaccumulation.

Logistic considerations

Because of the absence of redistribution or rapid washout, two separate injections of Tc-99m SestaMIBI or Tc-99m teboroxime are necessary to be able to distinguish ischemia from scar tissue. Tc-99m has a half-life of 6 hr and, therefore, 24–hr separations between the two injections would be ideal. If a two-day protocol is chosen the first study should be after exercise because, if this study is normal, the resting study is not needed. In clinical practice however physicians prefer to have all the information on a single day. In our clinic we use a one-day protocol and in those patients known with a previous myocardial infarction we start with a resting study and inject 5–8 mCi. Imaging starts 0.5–1 hour after injection and 4 hours later the second injection is given at peak exercise. Imaging starts 10–30 minutes after injection of 25–30 mCi. In patients in whom ischemia has to be proven or ruled out we start with the injection after exercise. If the exercise imaging is normal no resting study is done. Taillefer et al. [21] compared this one day protocol with a two-day protocol in 15 patients. Quantitative and qualitatitive comparisons between both studies showed the same number of ischemic and fixed defects. So they concluded that a one-day protocol can be done with reliable results.

Clinical applications

Chronic coronary artery disease

Planar imaging of perfusion of myocardial tissue using Tl-201 is a well-established clinical technique for the diagnosis and assessment of patients with definite or suspected coronary disease. However Tl-201 has two important disadvantages; first, soft tissue attenuation and scatter caused by the low photon energy emission (80 keV), and second, a relatively long half-life (68–73 hr). The new agents labeled to Tc-99m lack these disadvantages and several comparative studies between Tl-201 and Tc-99m SestaMIBI have been performed and have shown this agent to be at least as good as Tl-201 [9, 22–24]. Maisey et al. [25] used another distinguishing characteristic of Tc-99m SestaMIBI compared to Tl-201 to diagnose myocardial ischemia: The higher photon yield and myocardial fixation of Tc-99m SestaMIBI make it possible to obtain electrocardiographic gated images, thereby providing simultaneous global ventricular function and regional wall motion data. The acquisition of gated images also allows the examination of static perfusion images at different phases in the cardiac cycle so the loss of resolution imposed by cardiac motion can be avoided. Whether these techniques improve the detection of coronary artery disease has however still to be confirmed. Jones [26] et al. combined the myocardial perfusion images with data of ventricular function using a single tracer injection.

A first-pass radionuclide angiogram was recorded at rest followed by tomographic perfusion images one hour later. The same procedure was repeated thereafter with the tracer now injected on attainment of an exercise endpoint. Their data suggest that combining simultaneous assessment of perfusion and function can improve the diagnostic and prognostic information.

The other technetium based myocardial perfusion imaging agent used in clinical trials is Tc-99m teboroxime. Tc-99m teboroxime is in a class of neutral, lipophilic, technetium complexes known as boronic acid adducts of technetium dioxime (BATO) complexes and has very different pharmacokinetics compared to the cationic tracer Tl-201 and the cationic technetium complex Tc-99m SestaMIBI. Tc-99m teboroxime has the highest myocardial extraction but a very rapid myocardial washout. The rapid myocardial washout necessitates brief imaging protocols. Seldin et al. [11] compared Tl-201 and Tc-99m teboroxime in 30 patients of whom 20 had coronary artery disease documented by recent angiography and 10 were normal volunteers. Stress imaging with Tc-99m teboroxime was performed first, patients were in the upright position on a bicycle in front of the camera, and the stress test was followed 2 hours later with an injection at rest. No significant difference was found between the two techniques for detecting abnormal vessels or identifying coronary artery disease. However, the number of fixed defects on the Tc-99m teboroxime scintigrams was significantly higher. In our clinic we have also some experiences with Tc-99m teboroxime for detecting coronary artery disease and identifying abnormal vessels [27]. In 26 patients we compared Tl-201 and dynamic myocardial imaging with Tc-99m teboroxime. Dynamic myocardial imaging with Tc-99m teboroxime was performed with the patient in the upright position and 20 frames of 10 seconds were recorded, starting in the anterior position for 6 frames. After turning of the patient, 6 frames of 10 seconds were recorded in the 45° left anterior oblique position. Then the patient turned again 45° and 6 frames were recorded in the left lateral position. In the Tc-99m teboroxime part of the study we started with imaging at rest followed an hour later by imaging after exercise. Both in rest and after exercise 20 mCi Tc-99m teboroxime was injected and imaging was started 2 minutes after injection. Both Tl-201 and Tc-99m teboroxime studies were performed in a time interval of ≤ 48 hours. In 13 patients the Tl-201 as well as the Tc-99m teboroxime scintigrams showed the same defects while in seven patients no defects were seen on either scan. In three patients the Tl-201 scintigrams showed a reversible inferior wall defect, while the Tc-99m teboroxime scintigrams were considered to be normal. In three patients the Tc-99m teboroxime scintigrams showed a fixed defect, while the Tl-201 scan showed reversed redistribution. All 3 patients had had thrombolytic therapy. From these data we concluded that Tc-99m teboroxime generally yields comparable information to Tl-201 and that differences appear to be related to early blood pool activity (masked inferior wall defects in the first performed anterior view) and to different kinetics of the tracers after fibrinolysis.

Applications in the coronary care unit

A) Detection and localization of myocardial infarction and of myocardial ischemia

Tl-201 myocardial perfusion imaging at rest has long been used to detect and localize myocardial ischemia and/or necrosis [28–35]. However Tl-201, on top of its physical disadvantages, i.e. a low photon energy and relatively long half-life, shows redistribution occurring both at rest and during stress. So imaging must be performed shortly after injection. This can cause logistical problems of camera availability. Another problem is the fact that the patient can remain unstable and not transportable to the nuclear cardiology labora- tory for some time after the injection. Tc-99m SestaMIBI offers the potential of overcoming these problems while it shows no redistribution. Boucher et al. [36] reported the results of a multicenter phase III clinical trial in which the efficacy of Tc-99m SestaMIBI was investigated to localize and detect myocardial infarction. In this study 17 institutions in the United States and Canada were involved. A total of 122 patients were enrolled in the study, of whom 50 had a recent infarction (< 14 days old), 61 had an old infarction and 11 had both. The diagnosis of myocardial infarction was made on clinical grounds, based on clinical history, electrocardiographic and/or enzymatic documentation of a myocardial infarction and the 122 patients were com- pared to 24 clinically normal subjects [37]. Of the 122 patients, 115 had pathologic Q-waves on the electrocardiogram and 113 of them had a defect on the Tc-99m SestaMIBI study. Of the seven patients without pathologic Q-waves on the electrocardiogram, two patients had no defects on the scintig- rams. Also a 95 % concordance was found between defects on the Tc-99m SestaMIBI images and abnormal wall motion. From these data it can be concluded that resting Tc-99m SestaMIBI images can detect and localize infarction with a high degree of sensitivity and specificity.

Gregoire et al. [38,39] investigated the value of Tc-99m SestaMIBI as a noninvasive tool to diagnose myocardial ischemia in patients with spon- taneous chest pain. In a group of 45 patients with chest pain suggestive of myocardial ischemia, Tc-99m SestaMIBI was injected intravenously during chest pain. In all patients the study was repeated in a period when the patients were free of complaints. The patients were hospitalized with a presumed diagnosis of unstable angina and none had evidence of a previous myocardial infarction. In all patients a coronary angiogram was performed and a stenosis of ≥ 50 % was considered to be significant. A defect detected on single photon emission computed tomography after injection of Tc-99m SestaMIBI during chest pain had a sensitivity of 96 % and a specificity of 79 % for the detection of significant coronary disease. If the criterium was used that the defect(s) had to be larger during pain compared to control the sensitivity was 81 % and the specificity was 84 %. In contrast, transient electrocardiographic ischemic changes during pain had a sensitivity of 35 %

and a specificity of 68 %. Considering both electrocardiographic changes during and outside episodes of chest pain a sensitivity of 65 % and a specificity of 63 % was found for the diagnosis. The authors concluded that Tc-99m SestaMIBI single photon emission computed tomography represent a reliable noninvasive diagnostic tool that could aid in the diagnosis of myocardial ischemia in patients with spontaneous chest pain and provide additional information to that provided by the electrocardiogram.

B) Assessment of efficacy of thrombolytic therapy

In several studies the feasibility of Tc-99m SestaMIBI for the assessment of the myocardial area at risk and the effect of treatment with thrombolytic therapy in acute myocardial infarction has been reported [40,41]. In these studies Tc-99m SestaMIBI was injected intravenously within four hours of the onset of chest pain and before treatment with thrombolytic therapy. A second study was performed 6–14 days later. The control group consisted of a small number of patients in whom thrombolytic therapy was considered contra-indicated. The absence of redistribution of Tc-99m SestaMIBI permitted imaging with single photon emission computed tomography up to 6 hours later to assess the amount of myocardium at risk at the time of administration (Fig. 1). This initial area at risk varied greatly both in patients treated with thrombolytic therapy and in those treated conventionally, although there was a significant decrease in the area of hypoperfused myocardium between the initial and control studies in the patients who received thrombolytic therapy as compared with an insignificant increase in the patients who were treated conventionally. No data till now are available to support the hypothesis that in patients with large areas at risk the prognosis is worse or to justify interventions such as coronary angioplasty or bypass surgery.

Applications in the catheterization laboratory

As Tc-99m SestaMIBI does not redistribute, it can also be injected in the catheterization laboratory with later imaging to visualize its distribution.

In 13 patients in whom percutaneous coronary angioplasty was performed, 15–20 mCi Tc-99m SestaMIBI was administered intravenously during the first balloon inflation [42]. None of these patients had a documented myocardial infarction in the past and showed normal wall motion of the left ventricle. In 11 of 13 patients defects were seen on single photon emission computed tomography images corresponding to the area made ischemic during angioplasty. The occlusion period varied between 13 and 60 seconds. In the two patients in whom no defects were seen abundant collateral flow was present. From this study we conclude that Tc-99m SestaMIBI is able to demonstrate the area at risk of the myocardium during short episodes of ischemia.

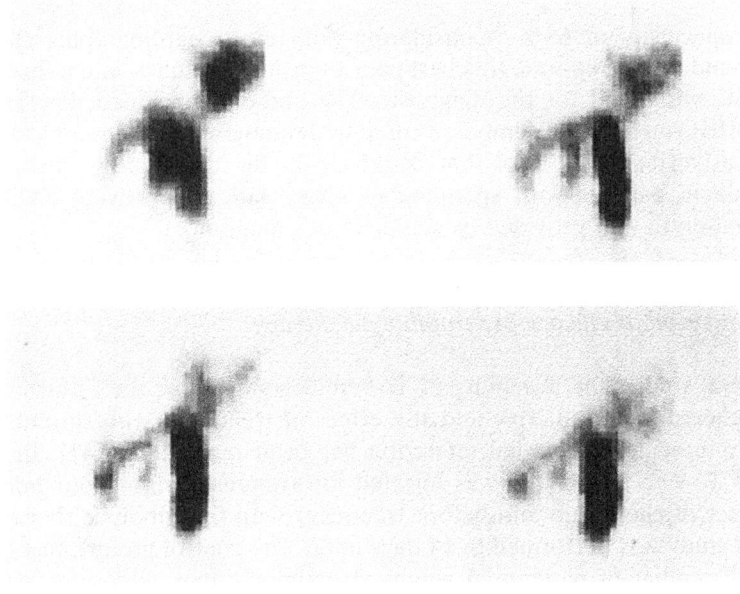

a

b

Figure 1. (a) Tc-99m SestaMIBI SPECT image of the horizontal long axis in a patient with an anteroseptal wall infarction before initiation of thrombolytic therapy. A large perfusion defect is visible in the anteroseptal area. (b) Similar image position 4 days after thrombolytic treatment. The initial perfusion defect has been completely resolved, indicating successful treatment.

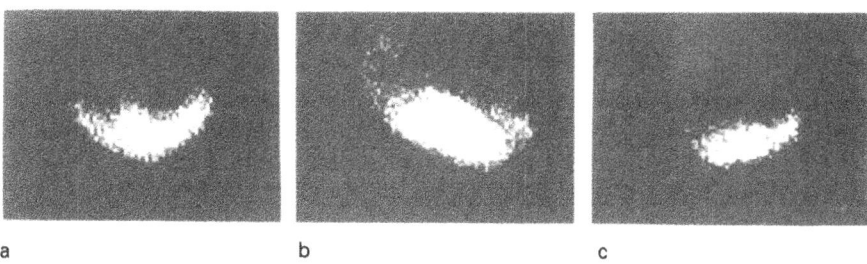

a   b   c

Figure 2. Selective administration of Tc-99m SestaMIBI into the right coronary artery; the myocardial tissue perfused by the right coronary artery is clearly delineated by planar imaging. (a) left anterior oblique view; (b) anterior view; (c) left lateral view.

In another study we also showed that selective intracoronary injection of Tc-99m SestaMIBI is able to demonstrate the size of the myocardium perfused by that artery [43] (Fig. 2).

Conclusions

Tl-201 has been used for more than 15 years for measuring of myocardial perfusion and viability. However, Tl-201 has important disadvantages such as soft tissue attenuation and scatter caused by the low photon energy emission (68–80 keV) and a relatively long half-life (68–73 hr), which limits the administered dose. On top of this, Tl-201 redistributes at rest as well as during exercise, so that imaging must be performed soon after injection and this can give rise to logistic problems. Since the introduction of Tl-201, perfusion agents labeled with Tc-99m have been sought to circumvent these limitations.

For a couple of years two groups of tracers, isonitriles and boronic acid adducts of technetium dioximes (BATO) compounds, labeled to Tc-99m have been available. Of the isonitriles, Tc-99m SestaMIBI has the best properties for myocardial imaging. It has minimal lung uptake, transient hepatic uptake and no myocardial redistribution. The combination of transient early hepatic uptake and no myocardial redistribution makes it an ideal tracer for single photon emission computed tomographic imaging. The uptake of Tc-99m SestaMIBI is proportional to blood flow, at low and medium flow rates. At higher flow rates it underestimates the myocardial flow, while with low flow rates the uptake is higher compared to the regional blood flow determined by microspheres. This is explained by an increased extraction. So, Tc-99m SestaMIBI uptake is proportional to regional blood flow in the physiologic flow range with enhanced extraction of the tracer in low flow regions where some tissue is still viable.

Tc-99m teboroxime has an uptake in the myocardium proportional to blood flow with an extraction which is higher than Tl-201 and Tc-99m Sesta-

MIBI and has a fairly rapid washout. This washout is also flow-related [18]. Both new tracers, one because of the absence of redistribution (Tc-99m SestaMIBI) and the other because of the rapid washout (Tc-99m teboroxime), have to be injected twice to be able to distinguish ischemic and scar tissue. The ideal situation would be to perform a resting and exercise study on different days. If however a one-day protocol has to be done it is advisable to start with a resting study. Tc-99m teboroxime and Tc-99m SestaMIBI have proven to be at least as good as Tl-201 for the diagnosis and assessment of patients with proven or suspected coronary artery disease. The rapid myocardial washout of Tc-99 teboroxime necessitates brief imaging protocols. Tc-99m SestaMIBI does not redistribute and it can therefore be injected in the coronary care unit or catheterization laboratorium. Imaging can be performed later at a suitable moment in the nuclear cardiology laboratory. Using this capability, Tc-99m SestaMIBI has been shown to be not only of value in detecting and localizing myocardial ischemia and infarction, but also to be capable of assessing the efficacy of thrombolytic therapy and to determine the size of the myocardial area perfused by a coronary artery.

References

1. Jones AG, Abrams MJ, Davison A, et al. Biological studies of a new class of technetium complexes: the hexakis(alkylisonitrile)technetium (I) cations. Int J Nucl Med Biol 1984;11:225–34.
2. Narra RK, Nunn AD, Kuczynski BL, Feld T, Wedeking P, Eckelman WC. A neutral technetium-99m complex for myocardial imaging. J Nucl Med 1989;30:1830–7.
3. Holman BL, Jones AG, Lister-James J, et al. A new Tc-99m-labeled myocardial imaging agent, hexakis(t-butyl-isonitrile)-technetium(I) (Tc-99m TBI): initial experience in the human. J Nucl Med 1984;25:1350–5.
4. Holman BL, Campbell CA, Lister-James J, Jones AG, Davison A, Kloner RA. Effect of reperfusion and hyperemia on the myocardial distribution of technetium-99m t-butylisonitrile. J Nucl Med 1986;27:1172–7.
5. Sia ST, Holman BL, McKusick K, et al. The utilization of Tc-99m-TBI as a myocardial perfusion agent in exercise studies: comparison with Tl-201 thallous chloride and examination of its biodistribution in humans. Eur J Nucl Med 1986;12:333–6.
6. McKusick K, Holman Bl, Jones AG, et al. Comparison of 3 Tc-99m isonitriles for detection of ischemic heart disease in humans (abstract). J Nucl Med 1986;27:878.
7. Holman BL, Sporn V, Jones AG, et al. Myocardial imaging with technetium-99m CPI: initial experience in the human. J Nucl Med 1987;28:13–8.
8. Okada RD, Glover D, Gaffney T, Williams S. Myocardial kinetics of Technetium-99m-hexakis-2–methoxy-2–methylpropyl-isonitrile. Circulation 1988;77:491–8.
9. Wackers FJ, Berman DS, Maddahi J, et al. Technetium-99m hexakis 2–methoxyisobutyl isonitrile: human biodistribution, dosimetry, safety and preliminary comparison to thallium-201 for myocardial perfusion imaging. J Nucl Med 1989;30:301–11.
10. Liu P, Houle S, Mills L, Dawood F. Kinetics of Tc-99m MIBI uptake and clearance in ischemia-reperfusion:comparison with Tl-201 (abstract). Circulation 1987;76 (suppl IV):IV-216.
11. Seldin DW, Johnson LL, Blood DK, et al. Myocardial perfusion imaging with technetium-

99m SQ30217: comparison with thallium-201 and coronary anatomy. J Nucl Med 1989;30:312–9.

12. Meerdink D, Moring A, Leppo J. Comparative myocardial transport of technetium-labeled SQ 30217 (Cardiotec) and thallium-201 [abstract(. J Am Coll Cardiol 1987;9:137A.

13. Canby RC, Silber S, Pohost GM. Relations of the myocardial imaging agents 99mTc-Mibi and 201Tl to myocardial blood flow in 2 canine model of myocardial ischemic insult. Circulation 1990;81:289–96.

14. Li QS, Frank TL, Franceschi D, Wagner HN Jr, Becker LC. Technetium-99m methoxyiso-butyl isonitrile (RP30) for quantification of myocardial ischemia and reperfusion in dogs. J Nucl Med 1988;29:1539–48.

15. Verani MS, Jeroudi MO, Mahmarian JJ, et al. Quantification of myocardial infarction during coronary occlusion and myocardial salvage after reperfusion using cardiac imaging with technetium-99m hexakis 2–methoxyisobutyl isonitrile. J Am Coll Cardiol 1988;12:1573–81.

16. Sinusas AJ, Watson DD, Cannon JM Jr, Beller GA. Effect of ischemia and postischemic dysfuntion on myocardial uptake of technetium-99m-labeled methoxyisobutyl isonitrile and thallium-201. J Am Coll Cardiol 1989;14:1785–93.

17. Glover DK, Okada RD. Myocardial kinetics of Tc-MIBI in canine myocardium after dipyridamole. Circulation 1990;81:628–37.

18. Leppo JA, Meerdink DJ. Comparative myocardial extraction of two technetium-labeled BATO derivatives (SQ302014, SQ32014) and thallium. J Nucl Med 1990;31:67–74.

19. Leppo JA, Meerdink DJ. Comparison of the myocardial uptake of a technetium-labeled isonitrile analoque and thallium. Circ Res 1989;65:632–9.

20. Meerdink DJ, Leppo JA. Comparison of hypoxia and ouabain effects on the myocardial uptake kinetics of technetium-99m hexakis 2–methoxyisobutyl isonitrile and thallium-201. J Nucl Med 1989;30:1500–6.

21. Taillefer R, Laflamme L, Dupras G, Picard M, Phaneuf DC, Leveille J. Myocardial per-fusion imaging with 99mTC-methoxy-isobutyl-isonitrile (MIBI): comparison of short and long time intervals between rest and stress injections. Eur J Nucl Med 1988;13:515–22.

22. Kiat H, Maddahi J, Roy LT, et al. Comparison of technetium 99m methoxy isobutyl isonitrile and thallium 201 for evaluation of coronary artery disease by planar and tomo-graphic methods. Am Heart J 1989;117:1–11.

23. Kahn JK, McGhie I, Akers MS, et al. Quantitative rotational tomography with 201Tl and 99mTc 2–methoxy-isobutyl-isonitrile. A direct comparison in normal individuals and pa-tients with coronary artery disease. Circulation 1989;79:1282–93.

24. Taillefer R, Lambert R, Dupras G, et al. Clinical comparison between thallium-201 and Tc-99m-methoxy isobutyl isontrile (hexamibi) myocardial perfusion imaging for detection of coronary artery disease. Eur J Nucl Med 1989;15:280–6.

25. Maisey MN, Mistry R, Sowton E. Planar imaging techniques used with technetium-99m SestaMIBI to evaluate chronic myocardial ischemia. Am J Cardiol 1990;66:47E-54E.

26. Jones RH, Borges-Neto S, Potts JM. Simultaneous measurement of myocardial perfusion and ventricular function during exercise from a single injection of technetium-99m Sesta-MIBI in coronary artery disease. Am J Cardiol 1990;66:68E-71E.

27. Braat SH, Rigo P, van Kroonenburg M, Wellens HJJ. Comparison between thallium 201 and dynamic myocardial imaging with technetium 99m teboroxime (abstract). J Nucl Med 1991;32.

28. Wackers FJ. Thallium-201 myocardial scintigraphy in acute myocardial infarction and is-chemia. Semin Nucl Med 1980;10:127–45.

29. Hamilton GW, Trobaugh GB, Ritchie JL, Williams DL, Weaver WD, Gould KL. Myocard-ial imaging with intravenously injected thallium-201 in patients with suspected coronary artery disease: analysis of technique and correlation with electrocardio-graphic, coronary anatomic and ventriculographic findings. Am J Cardiol 1977;39:347–54.

30. Wackers FJ, Buseman Sokole E, Samson G, et al. Value and limitations of thallium-201 scintigraphy in the acute phase of myocardial infarction. N Engl J Med 1976;295:1–5.

31. Wackers FJ, Becker AE, Samson G, et al. Location and size of acute transmural myocardial infarction estimated from thallium-201 scintiscans. A clinicopathological study. Circulation 1977;56:72–8.

32. Gibson RS, Taylor GJ, Watson DD, et al. Prognostic significance of resting anterior thallium-201 defects in patients with inferior myocardial infarction. J Nucl Med 1980;21:1015–21.

33. Perez-Gonzalez J, Botvinick EH, Dunn R, et al. The late prognostic value of acute scintigraphic measurement of myocardial infarction size. Circulation 1982;66:960–71.

34. Gewirtz H, Beller GA, Strauss HW, et al. Transient defects of resting thallium scans in patients with coronary artery disease. Circulation 1979;59:707–13.

35. Brown KA, Okada RD, Boucher CA, Philips HR, Strauss HW, Pohost GM. Serial thallium-201 imaging at rest in patients with unstable and stable angina pectoris:relationship of myocardial perfusion at rest to presenting clinical syndrome. Am Heart J 1983;106:70–7.

36. Boucher CA. Detection and location of myocardial infarction using technetium-99m Sesta-MIBI imaging at rest. Am J Cardiol 1990;66:32E-5E.

37. Kaul S, Newell JB, Chesler DA, Pohost GM, Okada RD, Boucher CA. Quantitative thallium imaging findings in patients with normal coronary angiographic findings and in clinically normal subjects. Am J Cardiol 1986;57:509–12.

38. Gregoire J, Theroux P. Detection and assessment of unstable angina using myocardial perfusion imaging: comparison between technetium-99m SestaMIBI SPECT and 12–lead electrocardiogram. Am J Cardiol 1990;66:42E-6E.

39. Bilodeau L, Grégoire J, Dupras G, Arsenault A, Gagnon D, Théroux P. Tc-99m-methoxy isobutyl isonitrile (MIBI) tomographies as a diagnostic help for spontaneously occurring chest pain (abstract). Circulation 1989;80 (suppl 2):II-620.

40. Gibbons RJ, Verani MS, Behrenbeck T, et al. Feasibility of tomographic 99mTc-hexakis-2–methoxy-2–methylpropyl-isonitrile imaging for the assessment of myocardial area at risk and the effect of treatment in acute myocardial infarction. Circulation 1989;80:1277–86.

41. Wackers FJ. Thrombolytic therapy for myocardial infarction: assessment of efficacy by myocardial perfusion imaging with technetium-99m SestaMIBI. Am J Cardiol 1990;66:36E-41E.

42. Braat SH, de Swart H, Rigo P, Koppejan L, Heidendal GAK, Wellens HJJ. Value of technetium Mibi to detect short lasting episodes of severe myocardial ischaemia and to estimate the area at risk during coronary angioplasty. Eur Heart J 1991;12:30–3.

43. Braat SH, de Swart H, Janssen JH, Brugada P, Rigo P, Wellens HJJ. Use of technetium-99m SestaMIBI to determine the size of the myocardial area perfused by a coronary artery. Am J Cardiol 1990;66:85E-90E.

14. Clinical application of antimyosin monoclonal antibody imaging in cardiology

JAMSHID MADDAHI

Summary

Indium-111 (In-111) labeled antimyosin monoclonal antibody is specific for myocardial necrosis since it binds to cardiac myosin which becomes exposed during the process of myocardial cell membrane disruption and death. Myocardial uptake of antimyosin is directly related to the amount of necrosis and does not depend on regional myocardial blood flow which is often severely reduced during acute myocardial infarction and its positive uptake is observed even when it is injected very early after the onset of myocardial infarction. In a multicenter clinical trial (16 sites in the United States and 9 in Europe), the clinical safety of antimyosin was documented and its utility was evaluated in 497 patients with chest pain. The overall sensitivity and specificity of antimyosin were 87.5 % and 95 %. Using the Bayesian approach to the diagnostic utility of antimyosin it becomes apparent that patients who have an intermediate (25 % to 75 %) likelihood of myocardial infarction will benefit most from this test. These include 1) patients with conflicting clinical and laboratory findings for presence of infarction, 2) patients with equivocal or nondiagnostic electrocardiograms and/or cardiac enzymes such as a) patients who have conduction disturbances on their electrocardiograms, b) those who might have suffered infarction during bypass surgery or coronary angioplasty, and c) those following thrombolysis therapy or with non-Q wave infarction in whom the size of necrosis cannot be accurately determined by the conventional methods, and 3) patients who present late after developing symptoms suspicious of myocardial infarction.

An important application of antimyosin is risk stratification early following myocardial infarction. In the multicenter trial, there was a linear relationship between the minimum number of segments of antimyosin uptake and the incidence of cardiac death, nonfatal myocardial infarction, or both. An antimyosin study demonstrating less than 10 segments of uptake or no uptake identified patients with a low risk of developing events (5 %) compared to those with 10 or more segments of antimyosin uptake who represented a high risk category with 25 % cardiac event rate. The presence of extensive antimyosin uptake had superior prognostic value and was independent of other variables such as Killip class, Q wave myocardial infarction, recurrent

Johan H.C. Reiber & Ernst E. van der Wall (eds.), Cardiovascular Nuclear Medicine and MRI, 207–221.
© 1992 *Kluwer Academic Publishers.*

ischemia and total creatine kinase. The intensity of regional myocardial uptake of antimyosin may be quantified which represents the degree of transmurality of infarction and correlates with the development of ischemic events following myocardial infarction. Furthermore, dual isotope imaging with In-111 antimyosin and thallium-201 (Tl-201) may identify the amount of necrotic and viable but jeopardized myocardium as markers of prognosis after myocardial infarction.

Antimyosin imaging has been helpful in identifying patients with a low risk for cardiac transplant rejection and decreases the total number of biopsies that are obtained in the post operative course. Similarly, in patients with dilated cardiomyopathy who are being evaluated for the presence of myocarditis, a negative antimyosin study effectively rules out this possibility and obviates the need for endomyocardial biopsy.

Introduction

In management of patients with or suspected of having myocardial infarction, the challenge to a cardiologist is to confirm the diagnosis, assess the size of the patient's infarction, determine prognosis and optimize patient care according to these data. In addition to clinical evaluation, several diagnostic modalities have been available for diagnosis and evaluation of myocardial infarction. The standard 12–lead electrocardiogram, though helpful in diagnosis of myocardial infarction, has well-recognized limitations. Prior infarction or left bundle branch block frequently invalidate interpretation of the standard electrocardiogram during myocardial infarction and infarct extent and location may not be accurately assessed especially in patients with inferoposterior wall myocardial infarction. Traditional creatine kinase-MB enzymes studies are useful in establishing development of myocardial infarction but are less reliable in assessing the extent of infarction especially in patients following thrombolysis. Successful reperfusion causes rapid, profound enzymes release even from quite small infarcts. When myocardial infarction is the result of intermittent coronary occlusion, enzyme release is erratic and routine protocols for obtaining blood samples for enzyme determination do not allow reliable analysis of creatine kinase-MB release to assess the size of necrosis. Furthermore, enzyme release is time dependent and patients who present late after the onset of their symptoms may present falsely negative enzymes levels. Two-dimensional echocardiography or radionuclide ventriculography may be used to demonstrate presence and size of myocardial infarction by presence and extent of regional wall motion abnormalities. However, ventricular function measurements, especially in the post-infarction assessment, are often artificially depressed in the presence of stunned or hibernating myocardium. In these circumstances, ventricular function may not improve for days or even months despite the presence of viable myocardium, making the early use of these measurements a less precise prognostic indicator for the assessment of longterm outcome. Tc-99m pyrophosphate imaging has been used for assessment of myocardial necrosis [1–3]. However, optimal uptake of Tc-99m pyrophosphate by the necrotic myocardial tissue occurs 48–72 hours after the onset of chest pain resulting in suboptimal sensitivity of this method to diagnose infarct within a clinically useful period after the onset of chest pain. Furthermore, the Tc-99m pyrophosphate technique is not very specific for myocardial necrosis, and may not be ideal for determining the size of infarction because it is not effectively taken up in areas with a most severe reduction of blood flow which contains the largest amount of necrotic myocardium.

Antimyosin monoclonal antibody imaging

Antimyosin monoclonal antibody (Myoscint, Centocor) is a Fab fragment of murine monoclonal antibody which binds specifically to an antigenic site on the heavy chain of human myosin. Myosin in an intracellular protein found in myocytes and is not exposed when the cell membrane is intact. Destruction of cell membrane during myocardial necrosis exposes myosin and allows its binding with antimyosin monoclonal antibody. This antibody was first developed by Dr. Khaw and his colleagues and has been well characterized in animal studies [4–6]. In these studies the specificity of interaction between antimyosin monoclonal antibody and myosin has been well demonstrated. Furthermore, they demonstrated that antimyosin monoclonal antibody is taken up by the necrotic tissue in proportion to the amount of necrosis with maximal uptake in areas with severely reduced myocardial blood flow, i.e. when necrosis is maximal. It appears that even in the presence of a totally occluded vessel, antimyosin monoclonal antibody reaches the infarcted tissue by way of diffusion. These features make In-111 radiolabeled antimyosin monoclonal antibody a suitable tracer for in vivo detection of myocardial necrosis in humans [7–13].

Clinical safety and dosemetry of antimyosin monoclonal antibody

The clinical safety of antimyosin has been extensively evaluated in multicenter clinical trials [9,14]. In over 1700 blood samples tested, there has been no evidence of human anti-murine antibody response in patients receiving single or multiple injections of antimyosin. This has been a major safety concern about antibody based drugs of murine origin. The only adverse experience related to antimyosin injection was pain at the site of injection occurring in 1.9 % of patients. No serious adverse effects were noted which were directly attributable to antimyosin. Furthermore, no significant effects on vital signs, laboratory chemistry parameters, or hematologic parameters of urine analysis were noted.

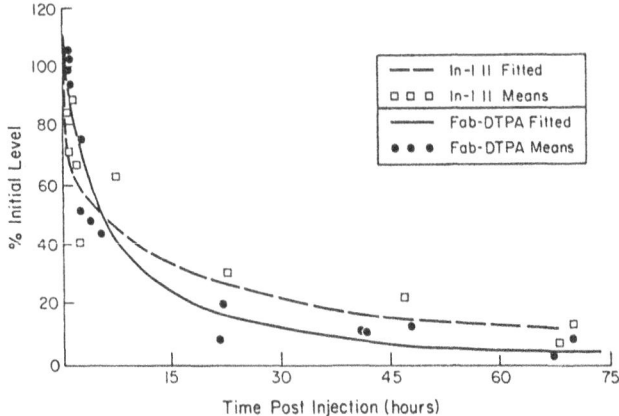

Figure 1. Plasma clearance curves of In-111 radiolabel and the antimyosin antibody showing no significant difference indicative of a stable in vivo complex. Blood activity is reduced to 20 % by 24 hr and 10 " by 48 hr.

After intravenous injection, In-111 labeled antimyosin clears from the blood exponentially such that blood activity is reduced to 20 % by 24 hours after injection, permitting a good target to background ratio at this time. Blood activity further drops to 10 % at 48 hours (Fig. 1). Since most of the circulating antimyosin is excreted through the urine, kidneys are the critical organ. The dose to the kidney is 9.35 rads per 2 mCi (74 MBq) of In-111 DTPA. The total body dose is 0.86 rads per 2 mCi (74 MBq) of In-111 DTPA. These doses represent exposures to the patients which are well within recognized radiation exposure limits.

Clinical application for detection of myocardial infarction

The unique features of antimyosin just described make this agent quite useful in patients presenting with ischemic chest pain for determining 1) whether or not infarction occurred, 2) where infarction is located, and 3) how extensive necrosis is. These issues were extensively evaluated in the antimyosin phase III clinical trial [14]. This trial consisted of 25 sites, 16 in the Unites States and 9 in Europe. A total of 497 patients were studied who presented with chest pain which was thought to be due to a myocardial infarction and who were admitted to the hospital for further evaluation. Two mCi (74 MBq) of In-111 antimyosin was injected within 72 hr of chest pain and three-view planar images were obtained 24 and 48 hr after injection of antimyosin. In all patients, serial creatine kinase-MB were taken every 6 hours for 36 hr and serial electrocardiograms were obtained every 12 to 24 hr for 5 days. These data were used to categorize patients into 4 groups: 1) Acute Q-wave myocardial infarction, 2) acute non-Q-wave myocardial infarction, 3) unstable angina pectoris, and 4) chest pain without myocardial necrosis or

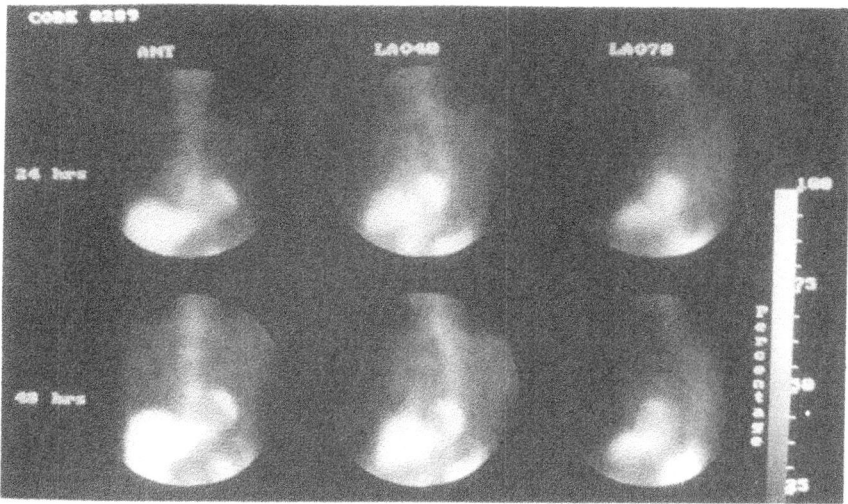

Figure 2. In-111 antimyosin antibody images obtained at approximately 24 and 48 hr after injection demonstrating abnormal focal myocardial uptake in the high anterolateral wall. Uptake by the liver and kidneys is also noted.

resting ischemia. Antimyosin images were evaluated by consensus interpretation of a blinded panel of nuclear cardiology experts.

The overall sensitivity of antimyosin for detection of myocardial necrosis was 87.5 % This was assessed in a total of 257 patients with a definitive diagnosis of myocardial infarction based on clinical, electrocardiographic or enzymatic criteria. The sensitivity of antimyosin for detection of Q-wave infarction was 91 % and for detection of non-Q-wave infarction was 76 %. The specificity of antimyosin was evaluated in 40 patients with chest pain but without myocardial infarction or ischemia and was 95 % (Figs. 2 and 3).

Utility of antimyosin imaging for diagnosis of myocardial necrosis in equivocal cases

Patients not infrequently present with equivocal or conflicting electrocardiograms or enzymatic findings that make the definitive diagnosis of myocardial infarction uncertain such as patients with conflicting clinical and laboratory findings for presence of infarction or those with equivocal or nondiagnostic electrocardiograms, and/or cardiac enzymes. The latter may be encountered in patients who have conduction disturbances on their electrocardiogram, those who might have suffered infarction during bypass surgery of coronary angioplasty, and those following thrombolysis therapy or with non-Q-wave infarction in whom the extent of necrosis may not be accurately assessed by the conventional methods. Other patients who pose a problem for diagnosis

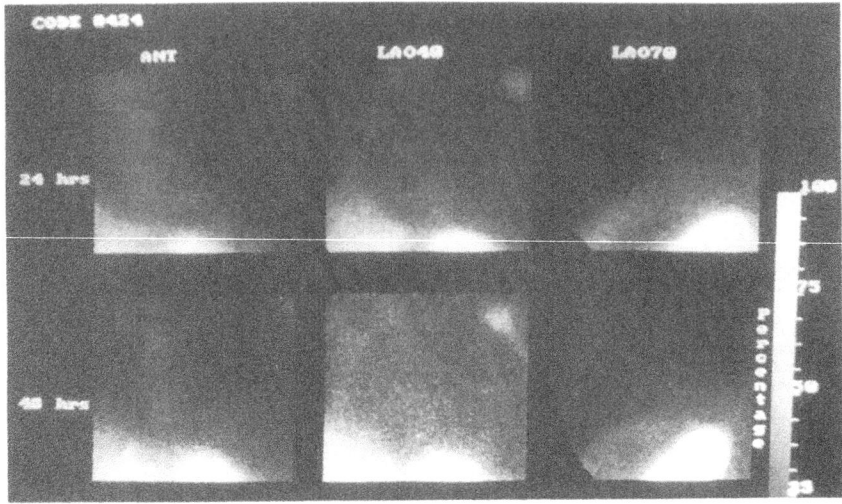

Figure 3. In-111 antimyosin antibody images obtained about 24 and 48 hr after injection showing faint blood pool activity at 24 hr with no focal myocardial uptake to suggest myocardial necrosis.

of infarction are those who present later after developing symptoms suspicious of an ischemic event.

In the multicenter trial [15], equivocal or conflicting electrocardiographic and/or enzymatic results were seen quite frequently in the 497 patients who were admitted to the study with chest pain of varying etiologies. Almost 1/3 of these patients could not be classified definitively as having acute myocardial infarction, unstable angina, or chest pain of nonischemic origin based on their electrocardiographic findings, clinical presentation and creatine kinase enzyme determinations. In order to assess the value of antimyosin imaging in these patients, all available data were used to attempt to best classify these patients into those who did and those who did not have a myocardial infarction. This 'best guess' classification for the presence of myocardial infarction was then correlated with the results of antimyosin images, with uptake of antimyosin interpreted as evidence of necrosis. In 73 % of these patients there was a correlation between the two classifications.

Bayes' theorem may also be used to address the question whether patients with a non-definitive diagnosis of myocardial necrosis may benefit from antimyosin study. Bayes' theorem states that the probability of disease after a given test depends on the pre-test likelihood of the disease, as well as the sensitivity and specificity of the test (Fig. 4). Using the sensitivity and specificity of antimyosin study determined from the multicenter trial, we observe that the greatest discrimination between positive test responders and those with a negative study is achieved in patients who have an intermediate likelihood (equivocal evidence) of necrosis. In such patients the presence of

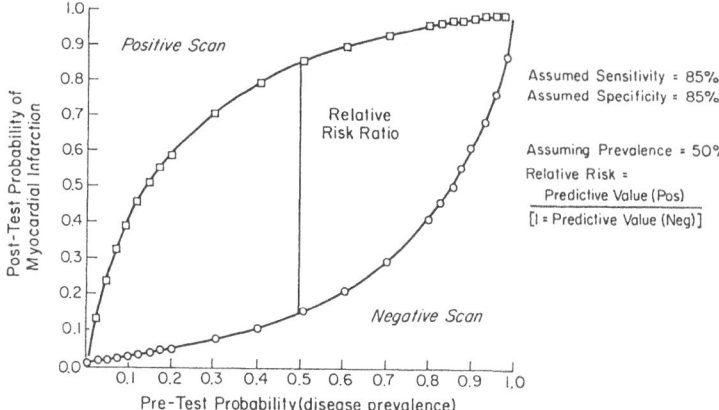

Figure 4. Influence of positive and negative antimyosin scan results on the post-test probability of myocardial infarction according to different pre-test probability levels. The greatest discrimination between the positive and negative test responders is achieved in patients who have an intermediate (25 % – 75 %) likelihood of myocardial infarction.

a positive study indicates a high likelihood of myocardial necrosis, whil a negative study essentially rules out the presence of myocardial necrosis.

Application of antimyosin imaging for prognosis of myocardial infarction

Prognosis of patients following acute myocardial infarction is related to the quantity of myocardium that has become necrotic, and the quantity that is in danger of becoming necrotic (jeopardized myocardium). It is of note that in acute ischemic syndromes (acute myocardial infarction and instable angina) and following thrombolysis, the amount of necrotic myocardium and the amount of viable but jeopardized myocardium is quite unpredictable and may not be accurately assessed based on the clinical, enzymatic and electrocardiographic findings. Antimyosin image results may be interpreted in several ways to assess the extent of necrotic and jeopardized myocardium to provide prognostic information.

Semi-quantitative method

Antimyosin images may be analyzed semi-quantitatively to assess the extent of myocardial necrosis on either planar or tomographic (SPECT) images. In the multicenter trial the extent of myocardial necrosis was evaluated from

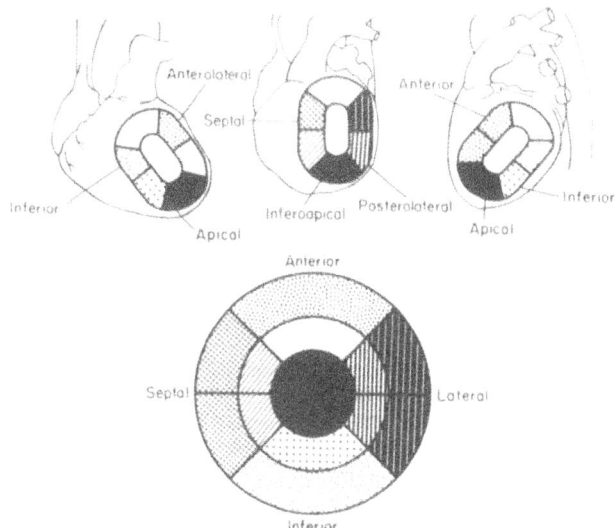

Figure 5. Diagrammatic representation of various myocardial regions observed in three standard planar views and their composite display in a polar map format.

the three view planar images by a method shown in Fig. 5. Each view of the left ventricle was divided intro six segments and each segment was visually scored for presence of antimyosin uptake as mild, moderate or intense. It is important to note that summing the number of involved segments from all three views may overestimate the extent of necrosis since specific regions of the left ventricular are visualized on more than one view. Furthermore, what may appear to be uptake in a specific wall of the left ventricle may be caused by 'shine-through' of In-111 antimyosin from an overlapping region. 'Shine-through' is caused by the transmission of the higher energy photons of In-111 through superimposed walls of the myocardium. Therefore, it is necessary to determine if uptake seen in a given planar view is anatomically correct in its location or represents shine-through from a more distal or overlaying region. This is best accomplished by confirming uptake location in at least two planar views. In order to more accurately assess the location and the extent of myocardial necrosis, the information from the three planar images were translated into a single composite image of the entire left ventricle using the polar map or bull's eye method that has been described for Tl-201 SPECT imaging. The polar map display not only demonstrated the location of antimyosin uptake but also allowed assessment of the percent of the entire left ventricular myocardium with antimyosin uptake expressed as the number of positive segments divided by 18, which is the total number of evaluable segments.

A linear relationship was noted between the number of segments with antimyosin uptake and the incidence of cardiac death, nonfatal myocardial

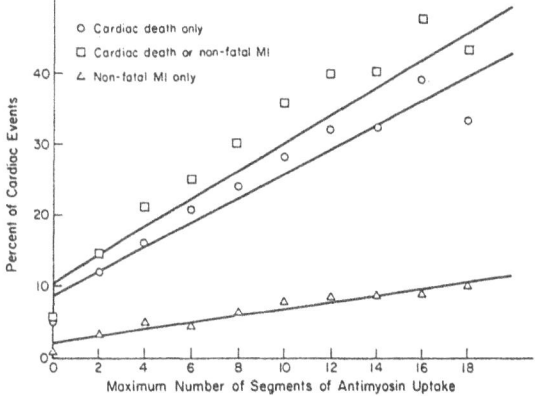

Figure 6. Linear relationship between the number of myocardial segments with antimyosin uptake and the incidence of cardiac death, nonfatal myocardial infarction, and either of the two events during the follow-up period.

infarction, and either of these two events during the 5–month follow-up period in the multicenter trial [16]. The cumulative cardiac death rate during the follow-up period ranged from 4 % in patients with a negative study to over 30 % in patients with extensive antimyosin uptake (Fig. 6). Receiver operating curve analysis demonstrated that > or = to 10 segments of antimyosin uptake best discriminated patients with low risk from those with high risk for developing cardiac events. An antimyosin study demonstrating <10 segment of uptake or no uptake identified patients with a low risk for developing events (5 %). However, patients with 10 or more segments of antimyosin uptake represented a high risk category with 25 % cardiac event rate. Of note, in patients who were classified as being nondefinitive for myocardial infarction (because of conflicting or equivocal clinical findings, nondiagnostic electrocardiograms, or cardiac enzyme results), the incidence of major cardiac events was 36 % in those with extensive uptake compared to 4 % in those without extensive uptake resulting in a relative risk of 9 to 1. The presence of extensive antimyosin uptake had superior and independent prognostic value compared with all of the other variables that were included in the multivariate analysis model such as Killip Class, age, presence of Q-waves, ischemia, peak creatine kinase, and prior myocardial infarction. Therefore, it appears that the information gained by assessing the extent of antimyosin uptake was independent of all other clinical variables evaluated, alone or in combination, and added new prognostic information. However, it should be pointed out that in the multicenter trial, left ventricular ejection fraction or extent of perfusion abnormality by Tl-201 imaging was not evaluated and thus, the relative role of antimyosin imaging versus these additional prognostic indicators is not yet determined.

Intensity of myocardial uptake of antimyosin

In quantifying the extent of myocardial necrosis, it is also important to determine whether necrosis involves the full thickness of the myocardium, or is interspersed with viable myocardium (i.e., nontransmural). One approach to assessing the degree of transmurality of necrosis is to quantify the intensity of regional antimyosin uptake. Van Vlies and associates [17] have developed a count density index (CDI), which is the ratio of myocardial and the left lung count densities. The lower the ratio, the less the volume of necrosis in a given region and the less likely that it is transmural. This group demonstrated that in 38 patients with their first myocardial infarction CDI correlated with two-dimensional echocardiographic estimates of regional wall motion 5–9 days after admission. In patients with mild asynergy in at least one segment, CDI was significantly lower than in those with severe asynergy (1.6 versus 2.5). In a subgroup of patients following thrombolytic therapy of their first myocardial infarction, similar observations were made [17].

Another evidence that CDI reflects the degree of transmurality of infarction was provided by Van Vlies and associates (personal communication) in a study of 55 patients with their first acute myocardial infarction who had an uncomplicated initial course defined as Killip Class I of II, no severe heart failure and no significant arrhythmias. There were 18 events with 6 months, 11/18 occurring within 6 weeks of the acute myocardial infarction. Events were defined as cardiac death, recurrent infarction, unstable angina, the need for bypass surgery or angioplasty, or recurrent ischemia (judged by symptoms and a positive Tl-201 study). In patients with an event, the mean CDI was 1.82 but in patients without an event, it was 2.2; a statistically significant difference ($p < 0.01$). The positive predictive value of a CDI of 2.0 was 57 % but the negative predictive value was 93 % suggesting that measurement of CDI allows identification of a subgroup of patients after acute myocardial infarction with a low chance of experiencing a recurrent ischemic event during follow-up.

Dual-isotope imaging

Another approach to determining the transmurality of necrosis and the presence and size of viable but jeopardized myocardium is dual isotope imaging. This involves the use of Tl-201 in conjunction with In-111 antimyosin to assess myocardial perfusion and viability. The perfusion images may be superimposed on the antimyosin images to discern the relationship between the two. Several patterns may be observed: 1) normal uptake of Tl-201 without antimyosin uptake indicating normal myocardium, 2) reduced Tl-201 uptake without antimyosin uptake suggesting resting ischemia (if defect is reversible) or infarction (if Tl-201 defect is nonreversible), 3) absence of

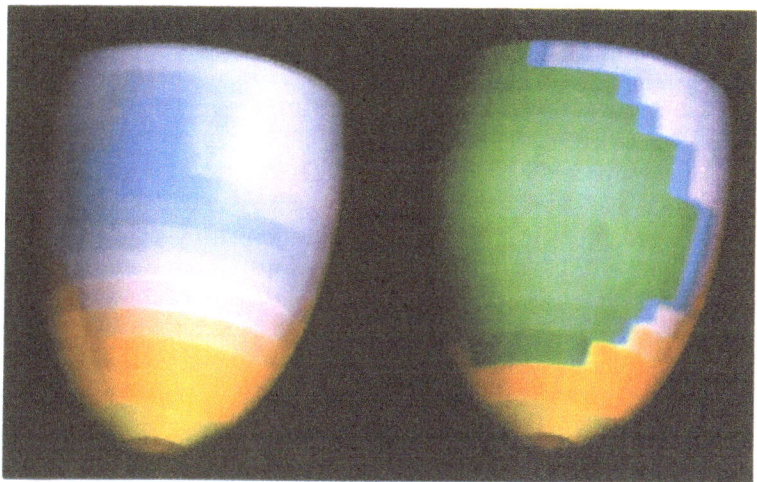

Figure 7. Three-dimensional display of myocardial distribution of Tl-201 (a) before and (b) after superimposition of the myocardial region with In-111 labeled antimyosin antibody uptake. The relationship between antimyosin uptake (green) and Tl-201 uptake patterns (yellow = normal, magenta = reduced, and blue = absent) implies the presence of transmural necrosis (green overlapping with blue), nontransmural necrosis (green overlapping with magenta), and viable but ischemic (magenta without green overlap) myocardium.

Tl-201 uptake in areas with antimyosin uptake suggesting transmural necrosis, and 4) presence of some Tl-201 uptake in an area of antimyosin uptake indicating nontransmural infarction. In a given patient, different extent of one or more of these regional patterns may be observed.

Studies performed in 42 patients by Dr. Johnson and her associates at Columbia University [18] have substantiated the concept that these patterns may have prognostic implications. In patients with matching areas of abnormality consistent with transmural infarction, there were no ischemic events. However, among the 23 patients with a mismatch pattern, i.e., areas of Tl-201 reduction without antimyosin uptake (suggesting the presence of ischemia), there were further ischemic manifestations in 16 patients. Furthermore, of five patients who showed antimyosin and Tl-201 overlap in the same areas, four patients had evidence of ischemia. Thus, it appears that dual isotope imaging early following acute myocardial infarction thrombolysis may be helpful in identifying patients who are at a higher risk for developing further ischemic events.

In a collaborative research between the University of California at Los Angeles (J. Maddahi) and Emory University (E. Garcia, J. Cullom, and D. Cook), three-dimensional display of dual isotope In-111 antimyosin antibody and Tl-201 are being developed to better assess the extent of nontransmural and transmural infarction as well as the extent of viable but jeopardized myocardium (Fig. 7).

Applications of antimyosin imaging for evaluation of patients after cardiac transplant

In 1989, there were 1,700 heart transplants in the United States and 2,400 worldwide. The current method for detecting transplant rejection is right ventricular endomyocardial biopsy which is generally performed 10–15 times during the first year after transplant in a given patient. On biopsy, severe rejection is highlighted by lymphocytic infiltrate and myocyte necrosis. The method of right ventricular endomyocardial biopsy is not only invasive, it is expensive and causes inconvenience to the patient. Several animal experimental studies showed that antimyosin monoclonal antibody may be used to detect myocardial necrosis caused by cardiac transplant rejection which led to its subsequent application, by several groups, in humans to assess its utility for noninvasive and more convenient detection of cardiac transplant rejection. In 1987, Frist et al. [19] published the first human series using antimyosin imaging. In 20 patients who were imaged 7 days to more than 9 years after cardiac transplantation, sensitivity was 80 % and specificity was 80 %. Carrio et al. [20, 21] have studied 52 patients from 7 days to 15 months after receiving heart transplants. In a subgroup of 32 patients, repeat studies were performed and a subgroup of 19 patients were studied beyond the first year of transplant. The findings demonstrated that initially after cardiac transplantation, there was evidence of antimyosin uptake in almost all patients. Thereafter, three different patterns may evolve: the first pattern is that the initial high heart to lung ratio tends to decrease with time and becomes normal within 6 months or a year after transplant; this has been associated with a favourable clinical course. The second pattern is that the initially high heart to lung ratio tends to decrease with time but it remains above the normal limits at 6 months to a year after transplantation; this pattern has been associated with the high probability of subsequent rejection. The third pattern is that the initial high heart to lung ratio persists over time which has been associated with a high likelihood of cardiac rejection. Therefore it appears that a negative or subsiding pattern of antimyosin uptake by the heart transplant suggests a low likelihood of rejection and thus endomyocardial biopsy may be avoided. However, a positive antimyosin uptake observed at one point of time during the first year of transplant does not necessarily indicate a high likelihood of rejection unless the uptake remains persistently high.

Application of antimyosin imaging for evaluation of myocarditis

Myocarditis is pathologically characterized by both an inflammatory cellular (generally lymphocytic) infiltrate within the myocardium and by associated myocyte necrosis (the Dallas criteria). The clinical features of active myocarditis are extremely varied ranging from asymptomatic electrocardiographic abnormalities during Coxsackie outbreaks in a community to fulminant congestive heart failure [22]. Since the introduction of endomyocardial biopsy, a key question has been how frequently myocarditis is the cause of dilated cardiomyopathy. The prognosis of idiophatic dilated cardiomyopathy remains poor with a 50 % mortality in 24 months. Myocarditis however has been associated with improvement in ventricular function during immunosuppressive treatment in over 50 % of patients. Thousands of patients with unexplained heart failure are currently undergoing endomyocardial biopsy each year in order to try to detect myocarditis and to institute appropriate therapy. However, the rate of detection of myocarditis in patients with symptomatic dilated cardiomyopathy varies widely ranging from 1 % to 67 %. It would be useful to have a noninvasive screening method to select those patients with symptomatic cardiomyopathy who should undergo biopsy.

Monoclonal antimyosin antibody imaging in a murine model [23] showed that antimyosin uptake ratio for the heart increased significantly by day 28. The uptake ratio paralleled the pathologic findings of cellular infiltration and myocyte necrosis suggesting that antimyosin scintigraphy may prove to be a reliable noninvasive method for the evaluation of patients with acute and subacute myocarditis. Antimyosin scintigraphy was evaluated by Dec et al. [24] in 72 patients with suspected myocarditis. All patients had dilated cardiomyopathy ≤ 12 months' duration and the mean left ventricular ejection fraction was 0.30 ± 0.02. Sixty-six patients presented with heart failure; the other six had life-threatening ventricular arrhythmias. All patients underwent planar and SPECT cardiac imaging after injection of 1.8 mCi of In-111 labeled antimyosin antibody fragments, as well as right ventricular biopsy within 48 hours of imaging. On the basis of the right ventricular histologic findings, the sensitivity of antimyosin imaging was 83 % and the specificity was 49 %. The low specificity resulted from a large number of false positive antimyosin scintigrams; some of these scintigrams may actually have detected myocarditis that was missed by right ventricular biopsy, due to sampling error. Improvement in left ventricular function occurred within 6 months of treatment in 54 % of patients with a positive antimyosin scintigrams, compared with only 18 % of those with a negative scintigram ($p < 0.001$). These findings suggest that antimyosin imaging is a useful technique for the initial noninvasive evaluation of patients with dilated cardiomyopathy and suspected myocarditis. A negative antimyosin scintigram is associated with a very low rate (8 %) of myocarditis detection and may obviate the need for biopsy in many such individuals.

Acknowledgements

The author wishes to thank Miss Mercedes Boccanegra for typing and preparation of the manuscript and Ms. Lee Griswald for preparation of figures.

References

1. Willerson JT, Parkey RW, Bonte FJ, Meyer SL, Atkins JM, Stokeley EM. Technetium stannous pyrophosphate myocardial scintigrams in patients with chest pain of varying etiology. Circulation 1975;51:1046–52.
2. Turi ZG, Rutherford JD, Roberts R, et al. Electrocardiographic, enzymatic and scintigraphic criteria of acute myocardial infarction as determined from study of 726 patients (A MILIS Study). Am J Cardiol 1985;55:1463–8.
3. Tamaki N, Yamada T, Matsumori A, et al. Indium-111–antimyosin antibody imaging for detecting different stages of myocardial infarction: comparison with technetium-99m-pyrophosphate imaging. J Nucl Med 1990;31:136–42.
4. Khaw BA, Beller GA, Haber E, Smith TW. Localization of cardiac myosin-specific antibody in myocardial infarction. J Clin Invest 1976;58:439–46.
5. Khaw BA, Beller GA, Haber E. Experimental myocardial infarct imaging following intravenous administration of iodine-131 labeled antibody (Fab')^2 fragments specific for cardiac myosin. Circulation 1978;57:743–50.
6. Khaw BA, Fallon JT, Beller GA, et al. Specificity of localization of myosin-specific antibody fragments in experimental myocardial infarction. Histologic, histochemical, autoradiographic and scintigraphic studies. Circulation 1979;60:1527–31.
7. Khaw BA, Gold HK, Yasuda T, et al. Scintigraphic quantification of myocardial necrosis in patients after intravenous injection of myosin-specific antibody. Circulation 1986;74:501–8.
8. Khaw BA, Yasuda T, Gold HK, et al. Acute myocardial infarct imaging with indium-111–labeled monoclonal antimyosin Fab. J Nucl Med 1987;28:1671–8.
9. Johnson LL, Seldin DW, Becker LC, et al. Antimyosin imaging in acute transmural myocardial infarctions: results of a multicenter clinical trial. J Am Coll Cardiol 1989;13:27–35.
10. Braat SH, de Zwaan C, Teule J, Heidendal G, Wellens HJJ. Value of indium-111 monoclonal antimyosin antibody for imaging in acute myocardial infarction. Am J Cardiol 1987;60:725–6.
11. Volpini M, Giubbini R, Gei P, et al. Diagnosis of acute myocardial infarction by indium-111 antimyosin antibodies and correlation with the traditional techniques for the evaluation of extent and localization. Am J Cardiol 1989;63:7–13.
12. Berger H, Lahiri A, Crawley J, et al. Indium-111–antimyosin imaging in patients with acute myocardial infarction: post-mortem correlation between histopathologic and autoradiographic extent of myocardial necrosis. Am J Card Imaging 1988;2:158–61.
13. Jain D, Crawley JC, Lahiri A, et al. Indium-111–antimyosin images compared with triphenyl tetrazolium chloride staining in a patient six days after myocardial infarction. J Nucl Med 1990;31:231–3.
14. Berger H, Lahiri A, Leppo J, et al. Antimyosin imaging in patients with ischemic chest pain; initial results of phase III multicenter trial (abstract). J Nucl Med 1988;29:805–6.
15. Berger HJ. Antimyosin imaging in patients with chest pain but without a definitive diagnosis of myocardial infarction or unstable angina (abstract). Circulation 1988;78(Suppl II):II493.
16. Berger HJ. Prognostic significance of the extent of antimyosin uptake in unstable ischemic heart disease: early risk stratification (abstract). Circulation 1988;78 (Suppl II):II131.
17. Van Vlies B, Baas J, Visser CA. Predictive value of indium-111 antimyosin uptake for improvement of left ventricular wall motion after thrombolysis in acute myocardial infarction. Am J Cardiol 1989;64:167–71.
18. Johnson LL, Seldin DW, Keller AM, et al. Dual isotope thallium and indium antimyosin SPECT imaging to identify acute infarct patients at further ischemic risk. Circulation 1990;81:37–45.
19. Frist W, Yasuda T, Segall G, et al. Noninvasive detection of human cardiac transplant rejection with indium-111 antimyosin (Fab) imaging. Circulation 1987;76:V81–5.

20. Carrio I, Berna L, Ballester M, et al. Indium-111 antimyosin scintigraphy to assess myocardial damage in patients with suspected myocarditis and cardiac rejection. J Nucl Med 1988;29:1893–900.
21. Carrio I, Berna L, Estorch M, Ballester M, Obrador D. Noninvasive follow-up of heart transplant patients with quantitative indium-111–antimyosin scintigraphy (abstract). J Nucl Med 1989;30:862.
22. Dec GW Jr, Palacios IF, Fallon JT, et al. Active myocarditis in the spectrum of acute dilated cardiomyopathies. Clinical features, histologic correlates, and clinical outcome. N Engl J Med 1985;312:885–90.
23. Ohkusa T, Matsumori A, Matoba Y, et al. Antimyosin monoclonal antibody Fab imaging of experimental viral myocarditis (abstract). Circulation 1988;78 (Suppl II):II492.
24. Dec GW, Palacios I, Yasuda T, et al. Antimyosin antibody cardiac imaging: its role in the diagnosis of myocarditis. J Am Coll Cardiol 1990;16:97–104.

15. Thallium-201 myocardial imaging

ABDULMASSIH S. ISKANDRIAN and JAEKYEONG HEO

Summary

The important clinical applications of thallium-201 include: diagnosis of coronary artery disease, risk stratification, selection of patients for surgical or non-surgical revascularizations, follow-up of patients after interventions and assessment of myocardial viability. These will be discussed in this chapter.

Introduction

During the past two decades, considerable advances have been realized in the application of nuclear imaging to the study of myocardial perfusion and function [1–11]. This paper will address the current clinical role of thallium imaging in patient management.

Although this discussion will not deal with physics, pharmacokinetics, imaging techniques and protocols, several points need to be considered: 1) The regional myocardial thallium concentration is dependent upon regional blood flow, the extraction fraction, ratio of coronary blood flow to cardiac output, and the partial volume effect, which simply means that the true tissue concentration is underestimated if the thickness of a region is less than the resolution of the imaging system; 2) the sensitivity of exercise thallium imaging is superior to the sensitivity of exercise ECG in detecting coronary artery disease (CAD) (Table 1) [12–18]; 3) SPECT imaging is superior to planar imaging because of the lack of superimposition and overlap of normal and abnormal areas. The image quality is also better (Table 2) [19–25]; 4) the sensitivity of exercise thallium imaging is lower if exercise is submaximal, and is lower in patients with one-vessel disease than patients with multivessel disease [2,8].

It is important to indicate that the ability of angiography to determine the hemodynamic significance of stenosis is not optimal. The following discussion may be important to the understanding of the role of thallium imaging in patient management. Traditionally, the severity of coronary stenosis has been done visually based on percent diameter stenosis. This method is plagued by two problems; 1) considerable inter- and intra-observer variability and 2)

Johan H.C. Reiber & Ernst E. van der Wall (eds.), Cardiovascular Nuclear Medicine and MRI, 223–238.
© 1992 *Kluwer Academic Publishers.*

Table 1. Previous reports of planar exercise thallium imaging

	No. of patients		Sensitivity		Specificity		Accuracy	
	CAD	no CAD	ECG	Tl	ECG	Tl	ECG	Tl
Botviniek [12]	27	19	67	93	63	89	65	91
Boucher [13]	162	48	51	87	77	75	57	84
Corne [14]	26	20	58	81	65	90	61	85
Iskandrian [15]	98	96	49	80	52	96	80	88
Ritchie [16]	132	42	73	76	86	88	76	79
Turner [17]	34	30	71	68	79	97	75	82
Verani [18]	35	21	65	77	62	95	64	84

Abbreviations: CAD, coronary artery disease; ECG, exercise ECG testing; No., number; Tl, exercise thallium imaging.

more fundamentally, the problem is related to the inaccuracy of the percent diameter stenosis as a measure of hemodynamic significance of coronary stenosis, even when such a measurement is obtained quantitatively using calibers or computer-guided edge detection method. The limitation of percent diameter stenosis is at least in part attributed to variation in the caliber of normal arteries.

For these reasons, the minimal stenosis dimension (or area) may be a better predictor of the severity of stenosis than percent diameter (or area) stenosis. It should be remembered that a 50 % diameter stenosis represents a 75 % area stenosis. In fact, we and others have found a better correlation between stress thallium results (using count density ratios from the abnormal and normal zones) with minimal diameter stenosis (or minimal area stenosis) than with percent diameter (or area) stenosis [26]. These studies were obtained in patients with one-vessel disease and the stenosis dimensions were measured by calibers from two orthogonal projections. Other investigators have observed that the pressure gradient across the coronary stenosis measured at the time of angioplasty to be a better predictor of the results of the thallium imaging than the percent diameter stenosis [15].

The resistance at site of coronary stenosis is affected by several factors; it is directly proportional to the length of stenosis and inversely proportional

Table 2. Comparison between planar and SPECT thallium imaging

	Type	No. of patients		Sensitivity		Specificity		Accuracy	
		CAD	no CAD	Plan	Tomo	Plan	Tomo	Plan	Tomo
Fintel [19]	Ex	96	39	84	91	90	90	86	91
Maublant [20]	Rest	64	15	89	98	93	93	90	97
Nohara [21]	Ex	48	10	92	96	80	70	90	92
Prigent [22]	Ex	19	14	89	84	79	71	85	78
Ritchie [23]	Ex	38	15	63	87	93	93	71	87
Schmitt [24]	Ex	19	15	66	84	–	93	–	88
Tamaki [25]	Rest	160	39	78	96	92	92	81	95

Abbreviations: CAD, coronary artery disease; Ex, exercise thallium imaging; No., number; Plan, planar technique; Tomo, tomographic technique; Rest, rest thallium imaging.

to the fourth power of the minimal stenosis dimension, it is also affected by the blood viscosity and possibly by the entrance and exit angles of the stenosis. Multiple stenoses are likely to have an additive effect. The resistance also increases as a function of flow and recent observations suggest that vasomotor changes at the stenosis site do occur and may contribute to the severity of stenosis. These principles are based on a stenosis model which is eccentric, implying the presence of the normal segment of an arterial wall. The modulator for the vasomotor changes is thought to be an endothelial dependent relaxing factor (EDRP), which is present in normal, but not in atherosclerotic areas. For example, in normal arteries an increase in flow results in an increase in EDRP and vasodilation of the artery. On the other hand, exercise in patients with CAD tends to augment the stenosis. Small thrombi may also add to the degree of stenosis. Finally when the coronary flow increases due to a decrease in distal resistance such as by pharmacologic vasodilatation, the pressure gradient across the stenosis increases; the lower distal pressure may result in a collapse of the segment at the stenosis site and hence an increase in stenosis severity.

One method to assess the hemodynamic significance of coronary stenosis is measurement of the coronary blood flow. This is now possible using a small sized doppler catheter at the time of coronary angiography. Maximal coronary vasodilatation with papaverine or adenosine has shown augmentation in the coronary blood flow in the range of 3–6 fold greater than the resting flow. The hyperemic flow decreases with increasing severity of coronary stenosis. The ratio between the peak flow and the resting flow, so-called 'reserve flow ratio' can be altered by either increasing the resting flow or decreasing the peak flow. An increase in the resting flow is seen in patients with left ventricular hypertrophy (due to pressure or volume overload), because of an increase in myocardial oxygen demand. A shift of the peak flow to the right (i.e. a decrease) is seen in patients with left ventricular hypertrophy, tachycardia, anemia, etc. The reserve flow ratio is also sensitive to changes in the coronary perfusion pressure; a decrease in pressure results in a decrease in the flow ratio. The reserve flow ratio is also different in subendocardial and sub-epicardial layers of the myocardium. This is especially true in patients with CAD, where autoregulation results in exhaustion of the reserve mechanism in the endocardial layer before the epicardial layer. It should also be mentioned that using coronary flow doppler catheter, flow velocity rather than flow is being measured, and unless the coronary dimension remains unchanged, changes in flow velocity may not directly represent actual flow changes. The doppler technique obviously cannot measure the contribution of collateral flow. Other methods of measuring the coronary blood flow, such as thermodilution, DSA, inert gas technique and positron emission tomography do not measure transmural flow variations or collateral flow [27].

In summary, coronary angiography may be an accepted 'gold standard' for assessing the presence or absence of coronary stenosis, but it has important

Table 3. Clinical application of thallium imaging in Coronary Artery Disease (CAD)

(1) Diagnosis of presence and extent of CAD.
(2) Diagnosis of mild or early CAD.
(3) Diagnosis of progression and regression of CAD.
(4) Assessment of viability.
(5) Risk stratification.
(6) Applications in acute myocardial infarction.
(7) Applications after percutaneous transluminal coronary angioplasty.
(8) Applications after coronary artery bypass surgery.

problems in assessing the hemodynamic significance of stenosis in many situations. The nuclear techniques may provide the link between the coronary anatomy and physiology.

The clinical applications of thallium imaging are summarized in Table 3. The recent approval by the Food and Drug Administration in U.S.A. of two technetium labelled perfusion agents: Cardiolite® (SestaMIBI) and Cardio-Tec® (Teboroxime) may quite well change the uses of thallium imaging in one or more of the listed indications. Any discussion comparing the three imaging agents is beyond the scope of this presentation.

Diagnosis of coronary artery disease (CAD)

The diagnosis of CAD in most patients can be reliably made by careful clinical assessment; roughly 90 % of patients with typical angina pectoris have CAD, while 90 % of patients with non-anginal chest pains and 50 % of patients with atypical angina pectoris have CAD. The demographics, coronary risk factors and family history of premature atherosclerosis are helpful markers for establishing the diagnosis. Treadmill exercise testing produces inconclusive results in 30 %–40 % of patients due to submaximal stress or baseline electrocardiographic changes. It has a low sensitivity of 50 %–60 %, is unable to predict the individual diseased artery or arteries, or to quantify the extent of CAD, and to assess myocardial viability. Major advantages of thallium imaging include a higher sensitivity, an ability to localize the site of the disease, and to assess the extent of the CAD and myocardial viability.

Should an exercise test be done in every patient with suspected CAD? And what type? In patients with a high pretest probability of CAD and stable symptoms, an exercise study is indicated, not for diagnosis, but to assess the extent of the perfusion abnormality which is a strong predictor of prognosis. In such patients, exercise thallium imaging is preferred over exercise treadmill testing alone. It should be recognized that the presence or absence of angina during exercise (symptomatic vs silent ischemia) is not a useful marker, either of the extent of the CAD or the extent and severity of thallium abnormality [1–11].

In patients with a low pretest probability of CAD, exercise testing may

Table 4. Indications for thallium imaging in percutaneous transluminal coronary angioplasty

(1) Patient selection
(2) Assessment of immediate results.
(3) Assessment of residual coronary artery disease.
(4) Assessment of re-stenosis.
(5) Assessment of myocardial viability.

not be necessary, but if it is done, treadmill exercise testing alone is sufficient. If the test result is negative, no further testing is necessary. However, if the test is positive or equivocal, or the exercise is submaximal, then exercise thallium imaging is required. In patients with intermediate pretest probability of CAD, stress thallium imaging is preferred not only to make the diagnosis, but also to assess the extent of CAD. In patients with normal thallium images, but with submaximal exercise, dipyridamole or adenosine thallium imaging is suggested if the pretest probability is intermediate or high. In patients with pre-existing baseline electrocardiographic changes, such as left bundle branch block, S-T segment depression, pacemaker rhythm and pre-excitation syndrome, exercise testing with thallium-201 is preferred. In patients who are not candidates for exercise testing, pharmacologic testing is suggested. Also in patients with left bundle branch block, pharmacologic testing with thallium-201 may be preferred.

Percutaneous transluminal coronary angioplasty (PTCA)

The indications of thallium imaging in patients undergoing PTCA are summarized in Table 4. In 1989, there were more PTCA procedures done in U.S. than coronary artery bypass grafting (CABG). Compared to ten years ago, PTCA is now being done in patients with multi-vessel disease, unstable angina and acute myocardial infarction. The technical advances in the field have been enormous and have included the use of better designed stearing wires, balloons, catheters, angioscopy, intracoronary ultrasound, laser, atherectomy, and stents to mention only few!

In patients with one-vessel disease, objective evidence of ischemia is important, especially in patients with stable symptoms or in patients in whom the hemodynamic significance of the coronary stenosis is not certain by coronary angiography (see previous discussion). In patients with multi-vessel disease, the need is even greater, because it is essential to prove that ischemia is present in the territory of the vessel considered for angioplasty.

A major problem in PTCA continues to be the high rate of re-stenosis which is estimated to be 30 %–50 %. In most patients, re-stenosis appears within six months, but not all re-stenoses are associated with recurrence of symptoms. Sudden occlusion is the complication most feared, especially in an artery that provides flow to a substantial area of the myocardium. Re-stenosis can not be predicted from the pre-PTCA or even the post-PTCA angiograms. The definition of re-stenosis also is subject to controversy. Some re-stenoses may actually be examples of incomplete dilatation. Several trials using a variety of medications or interventions – such as calcium blockers, nitrates, anticoagulants, antiplatelet agents, steroids, etc. – have not been helpful in decreasing the incidence of re-stenosis [28–30].

Post-PTCA stress testing (exercise or pharmacologic) has been done to predict re-stenosis. The presence of ischemia in these scans suggests the presence of re-stenosis; the lack of ischemia predicts patency of the artery. Scintigraphic results have been more sensitive and specific than the ECG changes or symptoms.

The optimal timing for such studies is unknown. It has been suggested that early after PTCA (within two weeks), peak reactive coronary blood flow is still subnormal, despite patency of the artery. The precise reason is unknown, but may be related to changes in autoregulation in microcirculation. As a corollary to that, some patients with patent arteries have abnormal thallium images early after PTCA. It has therefore been recommended that such studies should be postponed to approximately four weeks after PTCA. Some of these abnormal results may in fact be due to inadequate dilatation. It is often very difficult to determine the degree of residual stenosis from the angiographic appearance of the vessel, because of the presence of local dissection, eccentricity of the lesion and the presence of clots. We suspect that an early positive scan is a marker of incomplete dilatation and a predictor of re-stenosis. Hecht et al. found that exercise SPECT thallium imaging to be almost 90 % accurate in predicting re-stenosis or progression of disease in other vessels in 116 patients with previous PTCA [31]. These are remarkably excellent results. Since the tracer (thallium) concentration is flow dependent, quantitative assessment of the tracer uptake in normal and abnormal areas may be used in serial studies as a marker of progression of re-stenosis. Such studies may be more suitable with Cardiolite® or CardioTec®, because of the higher energy and better image contrast obtained with these agents. However, the lower extraction fraction of SestaMIBI at high flow rates may be a problem for quantitative assessment. This problem is not present with teboroxime which has an extraction ratio of over 90 % even at high flow rates. An algorithm for the use of thallium to predict re-stenosis is shown in Fig. 1.

Coronary artery bypass surgery (CABG)

In 1990, over 300,000 patients underwent CABG in USA. There is an initial 10–15 % re-occlusion rate of the grafts and after 5 years many patients have recurrence of symptoms, either due to graft closure or progression of the disease in the native arteries. The patency of the internal mammary artery graft is better than patency of the vein grafts. Further, patency of the vein grafts is better if grafted in arteries with good distal runoff than in arteries

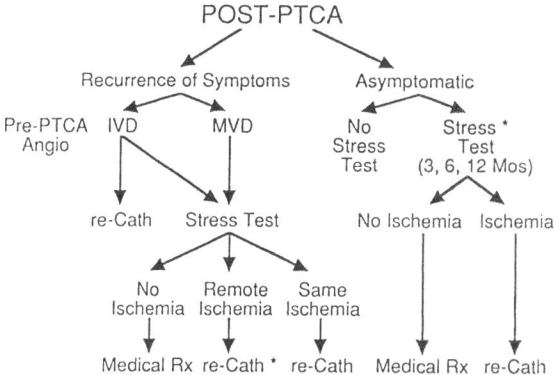

Figure 1. The algorithm for follow-up after PTCA.

with poor runoff. Treatment with aspirin (with and without dipyridamole) improves patency rate, while diabetes mellitus, hyperlipidemia, hypertension and smoking accelerate the rate of graft closure. As the number of PTCA is increasing, the patients who undergo CABG are older, sicker, have worse left ventricular function and more extensive CAD.

The recurrence of symptoms in patients after CABG requires the use of perfusion studies to determine the presence, location and the extent of the abnormality. The exercise ECG is often not helpful, further, these patients do not readily accept the idea of recatheterization. In patients with normal perfusion images or only mild abnormality, conservative management is satisfactory. On the other hand, for patients with large areas of ischemia, re-catheterization is necessary. Some of these patients may be candidates for laser angioplasty or PTCA of the vein graft, re-CABG or medical therapy depending on coronary anatomy. Laser angioplasty of the vein grafts has a very high initial success rate.

In our experience, radionuclide angiography during exercise has also provided important prognostic data in patients with previous CABG. The exercise left ventricular ejection fraction is a powerful predictor of the risk of cardiac events in these patients. Patients with normal exercise ejection fraction have a very low event rate, while the event rate (cardiac death or nonfatal myocardial infarction) increases proportionally as the exercise ejection fraction decreases. These results, therefore, appear to be very similar to patients without CABG [32].

The indications of thallium imaging in CABG are summarized in Table 5. In addressing recurrence of symptoms after CABG, one should consider completeness of revascularization (from the pre-operative coronary angiogram and the surgical note), the distal runoff (from the pre-operative angiogram), surgical skill, the number of grafts, the time elapsed since surgery,

Table 5. Indications of thallium imaging in conary artery bypass grafting

(1) Patient selection.
(2) Assessment of completeness of revascularization.
(3) Assessment of peri-operative infarction.
(4) Assessment of viability.
(5) Assessment of patients with recurrence of symptoms.

the pre-operative left ventricular function, the presence of peri-operative infarction and nature of symptoms. For example, in a patient with diffuse disease, poor distal runoff and incomplete revascularization, recurrence of symptoms is likely to be due to myocardial ischemia. On the other hand, in the case of a patient who had one vessel disease with excellent distal runoff and who had a mammary artery implantation, the recurrence of symptoms shortly after surgery is less likely to be due to myocardial ischemia.

In interpreting the thallium results, the conventional method of data reporting is not ideal or practical because of the multiple possibilities of diseases in the native arteries and grafts. A patient may have a patent graft, yet incomplete revascularization in that territory. For example, a patient with a patent graft to the left anterior descending artery, but an occluded graft to the diagonal branch. We suggest the use of 'complete revascularization', 'partial revascularization' and 'inadequate revascularization' for each of the three vascular territories (Fig. 2). Complete revascularization indicates either a normal vascular territory that requires no bypass grafting, or a diseased vessel with a patent graft (and no residual disease in the vessel or its branches). Partial revascularization indicates a disease in either the native artery or a graft in that vascular territory, provided the presence of at least another patent branch or another patent graft. Inadequate revascularization indicates the presence of native disease that could not be grafted or occluded graft (or grafts) within that vascular territory. We also suggest that the pre-operative angiogram and surgical report should be evaluated in addition to the thallium results. If the thallium abnormality, for example, shows ischemia in the territory of the left anterior descending artery and the pre-operative angiogram reveals that the distal left anterior descending artery had a good runoff, then a repeat angiography will be necessary because of the feasibility of re-revascularization (in the symptomatic patient). On the other hand, if the distal runoff of the left anterior descending artery was very poor, accounting for the graft closure, then angiography may not be necessary because re-revascularization is not ideal. Also, in patients who have recurrence of symptoms within two years after surgery, the most likely reason is graft occlusion or incomplete revascularization. In patients who have recurrence of symptoms five years or more after surgery, graft occlusion or progression of disease in previously normal or mildly diseased vessels may contribute to the recurrence of symptoms.

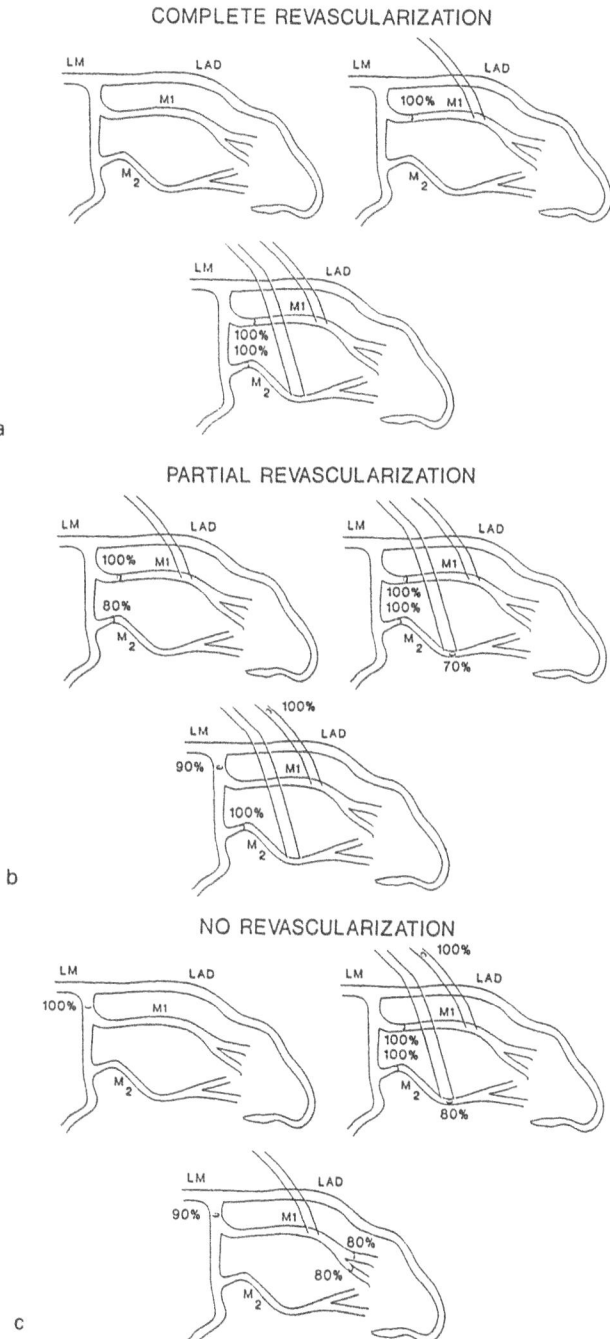

Figure 2. Examples of complete, partial and incomplete revascularization of the left circumflex artery.

Acute myocardial infarction (MI)

There are several reasons for nuclear imaging in acute MI; 1) diagnosis, 2) assessment of risk, 3) assessment of extent, 4) assessment of myocardial salvage after thrombolytic therapy. In most patients with acute MI, the diagnosis can be made using conventional methods of history, ECG and CK-MB iso-enzyme changes.

It should be noted that a rest perfusion defect seen on thallium (or Cardiolite®) image could be due to a recent infarction, old infarction, or severe ischemia. A redistribution image obtained 4 hours after the initial study may help determine the nature of the abnormality as reversible or fixed. Imaging with Tc-99m pyrophosphate or In-111 antimyosin antibody is more specific for the diagnosis of the acute MI than thallium imaging.

The determinants of prognosis after acute MI are: 1) left ventricular ejection fraction which by itself depends on the degree of myocardial necrosis. We have observed that the size of thallium abnormality in rest images is an excellent prognostic predictor [33], 2) residual ischemia in the infarct area or remote area which depends on the presence of residual stenosis or multi-vessel disease respectively, 3) the presence of ventricular arrhythmias. A consistent observation from thrombolytic trials is that the prognosis is better in patients treated with thrombolytic therapy, regardless of the thrombolytic agent. This finding has been observed even when there has been no significant improvement in left ventricular function! Improvement is often confined to patients in whom thrombolytic therapy resulted in recanalization. Therefore, the use of thrombolytic therapy may be an additional factor that should be added to the predictors of prognosis.

Stress thallium imaging using a submaximal exercise or pharmacologic testing with dipyridamole or adenosine are now increasingly being used for risk stratification. Other techniques for risk assessment include pre-discharge coronary angiography, exercise echocardiography, exercise radionuclide angiography and echocardiographic testing during dobutamine infusion [34].

The exercise study is either done at a sub-maximal level before hospital discharge or with maximal exercise 4–6 weeks after discharge. The arguments have been: 1) maximal exercise is more likely to elicit abnormal response than submaximal exercise, but may carry a higher risk when done shortly after acute MI, 2) most events occur in the first few weeks after MI and therefore early exercise can identify high risk patients who might otherwise die before undergoing maximal exercise. Some have therefore suggested the use of two exercise tests, a pre-discharge submaximal and a post-discharge maximal. There is yet another school of thought that a symptom-limited exercise can be done safely before patient discharge without additional risk, if patient selection is optimized to exclude patients with post-infarction angina, rest angina, congestive heart failure or malignant ventricular arrhythmias. It is in this context also that dipyridamole or adenosine thallium imaging has been used as early as two days after infarction to determine the presence of ischemia in the infarct zone and remote zones. The potential drawback from pharmacologic testing may be that some of the exercise variables which may have meaningful impact on patient management and prognosis are not available. These include the degree of S-T depression, blood pressure response, exercise heart rate, and exercise workload. It should however, be noted that the most important prognostic data appear to be derived from the perfusion or the ventricular function studies. The exercise treadmill data appear to provide much less important additional information. Comparison of pharmacologic studies and exercise studies to predict prognosis after acute MI have only been available in a small series of patients and both appear to be comparable, but more studies are necessary.

When one looks upon the events after MI, these events appear to be similar to those seen in patients with stable CAD, and they include hard events, such as death or recurrent MI or soft events, such as the development of unstable angina, and the need for PTCA or CABG. The common denominator for these events is the presence of ischemia and left ventricular function. Therefore, it is not surprising that perfusion imaging is better than ECG in risk assessment, and that the presence of ischemia, the extent of ischemia, and the extent of scar are reliable predictors of future events. These have been confirmed in virtually all studies. The bottom line from such a strategy is that patients after MI can be categorized into different risk groups. In the low risk group, a conservative management is sufficient, while in the high risk group, predischarge catheterization is necessary to select the patients for either PTCA or CABG. In the intermediate group of patients, the decision making process is more difficult, and should take into consideration other factors, such as patient's age, life style, etc. Needless to say, risk stratification using predischarge nuclear techniques is more cost effective than routine cardiac catheterization.

Risk stratification

Lessons learned from thrombolytic therapy suggest that 40 % of patients with acute MI may have sub-critical stenosis in one coronary artery after thrombolysis. The final event in these patients is coronary thrombosis. It is also clear that as high risk patients are identified and considered for surgical or nonsurgical revascularization, the remaining patients have only low or intermediate risk, which means that a larger number of patients and a longer follow-up period are necessary to determine the prognostic predictors in these patients. One can even suggest that in patients with sub-critical stenosis, none of the techniques may be applicable for risk stratification because these patients will fail to reveal evidence of ischemia on exercise testing. Nevertheless, the discussion to follow will be important to the understanding of how to interpret the results and data from exercise studies that deal with risk assessment [35].

Table 6. Thallium-201 predictors of risk of future cardiac events in medically treated patients with stable symptoms

(1) Presence of redistribution (reversible defects).
(2) Extent of ischemia.
(3) Extent of perfusion deficit (reversible and fixed).
(4) Severity of perfusion deficit.
(5) Increased lung thallium uptake.
(6) Number of vascular territories with abnormal thallium uptake.
(7) Left ventricular dilation during exercise.

It has been observed, however, that there is considerable variability in the extent of perfusion deficit in relation to anatomic severity of CAD. It is possible that the use of more precise measurements of coronary stenosis may tighten the observed correlation between coronary anatomy and physiologic assessment. Nevertheless, the above finding may explain the independent and complementary prognostic value of nuclear imaging techniques to coronary angiography.

During exercise the ischemic burden is primarily due to increased myo-cardial oxygen demand in the presence of a limited ability to augment the coronary blood flow. On the other hand, acute events such as cardiac death or nonfatal acute MI are primarily due to sudden interruption of coronary blood flow due to thrombus occlusion. The relationship between these two models, which results in demand/supply imbalance, is not well understood. The human model of transient coronary occlusion during PTCA is ideally suited to test this relationship using first-pass radionuclide angiography or thallium-201 imaging.

Thallium-201 derived variables shown to be important in risk stratification are listed in Table 6 [34]. To understand the use of clinical models in risk stratification, the issues shown in Table 7 need to be considered briefly. Studies with a large sample size and a large number of hard events (death and nonfatal MI) have more relevance than those with a small sample size and soft events (increasing angina pectoris, development of unstable angina, and the need for delayed coronary revascularization). Since CAD is a progressive disease, and since patients are followed-up on a regular basis, man-

Table 7. Appraisal of clinical prediction models

(1) Definition of events.
(2) Sample size.
(3) Number of events.
(4) Follow-up period.
(5) Presentation of results.
(6) Nature of variables analyzed.
(7) Method of statistical analysis.
(8) Low risk vs high risk.
(9) Patient selection.
(10) Clinical application.

agement strategies may change depending on the evolution of symptoms. Thus clinical models to be relevant should show differences in survival at 1 and 2 years; differences evident at 5 to 7 years only may be statistically significant but clinically irrelevant as they assume no progression or regression in the CAD and no change in exercise physiology.

The presentation of the data may at times be confusing and misleading. For example, assume there are two groups, each of 100 patients, and that at 1 year there were two deaths in group 1 and one death in group 2. These results represent a 1 % change in survival but a 50 %–100 % change in mortality! The performance of a model depends on the nature of the variables included in that model. For example, the age and history of previous MI are likely to be important risk factors on a univariate analysis, but if the model includes extent of CAD and left ventricular ejection fraction, the information by age and history of MI may not appear on a multivariate analysis, but that does not mean these factors are not important.

The Cox proportional hazard regression model is the preferred statistical method to express the results in prognostic models. However, when several factors are close to each other in univariate importance, the results of the multivariate analysis may be somewhat dependent on a few individual patients. A cross-validation (or 'bootstrapping') procedure for selection of independent variables should be considered. If repeat samples of a study population show the same consistent ranking of importance for the variables, the results should be strengthened. In a cost-conscious era, the cost of identifying a few additional patients should also be considered. In general, our ability to identify patients at low risk is better than our ability to determine patients at intermediate or high risk. Also, the group at the highest risk may constitute only a small subgroup of patients with a small number of events compared with the total number of patients and total events. Patient selection is important, not only in the interpretation of the results, but also in terms of their clinical application. If medically treated patients were selected on the basis of mild or inoperable CAD, the results would be irrelevant to most patients with CAD. Finally, mean group data cannot be translated to the management of an individual patient with a given problem.

Intuitively, the presence of myocardial ischemia (regardless of the size) may predispose to subsequent MI. It can even be argued that subcritical coronary stenosis with no evidence of ischemia may also be a harbinger of subsequent MI, since the final event in such patients is coronary thrombosis. Death, on the other hand, suggests a large MI or life-threatening ventricular arrhythmia that may be dependent on myocardial scar (with or without ischemia). Thus the presence of redistribution on thallium scans may be predictors of nonfatal MI, while the total perfusion abnormality may be a better predictor of death. The relative numbers of these two events in any sample may determine the relative importance of one or the other of these variables.

It is worth mentioning that there has been a notable decline in the use of rest/exercise radionuclide angiography in the past few years because of the recognition that diseases other than CAD may result in abnormal EF response. The newer technetium-labeled imaging agents can provide both perfusion and function information, and may therefore revive the interest in the use of first-pass radionuclide angiography. At the present time there are no sufficient data to suggest which of the two tests (thallium-201 or radionuclide angiography) is the method of choice in risk stratification. The results of thallium imaging are often interpreted subjectively, and quantitative data are not uniformly adopted, although a recent technique using the bull's-eye polar maps appears to be promising.

Myocardial viability

Detailed discussion of assessment of myocardial viability with thallium imaging is beyond the scope of this paper, but we now routinely use the reinjection technique in obtaining the delayed images. This in our experience, as well as those of others has decreased the prevalence of apparent fixed defects [36].

Acknowledgements

The authors would like to thank Barbara Clayton for preparing the manuscript.

References

1. Iskandrian AS. Thallium-201 myocardial imaging and radionuclide ventrioculography: theory, technical considerations, and interpretation. In: Iskandrian AS. Nuclear cardiac imaging: principles and applications. Philadelphia: F.A. Davis, 1986;81–161.
2. Iskandrian AS, Heo J, Kong B, Lyons E. Effect of exercise level on the ability of thallium-201 tomographic imaging in detecting coronary artery disease: analysis of 461 patients (see comments). J Am Coll Cardiol 1989;14:1477–86. Comment in: J Am Coll Cardiol 1989;14:1487–90.
3. Iskandrian AS, Heo J, Askenase A, Segal BL, Auerbach N. Dipyridamole cardiac imaging. Am Heart J 1988;115:432–43.
4. Iskandrian AS, Heo J, Kong B, Lyons E, Marsch S. Use of technetium-99m isonitrile (RP-30A) in assessing left ventricular perfusion and function at rest and during exercise in coronary artery disease, and comparison with coronary arteriography and exercise thallium-201 SPECT imaging. Am J Cardiol 1989;64:270–5.
5. Iskandrian AS, Heo J, Askenase A, Segal BL, Helfant RH. Thallium imaging with single photon emission computed tomography. Am Heart J 1987;114:852–65.
6. Iskandrian AS, Lichtenberg R, Segal BL, et al. Assessment of jeopardized myocardium in patients with one-vessel disease. Circulation 1982;65:242–7.
7. Iskandrian AS, Heo J, DeCoskey D, Askenase A, Segal BL. Use of thallium-201 imaging

for risk stratification of elderly patients with coronary artery disease. Am J Cardiol 1988;61:269–72.

8. Iskandrian AS, Hakki AH, Kane-Marsch S. Prognostic implications of exercise thallium-201 scintigraphy in patients with suspected or known coronary artery disease. Am Heart J 1985;110:135–43.

9. Iskandrian AS, Hakki AH, Goel IP, Mundth ED, Kane-Marsch SA, Schenk CL. The use of rest and exercise radionuclide ventriculography in risk stratification in patients with suspected coronary artery disease. Am Heart J 1985;110:864–72.

10. Iskandrian AS, Hakki AH. Thallium-201 myocardial scintigraphy. Am Heart J 1985;109:113–29.

11. Nguyen T, Heo J, Ogilby D, Iskandrian AS. Single photon emission computed tomography with thallium-201 during adenosine-induced coronary hyperemia: correlation with coronary arteriography, exercise thallium imaging and two-dimensional echocardiography (see comments). J Am Coll Cardiol 1990;16:1375–83. Comment in: J Am Coll Cardiol 1990;16:1384–6.

12. Botvinick EH, Taradesh MR, Shames DM, Parmley WW. Thallium-201 myocardial perfusion scintigraphy for the clinical classification of normal, abnormal and equivocal electrocardiographic stress tests. Am J Cardiol 1978;41:43–51.

13. Boucher CA, Zir LM, Beller GA, et al. Increased lung uptake of thallium-201 during exercise myocardial imaging: clinical, hemodynamic and angiographic implications in patients with coronary artery disease. Am J Cardiol 1980;46:189–96.

14. Corne RA, Gotsman MS, Weiss A, et al. Thallium-201 scintigraphy in diagnosis of coronary stenosis. Comparison with electrocardiography and coronary arteriography. Br He rt J 1979;41:575–83.

15. Iskandrian AS, Segal BL. Value of exercise thallium-201 imaging in patients with diagi ustic and nondiagnostic exercise electrocardiograms. Am J Cardiol 1981;48:233–8.

16. Ritchie JL, Trobaugh GB, Hamilton GW, et al. Myocardial imaging with thallium-201 at rest and during exercise: comparison with coronary arteriography and resting and stress electrocardiography. Circulation 1977;56:66–71.

17. Turner DA, Bettle NE, Deshmukh H, et al. The predictive value of myocardial perfusion scintigraphy after stress in patients without previous myocardial infarction. J Nucl Med 1978;19:249–55.

18. Verani MS, Marcus ML, Razzak MA, Erhardt JC. Sensitivity and specificity of thallium-201 perfusion scintigrams under exercise in the diagnosis of coronary artery disease. J Nucl Med 1978;19:773–82.

19. Fintel DJ, Links JM, Brinker JA, Frank TL, Parker M, Becker LC. Improved diagnostic performance of exercise thallium-201 single photon emission computed tomography over planar imaging in the diagnosis of coronary artery disease: a receiver operating characteristic analysis. J Am Coll Cardiol 1989;13:600–12.

20. Maublant J, Cassagnes J, Jeune JJ, et al. A comparison between conventional scintigraphy and emission tomography with thallium-201 in the detection of myocardial infarction: concise communication. J Nucl Med 1982;23:204–8.

21. Nohara R, Kambara H, Suzuki Y, et al. Stress scintigraphy using single-photon emission computed tomography in the evaluation of coronary artery disease. Am J Cardiol 1984;53:1250–4.

22. Prigent F, Friedman J, Maddahi J, et al. Comparison of rotational tomography with planar imaging for thallium-201 stress myocardial scintigraphy, (abstract). J Nucl Med 1983;24:p18.

23. Ritchie JL, Williams DL, Harp G, Stratton JL, Caldwell JH. Transaxial tomography with thallium-201 for detecting remote myocardial infarction. Comparison with planar imaging. Am J Cardiol 1982;50:1236–41.

24. Schmitt JM, Ritchie JL, Hamilton GW, Harp GD, Williams DL. Thallium-201 exercise tomography in the diagnosis of jeopardized myocardium. Am Heart Assoc Monogr 1982:II-149.

25. Tamaki S, Kambara H, Kadota K, et al. Improved detection of myocardial infarction by

emission computed tomography with thallium-201. Relation to infarct size. Br Heart J 1984;52:621–7.

26. Hadjimiltiades S, Watson R, Hakki AH, Heo J, Iskandrian AS. Relation between myocardial thallium-201 kinetics during exercise and quantitative coronary angiography in patients with one vessel coronary artery disease. J Am Coll Cardiol 1989;13:1301–8.

27. Demer L, Gould KL, Kirkeeide R. Assessing stenosis severity: coronary flow reserve, collateral functional, quantitative coronary arteriography, positron imaging, and digital subtraction angiography. A review and analysis. Prog Cardiovasc Dis 1988;30:307–22.

28. Waller BF, 'Crackers, breakers, stretchers, drillers, scrapers, shavers, burners, welders and melters' –The future treatment of atherosclerotic coronary artery disease? A clinical-morphologic assessment. J Am Coll Cardiol 1989;5:969–87.

29. Topol EJ, Emerging strategies for failed percutaneous transluminal coronary angioplasty. Am J Cardiol 1989;63:249–50.

30. Myler RK, Stertzer SH, Cumberland DC, Webb JG, Shaw RE: Coronary angioplasty: Indictions, contraindications, and limitations. J Intervent Cardiol 1990;2:179–85.

31. Hecht HS, Shaw RE, Bruce TR, Ryan C, Stertzer SH, Myler RK. Usefulness of tomographic thallium-201 imaging for detection of restenosis after percutaneous transluminal coronary angioplasty. Am J Cardiol 1990;66:1314–8.

32. Iskandrian AS, Hakki AH, Schwartz JS, Kay H, Mattleman S, Kane S. Prognostic implications of rest and exercise radionuclide ventriculography in patients with suspected or proven coronary heart disease. Int J Cardiol 1984;6:707–18.

33. Hakki AH, Nestico PF, Heo J, Unwala AA, Iskandrian AS. Relative prognostic value of rest thallium-201 imaging, radionuclide ventriculography and 24 hour ambulatory electrocardiographic monitoring after acute myocardial infarction. J Am Coll Cardiol 1987;10:25–32.

34. Brown KA. Prognostic value of thallium-201 myocardial perfusion imaging. A diagnostic tool comes of age. Circulation 1991;83:363–81.

35. Iskandrian AS. Appraisal of clinical models based on results of stress nuclear imaging in risk stratification. Am Heart J 1990;120:1487–90.

36. Iskandrian AS, Heo J, Nguyen T, et al. Assessment of coronary artery disease using single-photon emission computed tomography with thallium-201 during adenosine-induced coronary hyperemia. Am J Cardiol 1991;67:1190–4.

16. Tc-99m SestaMIBI: Will it replace Tl-201 in clinical cardiology?

FRANS J.Th. WACKERS

Summary

The development of technetium-99m (Tc-99m) labeled agents is a significant advance in myocardial perfusion imaging.

Worldwide, thousands of patients have been studied with Tc-99m Sesta-MIBI. There is a general consensus that as far as detection of coronary artery disease is concerned, this new perfusion imaging agent compares well with Tl-201 (better than 80 % agreement), employing either physical exercise or pharmacological vasodilatation. There is some concern about the lower extraction fraction of Tc-99m SestaMIBI (60 %) compared to that of Tl-201 (80 %). However at the present time it is unclear whether this difference is of clinical relevance. Because of the relatively high dose that can be administered, left ventricular function can be evaluated simultaneously by either first pass ejection fraction or ECG-gated regional wall motions studies. A unique application of Tc-99m SestaMIBI imaging is in patients with acute myocardial infarction. Because of the lack of significant redistribution, this imaging agent can be employed to assess the area at risk prior to initiation of thrombolytic therapy and later to assess the size of infarction as well as the extent of myocardial salvage. Myocardial imaging in this setting has been useful to predict patency of the infarct related artery.

Recent experimental data indicate that Tc-99m SestaMIBI may not only be an indicator of myocardial blood flow, but also an indicator of myocardial viability. In conclusion, Tc-99m SestaMIBI provides: 1) better quality images; 2) is better suited for SPECT imaging; 3) allows first-pass assessment left ventricular ejection fraction, and 4) assessment of regional wall motion by ECG-gated images. Clinical applications include; detection of 5) coronary artery disease and 6) myocardial ischemia by either physical exercise or pharmacological vasodilatation. Furthermore, 7) assessment of risk area of coronary occlusion and 8) assessment of ultimate size of infarction are both possible.

Introduction

The recent development of technetium-99m (Tc-99m) labeled myocardial perfusion imaging agents constitutes a significant advance in scintigraphic

Johan H.C. Reiber & Ernst E. van der Wall (eds.), Cardiovascular Nuclear Medicine and MRI, 239–248.
© 1992 *Kluwer Academic Publishers.*

imaging of the heart [1,2]. Although Tl-201 has been used for over 15 years with remarkable clinical success, this imaging agent has several physical characteristics that make it suboptimal for clinical imaging. The relatively long half-life of Tl-201 limits the dose of radionuclide that can be administered to 2–3 mCi per study. This results in suboptimal count density of Tl-201 images. In addition, Tl-201 images are substantially degraded by low energy background scatter. In spite of these limitations the published literature indicates a high diagnostic yield for detection of coronary artery disease by planar and tomographic (SPECT) Tl-201 imaging. Moreover, important prognostic information can be derived from Tl-201 stress images. It is realistic to state that these reports represent the best possible results in the hands of the most experienced investigators. In reality, many laboratories may not be capable of reproducing the same high quality images employing Tl-201. Consequently interpretation may fall short of achieving the same diagnostic accuracy as published in the literature. The inter and intraobserver variability of interpreting of Tl-201 images has been shown to vary considerably among various readers ranging from good to unacceptably low in certain instances. The *confidence* with which an image is interpreted is directly related to the *quality* of that image. Dissatisfied with the suboptimal quality of planar Tl-201 images and the realization that planar imaging is limited by superimposition and overlap of myocardial segments, many nuclear physicians turned in the mid-1980s to rotational tomographic or SPECT imaging. The more sophisticated image processing and display seemed a solution to the problems with planar imaging. This conversion was part irrational, since count density on Tl-201 SPECT images was usually *not* better, but rather the same or more frequently worse than that of planar Tl-201 images. Paradoxically, because of extensive filtering and more sophisticated image display, SPECT slices *appear* to be of better quality because of higher contrast, and seem to be easier to interpret than Tl-201 images. Although overlapping myocardial segments are well separated by reconstructed SPECT slices, the resolution of SPECT Tl-201 image is less than that of planar images (19 mm vs 12 mm).

Image quality

Employing technetium-99m labeled myocardial perfusion imaging agents 10–30 mCi of radioactivity can be administered per study, resulting in excellent count density, both in planar images and SPECT images (Figs. 1 and 2). Worldwide, thousands of patients have been studied with Tc-99m SestaMIBI. Initial validation studies indicated that sensitivity and specificity of rest exercise Tc-99m SestaMIBI imaging in patients with coronary artery disease is similar to that of Tl-201 [1–5]. Importantly, there is a general consensus that Tc-99m SestaMIBI images are of better quality and easier to interpret than those with Tl-201. Tc-99m SestaMIBI differs in several aspects from Tl-201. Although Tc-99m SestaMIBI is accumulated according to the distribution of

TI-201   **RP-30**

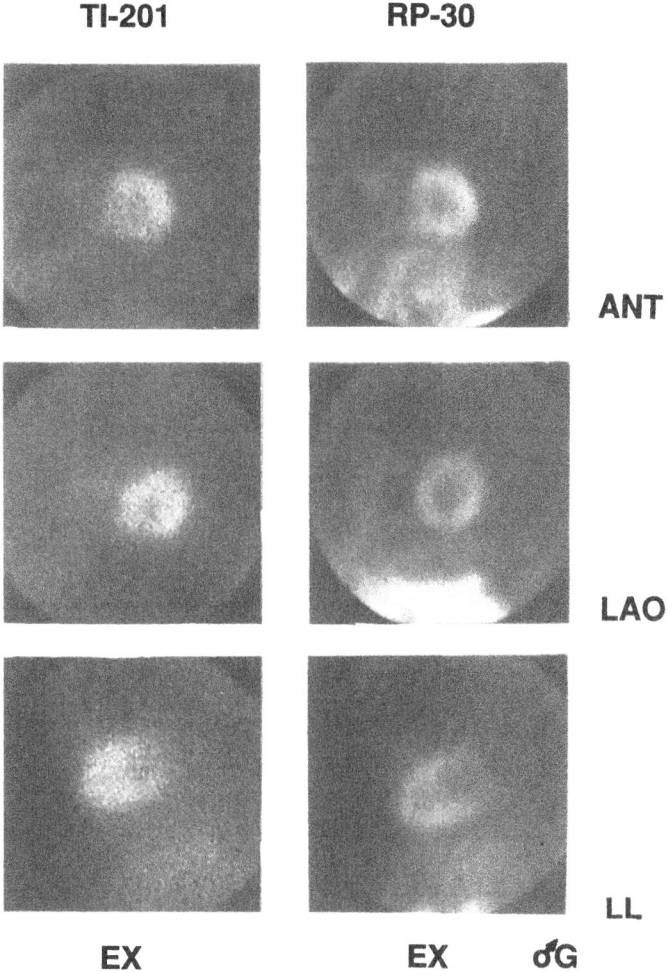

ANT

LAO

LL

EX   EX   ♂G

Figure 1. Thallium-201 (Tl-201) and Tc-99m SestaMIBI imaging (RP-30) after exercise in the same patient. Three views are shown, anterior (ANT) left anterior oblique (LAO), left lateral (LL). The better quality of the Tc-99m SestaMIBI images can be appreciated in comparison to the typical granular and fuzzy quality of Tl-201 images. The LAO and LL images are normal. The anterior views show reduced uptake in the inferoseptal area employing both agents.

regional myocardial blood flow [3], in contrast to Tl-201 no redistribution of significance occurs over time. The first-pass extraction fraction of Tc-99m is only 60 % compared to 80 % for Tl-201. This latter aspect of Tc-99m SestaM-IBI has been of some concern. It was feared initially that the relatively low extraction fraction might affect detection of small myocardial perfusion defects. However, clinical trials that compared Tl-201 with Tc-99m Sesta-MIBI in patients with coronary artery disease found no significant difference in the detection of significance coronary artery disease [1–5].

The superiority of Tc-99m SestaMIBI as an imaging agent is particularly

EX

R

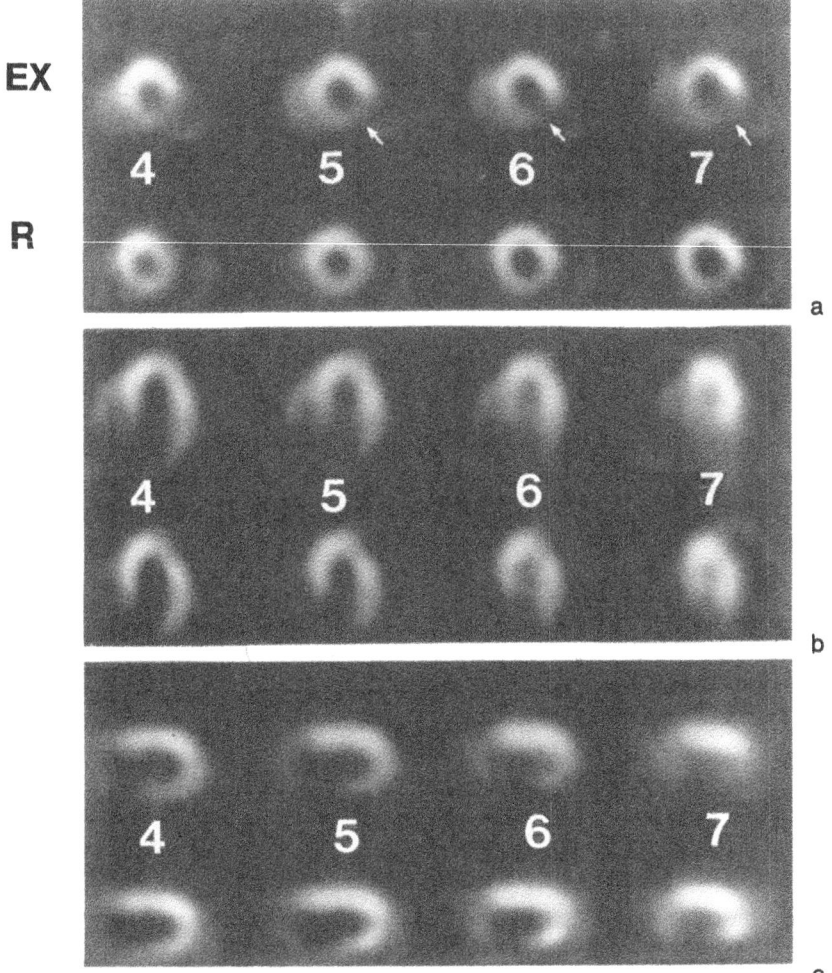

Figure 2. Tc-99m SestaMIBI SPECT images. (a) Short-axis slices; (b) horizontal long axis slices; (c) vertical long axis slices. After exercise (EX), an inferolateral defect is present which almost completely has normalized at rest (R). The high count density of these images can be appreciated.

striking when one compares Tl-201 and Tc-99m SestaMIBI tomography. Count density in Tc-99m SestaMIBI SPECT is approximately *four times higher* than with Tl-201. Moreover, considerably fewer problems with image artifacts appear to occur.

The relatively high dose of Tc-99m SestaMIBI that can be administered makes it feasible to combine evaluation of myocardial perfusion with *assessment of cardiac function*. This can be achieved in two ways: 1) the injection of the radiopharmaceutical can be utilized for first-pass radionuclide angiocardiography [6], 2) electrocardiographic synchronization or 'gating' of the perfusion images makes it possible to assess regional wall motion [7].

First-pass radionuclide angiocardiography

First-pass radionuclide angiocardiography at rest and exercise has been shown for over a decade to be a reliable method to detect patients with significant coronary artery disease. Although resting left ventricular ejection fraction has been shown to be an important prognostic parameter, in particular, in patients after myocardial infarction, *peak exercise left ventricular ejection fraction* was found to be an even more important prognostic indicator [8]. Patients with coronary artery disease who achieve a peak exercise left ventricular ejection fraction >50 % have excellent 5 year survival, whereas patients with a peak exercise ejection fraction <50 % had substantially greater 5 year mortality.

Preliminary studies have shown that when first-pass radionuclide angiocardiography is performed in combination with myocardial perfusion imaging, a substantial number of patients may demonstrate discordant results, i. e. a patient may have a reversible exercise-induced myocardial perfusion defect but normal peak exercise left ventricular ejection fraction and vice versa (Fig. 3). The clinical significance of this discordance is unclear at the present time. It is conceivable that this pattern has specific prognostic and functional significance, useful in the management of patients with coronary artery disease.

ECG-gated wall motion imaging

Electrocardiographic (ECG) gating of myocardial perfusion images allows cine display and assessment of regional wall motion. Since visual analysis is subjective, descriptive and lacks reproducibility, we developed a new count-based *functional image* that contains quantitative data with respect to endocardial motion and myocardial thickening [7]. From these images we derived a quantitative regional function index (QRFI), which correlates well with visual analysis of regional wall motion regional left ventricular ejection fraction on equilibrium radionuclide angiocardiography (Table 1).

Assessment of area at risk and effect of thrombolysis

A unique application of Tc-99m SestaMIBI imaging is in patients with acute myocardial infarction or unstable angina. Since Tc-99m SestaMIBI does not redistribute significantly after injection, the status of regional myocardial perfusion at the moment of injection can be 'frozen' over time and imaged

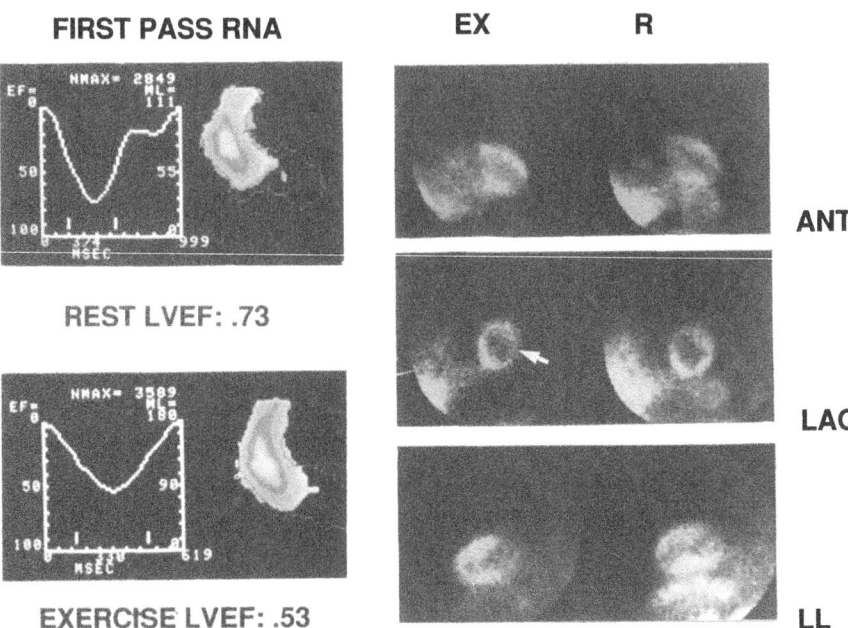

Figure 3. First-pass radionuclide angiocardiography (RNA) (left) at rest and exercise, and myocardial perfusion imaging (right) at rest (R) and after exercise (EX). Resting left ventricular ejection fraction (LVEF) was obtained by a rapid bolus injection of Tc-99m DPTA. Peak exercise LVEF was obtained by injection of 20 mCi of Tc-99m SestaMIBI. Exercise myocardial perfusion imaging was performed 1 hr later. The resting myocardial perfusion images were obtained 24 hr later after a repeat injection of 20 mCi Tc-99m SestaMIBI. Thus, one dose of Tc-99m SestaMIBI provided peak exercise LVEF, as well as images of myocardial perfusion at peak exercise. Resting LVEF and myocardial perfusion were normal. However, during exercise LVEF decreased, an abnormal LVEF response, but more important LVEF was still within the normal range. The myocardial perfusion images showed evidence of exercise-induced ischemia in the inferolateral wall (arrow).

Table 1. Segment by segment comparison of regional wall motion on Equilibrium Radionuclide Angiocardiography (ERNA) and ECG-gated Tc-99m SestaMIBI imaging (209 segments in 19 patients).

	ECG-GATED Tc-99m SestaMIBI			
	Endocardium		Epicardium	
	NL	ABN	NL	ABN
ERNA NL	94	4	73	25
ABN	63	48	17	94
McNemar Test	$p < 0.001$		$p = NS$	
agreement	68 %		80 %	

hours later. We utilized this unique characteristic of Tc-99m SestaMIBI in patients with acute myocardial infarction who underwent thrombolytic therapy [9,10]. Tc-99m SestaMIBI was administered in the emergency room *before* initiation of thrombolytic therapy and imaging was postponed until later when the patient was stable in the Coronary Care Unit. The latter images show the myocardial *area at risk* at the time *before* thrombolysis. Subsequent repeat administration of Tc-99m SestaMIBI reveals the distribution of myocardial blood flow *after* thrombolytic therapy and therefore the ultimate infarcted area. In patients with successful thrombolysis, i.e. reperfusion of the infarct artery, a significant decrease in myocardial perfusion defect size was observed (Fig. 4). Whereas, in patients with failure of thrombolytic therapy and occluded infarct arteries, no change in myocardial perfusion defect size occurred. Functional images of regional contraction on ECG-gated images showed that improvement of myocardial perfusion coincided with improvement of regional myocardial function, indicating not only restoration of blood flow, but also recovery of viable myocardium [11].

A similar protocol has been used in patients with unstable angina for objective assessment of the presence of acute myocardial hypoperfusion [12]. When Tc-99m SestaMIBI was administered during chest pain the presence of a myocardial perfusion defects indicated a high likelihood of having significant coronary artery disease. This was particularly true if patients had a smaller defect or a normal image, on repeat imaging in the absence of chest pain. Using this same concept Tc-99m SestaMIBI can also be employed in conjunction with coronary angioplasty for assessment of the extent of the myocardium at risk by a particular coronary artery.

In conclusion, Tc-99m SestaMIBI can be employed for a number of similar clinical applications as was practiced in the past with Tl-201. In addition, there are some new applications that are unique for Tc-99m SestaMIBI.

Should Tc-99m SestaMIBI replace Tl-201 for myocardial perfusion imaging?

Although for the detection of coronary artery disease the diagnostic information obtained by stress rest imaging with Tc-99m SestaMIBI appeared to be comparable to that with Tl-201, it is of clinical relevance that image quality with Tc-99m SestaMIBI is consistently superior to that with Tl-201. This in particular striking in SPECT imaging. Although high quality Tl-201 *planar images* may be equivalent to Tc-99m SestaMIBI images. We feel strongly that *for tomographic imaging Tc-99m SestaMIBI is a preferred agent.* Therefore, for tomographic imaging Tc-99m SestaMIBI could replace Tl-201.

For imaging in patients with acute myocardial infarction or acute myocardial ischemia, *resting* Tc-99m SestaMIBI images are of superior quality in comparison to resting Tl-201 images. Moreover, the lack of redistribution Tc-99m SestaMIBI allows flexible timing of imaging in these critically ill

THROMBOLYSIS

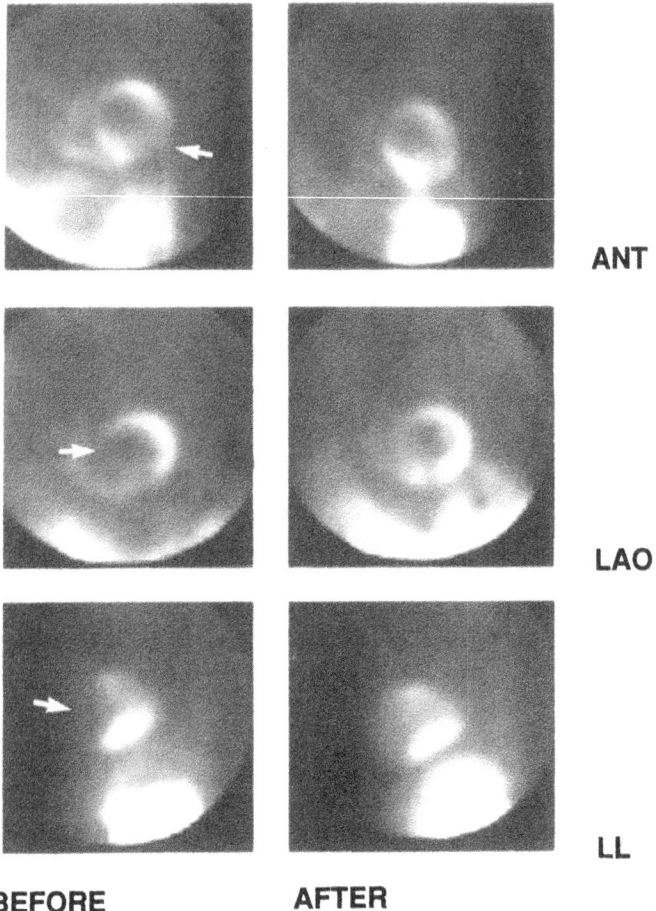

ANT

LAO

LL

BEFORE   AFTER

Figure 4. Tc-99m SestaMIBI imaging before and after thrombolytic therapy in a patient with acute anteroseptal infarction. The extensive anteroseptal defect (arrows) present before thrombolysis is significantly smaller after successful reperfusion of the infarct-related artery. (Reproduced with permission from ref. 9)

patients. For this application Tc-99m SestaMIBI is uniquely and better suited than Tl-201. One important issue remains at the present time still unresolved: are resting Tc-99m SestaMIBI images identical to resting Tl-201 imaging? This is of a particular importance for the evaluation of *myocardial viability*. Resting Tl-201 images are considered to be a reliable marker of myocardial viability. Reinjection of Tl-201 at rest has become a routine procedure in patients with fixed Tl-201 defects on delayed imaging, in whom the question of myocardial viability needs to be addressed [13]. Myocardial distribution of Tl-201 after an injection at rest has been shown to approximate information on myocardial viability derived from positron imaging with fluor(F)-18–deoxyglucose [14]. Preliminary experimental data suggest that accumulation of Tc-99m SestaMIBI in the myocyte is determined by cellular integrity and viability. No clinical studies have, as yet, definitively addressed this problem. As long as these issues are not resolved, Tl-201 imaging at rest will remain the only well accepted, although imperfect, single photon marker of myocardial viability.

We would anticipate that Tc-99m SestaMIBI indeed may replace Tl-201 as a myocardial *perfusion* imaging agent in particular for SPECT imaging. However, Tl-201 is likely to keep its unique value for assessment of one of the most important issues in patients with coronary artery disease: *myocardial viability*.

References

1. Wackers FJ, Berman DS, Maddahi J, et al. Technetium-99m hexakis 2–methoxyisobutyl isonitrile: human biodistribution, dosimetry, safety, and preliminary comparison to thallium-201 for myocardial perfusion imaging. J Nucl Med 1989;30:301–11.
2. Kiat H, Maddahi J, Roy LT, et al. Comparison of technetium99m methoxy isobutyl isonitrile with thallium 201 for evaluation of coronary artery disease by planar and tomographic methods. Am Heart J 1989;117:1–11.
3. Kahn JK, Henderson EB, Akers AS, et al. Prediction of reversibility of perfusion defects with a single post-exercise technetium-99m RP-30A gated tomographic image: the role of residual thickening. J Am Coll Cardiol 1988 (abstract);11 Suppl A:31A.
4. Iskandrian AS, Heo J, Kong B, Lyons E, Marsch S. Use of technetium-99m isonitrile (RP-30A) in assessing left ventricular perfusion and function at rest and during exercise in coronary artery disease, and comparison with coronary arteriography and exercise thallium-201 SPECT imaging. Am J Cardiol 1989;64:270–5.
5. Maddahi J, Kiat H, Van Train K, et al. Myocardial perfusion imaging with technetium-99m sestamibi SPECT in the evaluation of cononary artery disease. Am J Cardiol 1990;66:55E-62E.
6. Borges-Neto S, Coleman RE, Jones RH. Perfusion and function at rest and treadmill exercise using technetium-99m-SestaMIBI: comparison of one- and two-day protocols in normal volunteers. J Nucl Med 1990;131:1128–31.
7. Maniawski PJ, Allam AH, Wackers FJ, Zaret BL. A new non-geometric technique for simultaneous evaluation of regional function and myocardial perfusion from gated planar isonitrile images. Circulation 1989 (abstract);80(Suppl 2):II544.
8. Lee KL, Pryor DB, Pieper KS, et al. Prognostic value of radionuclide angiography in medically treated patients with coronary artery disease. A comparison with clinical and catheterization variables. Circulation 1990;82:1705–17.
9. Wackers FJ, Gibbons RJ, Verani MS, et al. Serial quantitative planar technetium-99m-isonitrile imaging in acute myocardial infarction: efficacy for noninvasive assessment of thrombolytic therapy. J Am Coll Cardiol 1989;14:861–73.
10. Gibbons RJ, Verani MS, Behrenbeck T, et al. Feasibility of tomographic 99mTc-hexakis-2–methoxy-2–methylpropyl-isonitrile imaging for the assessment of myocardial area at risk and the effect of treatment in acute myocardial infarction. Circulation 1989;80:1277–86.
11. Allam AH, Maniawski PJ, Verani MS, Gibbons RJ, Zaret BL, Wackers FJ. Simultaneous assessment of recovery of regional ventricular funtion and perfusion after thrombolysis using serial gated Tc-99m-isontrile imaging. Circulation 1989 (abstract);80 (4 Suppl 2):II620.

12. Gregoire J, Theroux P. Detection and assessment of unstable angina using myocardial perfusion imaging: comparison between technetium-99m SestaMIBI SPECT and 12–lead electrocardiogram. Am J Cardiol 1990;66:42E-7E.

13. Kiat H, Berman DS, Maddahi J, et al. Late reversibility of tomographic myocardial thallium-201 defects: an accurate marker of myocardial viability. J Am Coll Cardiol 1988;12:1456–63.

14. Bonow RO, Dilsizian V, Cuocolo A, Bacharach SL. Identification of viable myocardium in patients with chronic coronary artery disease and left ventricular dysfunction. Comparison of thallium scintigraphy with reinjection and PET imaging with 18F-Fluorodeoxyglucose. Circulation 1991;83:26–37.

17. Pharmacologic perfusion imaging: Similar to conventional radionuclide exercise stress testing?

GEORGE A. BELLER

Summary

Pharmacologic stress Tl-201 imaging utilizing either intravenous dipyridamole or adenosine is an acceptable alternative to exercise imaging for detection of coronary artery disease (CAD) and determining prognosis. Data from multiple published series indicate an 85 % sensitivity and 90 % specificity for CAD detection for dipyridamole imaging. Ischemia can be distinguished from scar with the same accuracy as achieved with exercise imaging. Several groups of investigators have shown that dipyridamole Tl-201 imaging is useful for preoperative risk stratification in patients with peripheral vascular disease scheduled for aortic or peripheral vascular surgery. Redistribution on dipyridamole Tl-201 scans identified high risk patients who experienced an increased incidence of perioperative ischemic events. Dipyridamole Tl-201 imaging is particularly useful in detection of occult CAD in diabetic patients. ST segment depression occurs in 15 % of patients undergoing dipyridamole imaging although chest pain is seen in more than 30 % of patients. Side effects from adenosine Tl-201 imaging are more prevalent than with dipyridamole imaging. Dipyridamole imaging appears safe when performed early after acute myocardial infarction and can identify a high risk subgroup.

In summary, pharmacological stress Tl-201 imaging with either dipyridamole or adenosine is useful for diagnosis and prognosis in patients with suspected or known CAD.

Introduction

Pharmacologic stress imaging has increasingly been employed as an alternative to exercise imaging for detection of coronary artery disease (CAD) and risk stratification [1–4]. Intravenous infusion of dipyridamole or adenosine is an acceptable alternative to exercise stress for detecting physiologically significant coronary artery stenoses utilizing planar or SPECT thallium-201 (Tl-201) myocardial perfusion imaging. Pharmacologic stress is of particular clinical value in patients judged unable to exercise adequately for a variety of noncardiac conditions. High- and low-risk CAD patients can be identified

Johan H.C. Reiber & Ernst E. van der Wall (eds.), Cardiovascular Nuclear Medicine and MRI, 249–269.
© 1992 *Kluwer Academic Publishers.*

by pharmacologic stress imaging similar to what has been described for exercise scintigraphy.

Physiologic effects of dipyridamole and adenosine

Intravenously administered dipyridamole or adenosine produces marked arteriolar vasodilation [5]. Dipyridamole prevents the cellular uptake of adenosine, thereby potentiating its vasodilator effect [6,7]. It inhibits adenosine uptake in both endothelium and myocardial cells, permitting greater concentration of the endogenous vasodilator at the receptor site mediating vasodilation. The systemic effects of intravenous dipyridamole infusion include a mild decrease in systemic blood pressure and a slight reflex increase in heart rate with no net change in myocardial oxygen consumption [8,9]. In myocardium supplied by normal coronary arteries, dipryidamole or adenosine causes a greater increase in subepicardial blood flow compared to endocardial flow, suggesting that total coronary vasodilator reserve is greater in the epicardium [10–12].

When dipyridamole or adenosine is administered in the setting of a critical coronary artery stenosis, significant regional flow alterations distal to the stenosis are observed [10,13–19]. Flow is redistributed away from the endocardium to epicardial layers, resulting in a transmural 'coronary steal.' Figure 1 shows the regional flow alterations consequent to intravenous dipyridamole administration in dogs with a critical coronary stenosis [10]. Flow may actually fall in the subendocardium to levels significantly lower than baseline flow which results in clinical manifestations of ischemia [9]. This transmural coronary steal is associated with a fall in the distal coronary perfusion pressure secondary to the diminution in coronary vascular resistance. Another type of 'steal' is the redistribution of blood flow away from a bed perfused by a stenotic artery to a normally perfused bed that becomes hyperemic after vasodilator infusion.

Dipyridamole-induced vasodilation and Thallium-201 kinetics

Dipyridamole-induced vasodilation in the presence of a partial coronary stenosis results in diminished uptake and delayed clearance of intravenously administered Tl-201, compared with increased uptake and more rapid clearance in normally perfused myocardium [10,13,20–22]. This produces an initial Tl-201 defect with subsequent delayed redistribution (Fig. 2). In clinical imaging studies, redistribution defects observed on myocardial scintigrams in patients with CAD receiving dipyridamole before administration of Tl-201 are similar in incidence and extent to what is observed following exercise scintigraphy [23].

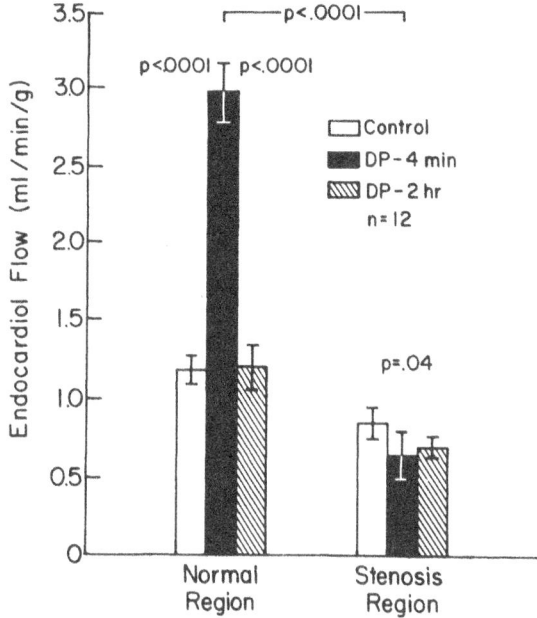

Figure 1. Endocardial blood flow in normal myocardium and in myocardium perfused by a stenotic coronary artery during control conditions (open bars), 4 min after intravenous dipyrida-mole (DP) infusion (solid bars) and 2 hr after dipyridamole administration (hatched bars) in 12 dogs. (From Beller GA et al, Circulation 1983;63:1328–38. Reprinted with permission from the American Heart Association.)

Clinical imaging protocol

Dipyridamole

The dipyridamole Tl-201 perfusion stress test is performed in the following manner: First, no caffeinated beverages or tea are permitted for 12 hr prior to imaging. Patients receiving theophylline-type drugs (e.g. for bronchospasm) cannot be considered for testing unless these drugs are discontinued [24]. After baseline hemodynamics are obtained, 0.56 mg/kg of dipyridamole is infused over a period of 4 min. A dose of 2.0 to 3.0 mCi of Tl-201 is injected at 9 min and initial images are obtained 5 min later. As with exercise scintigraphy, delayed images are obtained 2.5–4 hr later to evaluate for presence or absence of redistribution. Handgrip exercise [25,26] or low-level treadmill exercise [27,28] can be combined with dipyridamole imaging to attenuate systemic hypotension and to further enhance the increase in coronary blood flow. Vital signs and serial 12–lead electrocardiograms are obtained prior to dipyridamole infusion, at every minute during infusion and for at least 5 min after the infusion is completed.

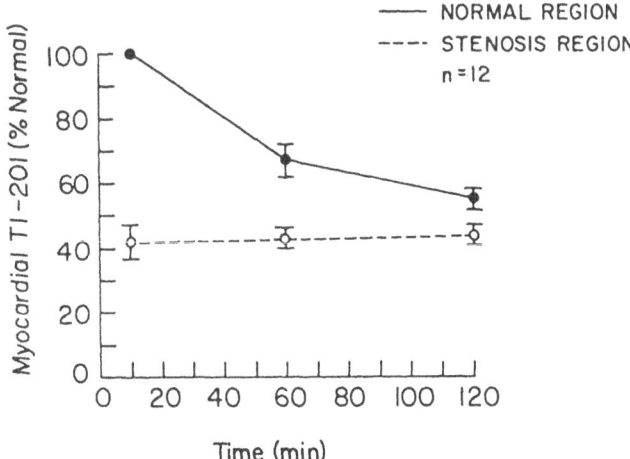

Figure 2. Serial changes in myocardial Tl-201 activity in normal (solid line) and stenotic (dotted line) regions in 12 dogs receiving intravenous dipyridamole before Tl-201 administration. Values are expressed as percent of initial normal myocardial Tl-201 activity which was designated as 100 %. Note the initial reduction in activity in the stenosis region with subsequent redistribution at 120 min (From Beller GA et al, Circulation 1983;68:1328–38. Reprinted with permission from the American Heart Association.)

Adenosine

Adenosine is infused in a peripheral vein with stepwise dose increments every minute [29]. The infusion rate begins with a dose of 50 μg/kg/min followed by 75, 100 and then 140 μg/kg/min [2]. After 1 min at the highest dose, 3 mCi of Tl-201 is injected as a bolus in a contralateral vein and flushed with normal saline. The adenosine infusion is maintained for 3 additional minutes after thallium administration. Vital signs are obtained and electrocardiographic monitoring performed during and for 5 min after adenosine infusion. Early and delayed images are acquired in a manner similar to what is undertaken after exercise or dipyridamole imaging.

Aminophylline, which is an adenosine antagonist, can be administered to reverse dipyridamole-associated side effects such as systemic hypotension, chest pain, significant ST-segment depression and nausea [9,30–32]. In a canine model of partial coronary stenosis, systemic hypotension, adverse regional flow effects (coronary steal) and prolonged Tl-201 washout consequent to intravenously administered dipyridamole are promptly reversed by intravenous aminophylline administration [31]. Reversal of angina and ST depression in clinical imaging studies with aminophylline reflects the reversal of coronary steal produced by intravenous dipyridamole or with adenosine imaging. Merely stopping the infusion will result in reversal of ischemic symptoms because of the short biologic half-life of exogenous adenosine.

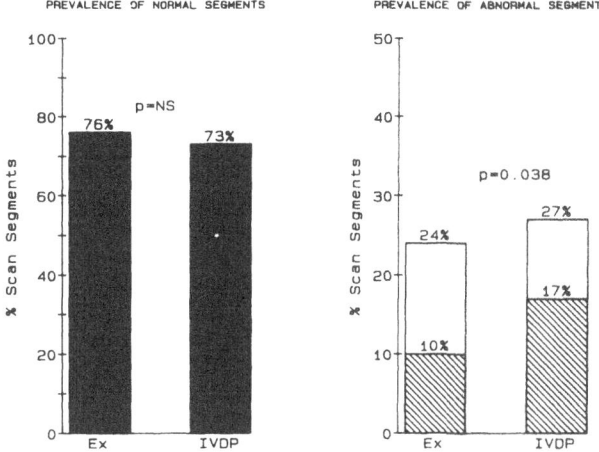

Figure 3. The prevalence of normal and abnormal Tl-201 scan segments after exercise (Ex) and after intravenous dipyridamole (IVDP) in 21 patients presenting with chest pain. The frequency of normal and abnormal segments on the two studies is similar but the frequency of redistribution defects (cross-hatched bars) was higher on the dipyridamole scan study. (From Varma SK et al, Am J Cardiol 1989;64:871–7.)

Detection of coronary artery disease

The sensitivity and specificity of dipyridamole and adenosine Tl-201 imaging for CAD detection are comparable to that observed with Tl-201 exercise scintigraphy [8,28,29,33–48]. Both exercise and dipyridamole infusion induce heterogeneity of blood flow at the time of tracer administration and therefore it is not surprising that the patterns of Tl-201 uptake on initial images after either stress are similar. In a recent study, segmental Tl-201 uptake and washout were comparable after exercise scintigraphy and dipyridamole Tl-201 scintigraphy performed 2 weeks apart in 21 patients with chest pain [23]. Agreement between the two tests was observed in 92 % (61 of 63) of coronary supply regions determined to be normal (41 of 41) or abnormal (20 of 22). In this group of patients, exercise and dipyridamole Tl-201 scintigraphy each detected 61 % of stenotic vessels. The prevalence of redistribution was slightly but significantly more prevalent on the dipyridamole scintigrams (Fig. 3). These data indicate that exercise and dipyridamole Tl-201 imaging when performed in the same patients are comparable in detecting and localizing regions of abnormal myocardial perfusion. Dipyridamole imaging may, however, better identify zones of jeopardized myocardium that are still viable.

In a review of five series in the literature comprising 215 patients who underwent both exercise and dipyridamole Tl-201 scintigraphy for the detection of CAD, the sensitivity was 79 % for both tests, with a 95 % specificity for dipyridamole imaging and a 92 % specificity for exercise imaging [3].

In a pooled analysis of data from 12 published series, [8,28,29,33–41] the sensitivity and specificity of dipyridamole Tl-201 scintigraphy for CAD

Table 1. Sensitivity and specificity of dipyridamole Thallium-201 scintigraphy for detection of coronary artery disease

Author	No. of Patients With CAD	Without CAD	Sensitivity (%)	Specificity (%)
Albro [8]	51	11	67	91
Leppo [33]	40	20	93	80
Schmoliner [34]	60	–	95	–
Francisco [35]	51	35	90	96
Timmis [40]	20	–	85	–
Narita [39]	35	15	69	100
Machecourt [41]	58	10	90	90
Okada [36]	23	7	91	100
Sochor [37]	149	45	92	81
Ruddy [38]	53	27	85	93
Taillefer [29]	19	6	79	86
Walker [28]	57	30	88	87
Total	616	206	85.3 %	90.4 %

detection averaged 85.3 % and 90.4 %, respectively (Table 1). Quantitative image analysis of Tl-201 uptake and clearance can be applied to dipyridamole Tl-201 scintigraphy similar to what has been employed for exercise imaging. However, one must be wary of interpreting isolated washout abnormalities without defects elsewhere on dipyridamole Tl-201 scans as abnormal. Several groups have shown that Tl-201 clearance between the initial and delayed images is slower after dipyridamole-induced vasodilation compared to exercise testing [23,49,50].

Ruddy et al. [38] showed by stepwise logistic regression analysis that the best quantitative Tl-201 correlate of the presence of CAD on serial dipyridamole imaging was a combination variable of "either abnormal uptake or abnormal linear clearance, or both," using a model comprising of three segments per view. This yielded a sensitivity of 85 % and specificity of 93 % for detection of CAD. Borges-Neto et al., [43] employing quantitative tomographic dipyridamole Tl-201 imaging, reported an overall sensitivity of 92 % with a corresponding specificity of 84 %. In that study, patients with severe multivessel disease ($\geq$70 % stenoses) were identified with a sensitivity of 79 % and a specificity of 87 %.

Some data are now available for adenosine Tl-201 scintigraphy with respect to detection of CAD. Verani et al. [29] reported a sensitivity of 83 % and specificity of 94 % for SPECT adenosine Tl-201 scintigraphy in detecting CAD in 89 patients who were unable to perform an exercise test. Nguyen et al. [48] reported a 92 % sensitivity and 100 % specificity for SPECT adenosine scintigraphy. In that study, 61 % of patients with multivessel CAD were also correctly identified. In a subgroup of patients, the predictive accuracy of adenosine Tl-201 scintigraphy was slightly higher than that of exercise SPECT Tl-201 imagine (90 vs 80 %, p = NS).

Assessment of myocardial viability

As with exercise imaging, dipyridamole Tl-201 scintigraphy can be employed to differentiate between ischemia and scar on perfusion scans. Okada and coworkers [42] compared various dipyridamole Tl-201 scan patterns with global and regional left ventricular function changes on exercise radionuclide angiography in 68 patients undergoing both dipyridamole Tl-201 imaging and exercise cardiac blood pool imaging. Redistribution defects on dipyridamole scans were associated with normal regional wall motion. Mild persistent Tl-201 defects were associated with normal regional wall motion at rest but with deterioration of both during exercise. Severe persistent Tl-210 defects were associated with a reduced ejection fraction and abnormal regional wall motion at rest but no further deterioration with exercise.

Dipyridamole Tl-201 perfusion imaging can also be used for distinguishing between ischemic and nonischemic cardiomyopathy. Eichhorn et al. [51] correctly classified 20 of 22 patients (91 %) using dipyridamole scanning when a perfusion defect of $\geq$ 15 % was used as an indication of nonischemically-induced left ventricular dysfunction. Patients with nonischemic cardiomyopathy demonstrated more homogeneous myocardial perfusion compared to those with ischemic cardiomyopathy. In the Eichhorn study, the mean perfusion defect was 25 $\pm$ 11 % in ischemic cardiomyopathy and 6 $\pm$ 6 % in those with idiopathic cardiomyopathy.

Leppo et al. [33] found that the segmental Tl-201 defect patterns on dipyridamole images predicted abnormal wall motion by angiography better than electrocardiographic Q waves. In that study, 74 % of myocardial scan segments demonstrating complete redistribution of an initial dipyridamole-induced perfusion defect had normal wall motion on ventriculography. Conversely, 71 % of scan segments demonstrating persistent Tl-201 defects had akinetic or dyskinetic wall motion. Thus, assessment of myocardial viability can be accomplished with dipyridamole Tl-201 scintigraphy in a manner comparable to what has been undertaken using exercise stress. It should be pointed out that as many as 20–25 % of mild persistent defects may represent viable myocardium rather than scar on either dipyridamole or exercise scintigraphy. Late redistribution imaging at 18–24 hr or reinjection of a second Tl-201 dose after the redistribution images have been acquired may enhance the ability to differentiate between mild persistent defects that represent predominantly scar from those which represent ischemia. Quantitation of Tl-201 uptake and washout is superior to visual scan interpretation alone for identifying scan segments that exhibit redistribution.

Tl-201 scintigraphy after the oral injection of 300–400 mg of dipyridamole in tablet form made into a suspension can be performed as an alternative to intravenous dipyridamole scintigraphy [44,47]. The peak level of serum dipyridamole concentration after oral ingestion is attained at 45 min, requiring a substantial delay before Tl-201 can be administered. Oral dipyridamole scintigraphy is associated with a greater incidence of nausea than intravenous dipyridamole imaging and often is not well tolerated.

Risk stratification and prognostication

Tl-201 scintigraphy performed in conjunction with dipyridamole stress has been reported to provide useful prognostic information in patients with CAD [52–57], particularly those who are undergoing risk assessment prior to peripheral vascular or aortic surgery [58–66]. Leppo et al. [52] reported that the presence of Tl-201 redistribution on serial dipyridamole scintigrams performed before hospital discharge in acute myocardial infarction survivors was the best predictor of subsequent cardiac events. In that study, exercise stress electrocardiography was a less sensitive predictor of events than was dipyridamole imaging. Brown et al. [56] evaluated the prognostic utility of dipyridamole Tl-201 scintigraphy performed very early (62 ± 21 hr) during hospitalization after acute myocardial infarction. There were no serious adverse reactions experienced during the dipyridamole protocol. Using stepwise multi-variate logistic regression analysis, the best and only statistically significant predictor of in-hospital ischemic cardiac events was the presence of Tl-201 redistribution within the infarct zone (p = 0.0001). Forty-five percent of patients demonstrating infarct zone redistribution developed in-hospital cardiac events. No patients without infarct zone redistribution had events. In postinfarction patients, Gimple et al. [55] reported that dipyridamole-induced Tl-201 redistribution outside of the infarct zone had a 63 % sensitivity and 75 % specificity for subsequent cardiac events. Redistribution outside the infarct zone was seen in 40 % of patients undergoing testing.

Increased lung Tl-201 uptake and left ventricular dilatation on the anterior view scintigram are high-risk scintigraphic variables on dipyridamole scans and may have similar prognostic implications as when seen on exercise scintigraphy [67,68]. Lette et al. [68] found that transient left ventricular cavity dilatation was seen in 9 % of 510 consecutive patients referred for dipyridamole Tl-201 imaging. Coronary angiography revealed high-risk CAD in the majority of those catheterized who exhibited transient left ventricular dilatation. The postoperative cardiac event rate was 2 % in the 101 patients with normal scans, 19 % in the 75 patients with redistribution defects and 58 % in the 12 patients with reversible cavity dilatation. Chouraqui et al. [69] found that patients with dipyridamole-induced transient dilation of the left ventricle on serial Tl-201 scintigrams had a significantly higher frequency of ≥ 90 % coronary stenoses (33 % vs 5 %), more extensive myocardial reversible defects on planar (71 vs 10 %) and SPECT (87 vs 35 %) images and a higher incidence of anginal chest pain (53 vs 22 %) compared to patients with transient dilation. Left ventricular cavity dilation and increased lung Tl-201 uptake are also markers of high-risk CAD on adenosine Tl-201 scintigrams correlating with extent and severity of SPECT perfusion

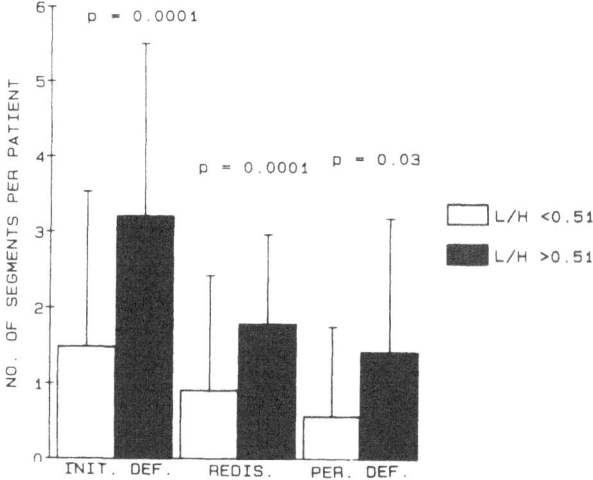

Figure 4. Comparison between patients with and without an increased lung/heart ratio (L/H) of Tl-201 in terms of the number of initial (INIT) defects (DEF), redistribution (REDIS) and persistent (PER) defects. Note that patients with a L/H ratio of > 0.51 had a greater frequency of perfusion abnormalities indicating a more severe ischemic response. (From Villanueva FS et al, Am J Cardiol 1990;66:1324–8.)

abnormalities [70]. Increased lung Tl-201 uptake on dipyridamole images has been shown to correlate with extent of myocardial perfusion abnormalities [67]. Figure 4 shows that patients with an increased lung/heart (>0.51) Tl-201 ratio on dipyridamole scintigrams had significantly more redistribution and more persistent defects than patients with a normal ratio (<0.51) [67].

Younis et al. [54] reported on the prognostic utility of dipyridamole Tl-201 imaging in 107 asymptomatic patients, including 33 who had a prior infarction and 47 who had undergone previous bypass surgery or angioplasty. These authors found that by stepwise logistic regression analysis, a reversible Tl-201 defect was the only significant predictor of subsequent cardiac events during follow-up. Of the 13 patients who subsequently died or experienced a nonfatal infarction, 12 had a redistribution defect at the time of the imaging study. None of the 36 patients with a normal dipyridamole Tl-201 scan experienced death or nonfatal infarction during follow-up. In an earlier study, Younis et al. [53] found that a reversible Tl-201 defect and the extent of angiographic CAD were the only independent predictors of cardiac events in patients recovering from unstable angina or a recent acute myocardial infarction who underwent dipyridamole Tl-201 imaging.

More recently, Hendel et al. [57] examined the prognostic utility of dipyridamole Tl-201 imaging in 516 consecutive patients undergoing the test for a variety of clinical indications (Fig. 5). By logistic regression analysis, an abnormal scan was an independent and significant predictor of subsequent infarction or death and increased the relative risk of any event more than threefold. The presence of redistribution on Tl-201 scintigraphy further increased the risk of a cardiac event. In patients with an abnormal scan, the

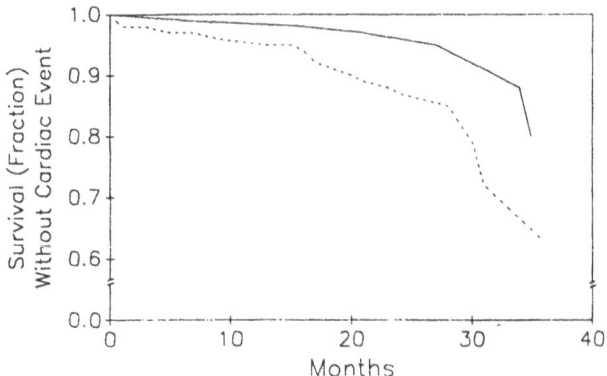

Figure 5. Life table analysis comparing event-free survival of 172 patients with a normal dipyridamole Tl-201 scan (solid line) with that of 332 patients with an abnormal scan (dashed line). Cardiac death or infarction occurred more frequently in patients with an abnormal scan (p < 0.005). (Reprinted with permission from the American College of Cardiology. J Am Coll Cardiol 1990;15:109–16.)

presence of more than one segment demonstrating redistribution, as well as persistent abnormalities (71 vs 45 %), was found significantly more often in the group that experienced cardiac events. In that study, the combination of diabetes mellitus, congestive heart failure and an abnormal dipyridamole Tl-201 study resulted in the highest predicted probability of having myocardial infarction or death and raised the relative risk of a cardiac event more than 26–fold.

Boucher et al. [58] were the first to report the clinical utility of dipyridamole Tl-201 imaging for preoperative risk stratification in patients undergoing vascular surgery for peripheral vascular or aortic disease. They reported that in patients with a prior history of angina or myocardial infarction, the presence of Tl-201 redistribution on dipyridamole scintigrams preoperatively was superior to any other clinical variable in predicting perioperative cardiac death, infarction, unstable angina or pulmonary edema. No cardiac events were observed in 32 patients whose perfusion scan was either normal or showed only persistent defects. Further studies from the Massachusetts General Hospital group [59,60] showed that one could be selective with respect to which patients with vascular disease would benefit most from preoperative dipyridamole Tl-201 scintigraphy for detection of underlying asymptomatic high-risk CAD (Fig. 6). They found that patients with no prior infarction, congestive heart failure, angina pectoris, diabetes mellitus or Q waves on the resting ECG have a low likelihood of a perioperative cardiac event and therefore dipyridamole Tl-201 imaging would not be of great additional value for risk stratification in this group. These patients can be expected to be in a low-risk status based upon these clinical criteria alone. In contrast, they found that among patients exhibiting one or more of these clinical high-risk variables, 50 % demonstrated a reversible Tl-201 defect on the preoperative

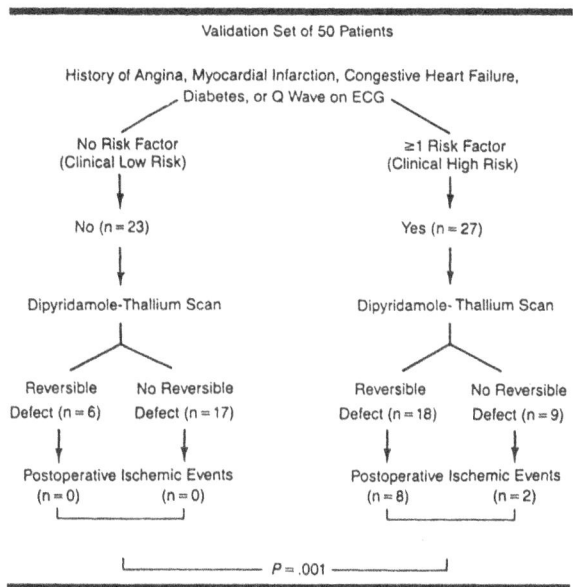

Validation Set of 50 Patients

History of Angina, Myocardial Infarction, Congestive Heart Failure, Diabetes, or Q Wave on ECG

No Risk Factor (Clinical Low Risk) — No (n = 23) — Dipyridamole-Thallium Scan

≥1 Risk Factor (Clinical High Risk) — Yes (n = 27) — Dipyridamole-Thallium Scan

Reversible Defect (n = 6)   No Reversible Defect (n = 17)   Reversible Defect (n = 18)   No Reversible Defect (n = 9)

Postoperative Ischemic Events (n = 0)   (n = 0)   Postoperative Ischemic Events (n = 8)   (n = 2)

P = .001

Figure 6. Cardiac postoperative event rate in 23 patients with a clinical low-risk status (absence of angina, myocardial infarction, congestive heart failure, diabetes or Q wave on the ECG) and 27 patients with ≥ 1 of these clinical risk factors. Note the high event rate in patients with clinical risk factors and redistribution defects on preoperative dipyridamole scintigraphy. (From Eagle KA et al, JAMA 1987;257:2185–9.)

dipyridamole scan. Nearly one-half of these patients experienced a postoperative ischemic event. In clinically high-risk patients with no evidence for a redistribution defect on scintigraphy, none experienced a postoperative event.

Cutler and Leppo [61] found that Tl-201 redistribution showed the best statistical correlation with postoperative myocardial infarction in 116 consecutive patients who were referred for aortic reconstructive surgery. The odds of a patient with Tl-201 scintigraphic abnormalities on dipyridamole imaging of having a postoperative infarction in this group of patients was 12 times greater than for those with a normal scan. Of interest, the incidence of postoperative infarction was similar in those with previous symptomatic or asymptomatic CAD. Lette et al. [62], employing a scintigraphic scoring system that took into account dipyridamole-induced reversible left ventricular dilatation on serial initial and delayed scans with indices of severity and extent of redistribution, found that patients could be successfully classified into low-, intermediate- and high-risk subgroups. Patients classified as low risk underwent noncardiac surgery uneventfully. In contrast, 8 of 10 patients with high-risk scintigraphic abnormalities had a postoperative event (7 deaths and 1 myocardial infarction).

Not all studies have shown dipyridamole Tl-201 imaging to be a reliable screening test for CAD in patients undergoing vascular surgery. Marwick and Underwood [64] reported and 11 % ischemic event rate in 64 patients with a normal preoperative Tl-201 scan compared with a 16 % event rate in patients undergoing surgery with persistent or redistribution Tl-201 defects.

The incidence of dipyridamole-induced Tl-201 scan abnormalities is extremely high in diabetic patients undergoing vascular surgery. Lane et al. [65] found an 80 % incidence of Tl-201 abnormalities in 101 diabetic patients undergoing dipyridamole scintigraphy prior to vascular surgery. Cardiac complications occurred in 10 of the 71 patients (14 %) who showed $\geq$ 1 reversible defect as compared to 1 of 30 (3.3 %) who demonstrated no reversibility. In that study for more optimum predictive accuracy for predicting cardiac events, quantification of the total number of redistribution defects, as well as assessment of ischemia in the distribution of the left anterior descending coronary artery were required. In a study by Brown et al. [66], the ability of dipyridamole Tl-201 scintigraphy and rest radionuclide angiography to predict perioperative and long-term cardiac events were evaluated in 36 uremic diabetic and 20 nondiabetic candidates for renal allograft surgery. By logistic regression analysis of multiple clinical and radionuclide variables, presence of Tl-201 redistribution and the left ventricular ejection fraction were the only significant predictors of future cardiac event. No other patient variables, including diabetes or receiving a renal allograft, had either univariate or multivariate predictive value. Overall, 5 of 6 patients with cardiac events had either Tl–201 redistribution defects or depressed left ventricular ejection fraction.

Dipyridamole Tl-201 scintigraphy has been successfully employed to identify patients prone to develop recurrent angina due to restenosis following coronary angioplasty. Jain et al. [71] found that restenosis developed in 71 % of patients who demonstrated a dipyridamole Tl-201 redistribution defect after angioplasty. Restenosis was seen in only 11.5 % of patients without an ischemic defect in that study.

Clinical indications for dipyridamole or adenosine Thallium-201 scintigraphy

Because sensitivity and specificity values for detecting CAD and the ability to separate high- and low-risk patients are comparable to results obtained with exercise scintigraphy, the pharmacologic 'stress test' should be strongly considered in patients who are judged to be unable to perform an exercise test. Presence of such noncardiac abnormalities as peripheral vascular disease with claudication, arthritis, disabling cerebral vascular disease and a variety of orthopaedic problems may preclude adequate exercise. Patients referred for elective peripheral vascular or aortic surgery are most appropriate candidates for pharmacologic stress scintigraphy. Dipyridamole or adenosine scintigraphy might also be considered in individuals who are strongly suspected to have underlying CAD despite a normal exercise myocardial perfusion scan at suboptimal heart rate responses. Some patients have poor motivation to exercise or are significantly deconditioned and, thus, may not attain a rate-pressure product sufficient to stress coronary reserve capacity. Perhaps patients who cease exercising at subopitmal heart rates and workloads with no symptoms or ST depression should not have Tl-201 injected on the treadmill of bicycle. Such patients could undergo dipyridamole or adenosine imaging immediately following the inadequate exercise stress test.

Side effects of dipyridamole

Ranhosky and Kempthorne-Rowson [9] reported the dipyridamole safety data from 3,911 patients collected from 64 investigators and which comprised the Boehringer Ingelheim Pharmaceuticals registry. All adverse events occuring within 24 hr after administration of dipyridamole were recorded. Ten patients (0.26 %) had major adverse events, and 1,820 (46.5 %) had minor side effects. Two patients (0.05 %) died as a consequence of myocardial infarctions, and two (0.05 %) had nonfatal infarctions. One of the two patients who had a fatal infarction and both patients who had a nonfatal infarction had unstable angina before dipyridamole Tl-201 imaging. It is not stated whether these three patients had 'stabilized' with resolution of ischemic rest pain before the dipyridamole study was conducted. Six patients (0.15 %) developed acute bronchospasm, which was reversed in all instances with intravenous aminophylline. Lesser side effects included chest pain (19.7 %), headache (12.2 %), dizziness (11.8 %), nausea (4.6 %) and hypotension (4.6 %). ST-segment depression was seen in 7.5 %, and chest pain developed in 19.7 %. Ninety-seven percent of patients receiving aminophylline to treat side effects experienced complete relief of symptoms.

Reports published since 1985 have suggested that with appropriate patient selection and adequate monitoring, the incidence of life-threatening adverse reactions is negligible. Homma et al. [72] reported no deaths or infarction in 293 consecutive patients undergoing dipyridamole imaging. Hendel et al. [57] reported no life-threatening reactions in more than 500 procedures. In that study, chest pain occured in 18 % of patients during dipyridamole infusion, and ST-segment depression was reported in only 7 %. Aminophylline was required in only 17 % of patients for treatment of side effects. Lewen et al. [73] reported a single patient who developed severe myocardial ischemia which persisted for 90 min and required emergency coronary angioplasty after dipyridamole imaging.

Dipyridamole Tl-201 imaging also appears to be safe in elderly patients. Lam et al. [46] found the side-effect profile comparable between 101 patients who were 70 years of age or greater compared to 235 patients less than 70 years of age. No deaths or infarctions were observed in this total group of 337 patients undergoing testing. Similarly, Gerson et al. [74] found a comparable side-effect incidence between patients less than and greater than 65 years of age.

It is apparent that more and more patients who have recovered from an uncomplicated myocardial infarction are undergoing dipyridamole Tl-201 imaging for purposes of prognostication. In five such studies comprising 247 patients undergoing intravenous dipyridamole stress testing within several weeks of the onset of acute infarction, no major adverse cardiac events were reported [53,55,56,75,76].

Most reports in the literature show that the incidence of chest pain is significantly higher than the incidence of ST-segment depression after dipyri-damole infusion [9,71,77]. It is apparent that some instances of chest pain after dipyridamole infusion are not secondary to ischemia from epicardial CAD. Angina-like chest pain can be provoked by intravenous adenosine administration and subsequently reversed by aminophylline in normal healthy volunteers [78]. Pearlman and Boucher [79] reported that 9 % of patients with angiographically normal coronary arteries developed chest pain during dipyridamole administration. Ischemic ST-segment depression is most likely secondary to the 'coronary steal' which results in an absolute decrease in nutrient subendocardial blood flow in the distribution of a stenotic vessel. This coronary steal is promptly reversed with administration of aminophylline as is the dipyridamole-induced hyperemia in the normal myocardium (Fig. 7). Chambers and Brown [80] found that only the presence of 'good' coronary collateral vessels and an increase in rate-pressure product after dipyridamole infusion were significant predictors of vasodilator-induced ST-segment de-pression. These investigators speculated that coronary collaterals facilitate steal when hyperemia occurs in the feeder vessel. Blood is directed away from the ischemic zone to the normal zone, resulting in diminished collateral flow and subendocardial hypoperfusion.

Caution should be exercised in performing dipyridamole Tl-201 imaging in patients with pulmonary disease and a history of recent bronchospasm. Lette et al. [81] reported a case of patient with chronic obstructive lung disease who developed sudden bronchospasm and respiratory arrest following dipyridamole infusion. This patient had aminophylline preparations with-drawn 48 hours prior to testing.

Thus, with respect to side effects, it appears that dipyridamole scintigraphy is relatively safe when patients with acute unstable angina or recent manifes-tations of bronchospasm are not studied. Aminophylline is effective in rapidly reversing both minor and major side effects. All patients receiving either intravenous or high-dose oral dipyridamole for perfusion imaging should be continuously monitored. If chest pain, ischemic ST depression or hemody-namic instability occur, then aminophylline should promptly be administered intravenously. The incidence of minor side effects with adenosine Tl-201 scintigraphy is higher than observed with dipyridamole scintigraphy [29]. Chest pain was provoked in 57 % of patients receiving intravenous adenosine [29]. However, only 12 % had ST-segment depression. Transient atrioventri-

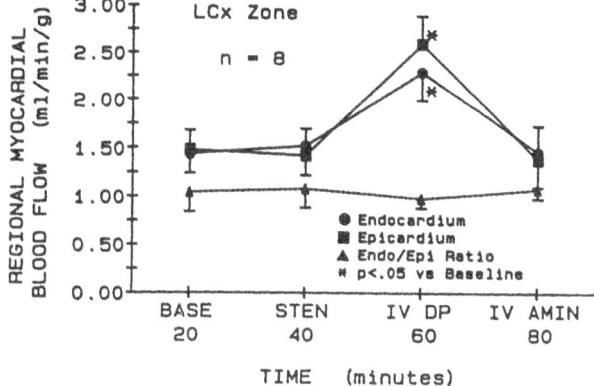

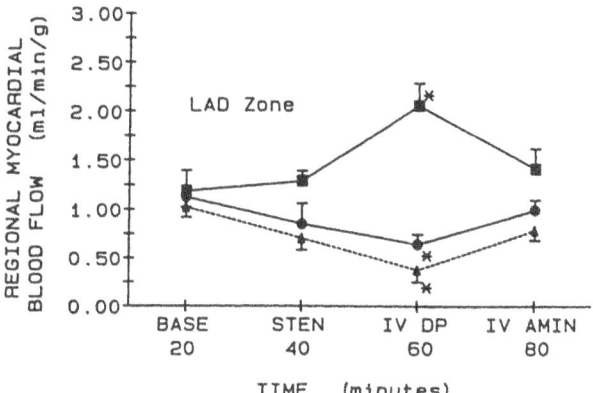

Figure 7. Serial changes in myocardial blood flow in the normal left circumflex (LCx) coronary artery zone (upper panel) and in the stenotic (STEN) left anterior descending coronary artery (LAD) zone at baseline (BASE), after creation of the LAD stenosis, after intravenous dipyrida- mole (IV DP) and after intravenous aminophylline (IV AMIN) in 8 dogs. Note that aminophyl- line reverses the dipyridamole-induced hyperemia in the LCx zone and the coronary steal in the LAD zone. (Reprinted with permission from the American College of Cardiology. J Am Coll Cardiol 1990;16:1760–70.)

cular block occurs in approximately 10 % of patients. Atrioventricular block is more often seen after intravenous adenosine and intravenous dipyridamole infusion.

Limitations of dipyridamole Thallium-201 scintigraphy

There are some limitations in performance of Tl-201 scintigraphy in conjunc- tion with either dipyridamole or adenosine infusion which are similar to those encountered with exercise stress. First, visual interpretation of unprocessed Tl-201 scintigrams can be quite difficult if the interpreter is not familiar with the various attenuation artifacts or variants of normal that can be encountered. An overlying breast shadow, an altered position of either the inflow or outflow tracks of the left ventricle, a greater than normal degree of apical thinning, and enlarged right ventricular blood pool overlying the inferior wall on the planar anterior image or a high diaphragm overlying the posterior wall on a steep left anterior oblique image can all result in false-positive interpretations. In certain patients, the upper septum and upper posterolateral wall (basal portions of the left ventricle) may be thin, which could be misinterpreted as representing left anterior descending and circumflex defects, respectively. In markedly obese individuals, Tl-201 images of the heart may be of such poor quality because of attenuation to make the studies uninterpretable. Quantitative scan analysis is recommended to maximize detection of redistribution and to enhance sensitivity and specifity for CAD detection.

In contrast to positron imaging techniques, absolute quantitation of myocardial blood flow in ml/min/g of myocardium cannot be obtained with Tl-201 scintigraphy in gamma scintillation techniques.

It has been suggested that SPECT thallium imaging should enhance both sensitivity and specificity of the myocardial perfusion technique. Unfortunately, SPECT imaging is also associated with problems that may diminish specificity in certain laboratories. Patient motion is a source of artifactual defects on tomographic reconstruction.

A new class of myocardial perfusion agents, the technetium-99m isonitriles, is being evaluated as an alternative to Tl-201 for myocardial perfusion imaging. These radiopharmaceuticals have superior physical characteristics to Tl-201 for imaging with a gamma scintillation camera. Initial clinical results with one of these agents, technetium-99m SestaMIBI, are encouraging. This agent could also potentially be utilized with pharmacologic stress.

Dipyridamole positron emission tomography (PET)

Dipyridamole perfusion imaging employing rubidium-82 or nitrogen-13 ammonia have also yielded high sensitivity and specificity values for CAD detection. Demer et al. [82] found that with increasing stenosis severity, PET defect severity induced by dipyridamole increased. In an earlier study of 50 patients by Gould and coworkers [83], where the PET scan results were compared with quantitative arteriographic stenosis flow reserve, both the sensitivity and specificity for CAD detection exceeded 90 %.

Conclusion

In conclusion, pharmacologic stress may be an attractive alternative to exercise stress imaging for detection of myocardial ischemia and determining its extent in patients with suspected or known CAD, or those who have recovered from a recent myocardial infarction. Dipyridamole infusion is the most commonly employed pharmacologic stress and is utilized in conjunction with Tl-201 scintigraphy or positron emission tomography. Sensitivity, specificity and predictive accuracy for CAD detection for dipyridamole or adenosine Tl-201 scintigraphy are comparable to values achieved with exercise stress. Similarly, the prognostic value of this technique for the detection of high-risk coronary disease patients has been demonstrated. High-risk patients have multiple defects in more than one coronary supply region, a high prevalence of redistribution-type perfusion abnormalities, increased lung Tl-201 uptake and transient left ventricular cavity dilation. High-risk patients by dipyridamole scan criteria who also have clinical risk factors for CAD are prone to an increased incidence of perioperative complications with vascular surgery. Both dipyridamole and adenosine scintigraphy are relatively safe, and most side effects are minor and transitory.

References

1. Gould KL. Pharmacologic intervention as an alternative to exercise stress. Semin Nucl Med 1987;17:121–30.
2. Iskandrian AS, Heo J, Askenase A, Segal BL, Auerbach N. Dipyridamole cardiac imaging. Am Heart J 1988;115:432–43.
3. Leppo JA. Dipyridamole-thallium imaging: the lazy man's stress test. J Nucl Med 1989;30:281–7.
4 Beller GA. Pharmacologic stress imaging. JAMA 1991;265:633–8.
5. Gould KL. Noninvasive assessment of coronary stenoses by myocardial perfusion imaging during pharmacologic coronary vasodilation. I. Physiologic basis and experimental validation. Am J Cardiol 1978;41:267–78.
6. Sparks HV Jr, Bardenheuer H. Regulation of adnosine formation by the heart. Circ Res 1986;58:193–201.
7. Knabb RM, Gidday JM, Ely SW, Rubio R, Berne RM. Effects of dipyridamole on myocardial adenosine and active hyperemia. Am J Physiol 1984;247:H804–10.
8. Albro PC, Gould KL, Westcott RJ, Hamilton GW, Ritchie JL, Williams DL. Noninvasive assessment of coronary stenoses by myocardial imaging during pharmacologic coronary vasodilation. III. Clinical trial. Am J Cardiol 1978;42:751–60.
9. Ranhosky A, Kempthorne-Rawson J. The safety of intravenous dipyridamole thallium myocardial perfusion imaging. Intravenous Dipyridamole Imaging Study Group. Circulation 1990;81:1205–9.
10. Beller GA, Holzgrefe HH, Watson DD. Effects of dipyridamole-induced vasodilation on myocardial uptake and clearance kinetics of thallium-201. Circulation 1983;68:1328–38.
11. Warltier DC, Gross GJ, Brooks HL. Pharmacologic- vs ischemia- induced coronary artery vasodilation. Am J Physiol 1981;240:H767–74.
12. Leppo JA, Simon M, Hood WB Jr. Effect of adenosine on transmural flow gradients in normal canine myocardium. J Cardiovasc Pharmacol 1984;6:1115–9.
13. Beller GA, Holzgrefe HH, Watson DD. Instrinsic washout rates of thallium-201 in normal and ischemic myocardium after dipyridamole-induced vasodilation. Circulation 1985;71:378–86.
14. Fam WM, McGregor M. Effect of nitroglycerin and dipyridamole on regional coronary resistance. Circ Res 1968;22:649–59.

15. Nakamura M, Nakagaki O, Nose Y, Fukuyama T, Kikuchi Y. Effects of nitroglycerin and diypridamole on regional myocardial flow. Basic Res Cardiol 1978;73:482–96.

16. Becker LC. Conditions for vasodilator-induced coronary steal in experimental myocardial ischemia. Circulation 1978;57:1103–10.

17. Okada RD, Jacobs ML, Daggett WM, et al. Thallium-201 kinetics in nonischemic canine myocardium. Circulation 1982;65:70–7.

18. Fung AY, Gallagher KP, Buda AJ. The physiologic basis of dobutamine as compared with dipyridamole stress interventions in the assessment of critical coronary stenosis. Circulation 1987;76:943–51.

19. Gewirtz H, Williams DO, Ohley WH, Most AS. Influence of coronary vasodilation on the transmural distribution of myocardial blood flow distal to a severe fixed coronary artery stenosis. Am Heart J 1983;106:674–80.

20. Okada RD, Leppo JA, Boucher CA, Pohost GM. Myocardial kinetics of thallium-201 after dipyridamole infusion in normal canine myocardium and in myocardium distal to a stenosis. J Clin Invest 1982;69:199–201.

21. Mays AE Jr, Cobb FR. Relationship between regional myocardial blood flow and thallium-201 distribution in the presence of coronary artery stenosis and dipyridamole-induced vasodilation. J Clin Invest 1984;73:1359–66.

22. Strauss HW, Pitt B. Noninvasive detection of subcritical coronary arterial narrowings with a coronary vasodilator and myocardial perfusion imaging. Am J Cardiol 1977;39:403–6.

23. Varma SK, Watson DD, Beller GA. Quantitative comparison of thallium-201 scintigraphy after exercise and dipyridamole in coronary artery disease. Am J Cardiol 1989;64:871–7.

24. Daley PJ, Mahn TH, Zielonka JS, Krubsack AJ, Akhtar R, Bamrah VS. Effect of maintenance oral theophylline on dipyridamole-thallium-201 myocardial imaging using SPECT and dipyridamole-induced hemodynamic changes. Am Heart J. 1988;115:1185–92.

25. Rossen JD, Simonetti I, Marcus ML, Winniford MD. Coronary dilation with standard dose dipyridamole and dipyridamole combined with hand-grip. Circulation 1989;79:566–72.

26. Huikuri HV, Korhonen UR, Airaksinen KEJ, Ikäheimo MJ, Heikkilä J, Takkunen JT. Comparison of dipyridamole-handgrip test and bicycle exercise test for thallium tomographic imaging. Am J Cardiol 1988; 61:264–8.

27. Casale PN, Guiney TE, Strauss HW, Boucher CA. Simultaneous low level treadmill exercise and intravenous dipyridamole stress thallium imaging. Am J Cardiol 1988:799–802.

28. Walker PR, James MA, Wilde RP, Wood CH, Rees JR. Dipyridamole combined with exercise for thallium-201 myocardial imaging. Br Heart J 1986;55:321–9.

29. Verani MS, Mahmarian JJ, Hixson JB, Boyce TM, Staudacher RA. Diagnosis of coronary artery disease by controlled coronary vasodilation with adenosine and thallium-201 scintigraphy in patients unable to exercise. Circulation 1990;82:80–7.

30. Afonso S. Inhibition of coronary vasodilating action of dipyridamole and adenosine by aminophylline in dog. Circ Res. 1970;26:743–52.

31. Granato JE, Watson DD, Belardinelli L, Cannon JM, Beller GA. Effects of dipyridamole and aminophylline on hemodynamics, regional myocardial blood flow and thallium-201 washout in the setting of a critical coronary stenosis. J Am Coll Cardiol 1990;16:1760–70.

32. Sollevi A, Ostergren J, Fagrell B, Hjemdahl P. Theophylline antagonizes cardiovascular responses to dipyridamole in man without affecting increases in plasma adenosine. Acta Physiol Scand 1984;121:165–71.

33. Leppo J, Boucher CA, Okada RD, Newell JB, Strauss HW, Pohost GM. Serial thallium-201 myocardial imaging after dipyridamole infusion: diagnostic utility in detecting coronary stenoses and relationship to regional wall motion. Circulation 1982;66:649–57.

34. Schmoliner R, Dudczak R, Kronik G, Hutterer B, Kletter K, Mösslacher H, et al. Thallium-201 imaging after dipyridamole in patients with coronary multivessel disease. Cardiology 1983;70:145–51.

35. Francisco DA, Collins SM, Go RT, Ehrhardt JC, Van Kirk OC, Marcus ML. Tomographic thallium-201 myocardial perfusion scintigrams after maximal coronary artery vasodilation with intravenous dipyridamole. Comparison of qualitative and quantitative approaches. Circulation 1982;66:370–9.

36. Okada RD, Lim YL, Rothendler J, Boucher CA, Block PC, Pohost GM. Split dose thallium-201 dipyridamole imaging: a new technique for obtaining thallium images before and immediately after an intervention. J Am Coll Cardiol 1983;1:1302–10.
37. Sochor H, Pachinger O, Ogris E, Probst P, Kaindl F. Radionuclide imaging after coronary vasodilation: myocardial scintigraphy with thallium-201 and radionuclide angiography after administration of dipyridamole. Eur Heart J 1984;5:500–9.
38. Ruddy TD, Dighero HR, Newell JB, et al. Quantitative analysis of dipyridamole-thallium images for the detection of artery heart disease. J Am Coll Cardiol 1987;10:142–9.
39. Narita M, Kurihara T, Usami M. Noninvasive detection of coronary artery disease by myocardial imaging with thallium-201 – for the significance of pharmacologic interventions. Jpn Circ J 1981;45:127–40.
40. Timmis AD, Lutkin JE, Fenney LJ, et al. Comparison of dipyridamole and treadmill exercise for enhancing thallium-201 perfusion defects in patients with coronary artery disease. Eur Heart J 1980;1:275–80.
41. Machecourt J, Denis B, Wolf JE, Comet M, Pellet J, Martin-Nöel P. Sensibilité et spécificité respective de la scintigraphie myocadique réalisée après injection de 201 Tl au cours de l'effort, après injection de dipyridamole et au respos. Comparaison chez 70 sujets coronaro-graphiés. Arch Mal Coeur 1981;74:147–56.
42. Okada RD, Dai YH, Boucher CA, Pohost GM. Serial thallium-201 imaging after dipyridamole for coronary disease detection: quantitative analysis using myocardial clearance. Am Heart J 1984;107:475–81.
43. Borges-Neto S, Mahmarian JJ, Jain A, Roberts R, Verani MS. Quantitative thallium-201 single photon emission computed tomography after oral dipyridamole for assessing the presence, anatomic location and severity of coronary artery disease. J Am Coll Cardiol 1988;11:962–9.
44. Gould KL, Sorenson SG, Albro P, Caldwell JH, Chaudhuri T, Hamilton GW. Thallium-201 myocardial imaging during coronary vasodilation induced by oral dipyridamole. J Nucl Med 1986;27:31–6.
45. DePuey EG, Guertler-Krawczynska E, D'Amato PH, Patterson RE. Thallium-201 single-photon emission computed tomography with intravenous dipyridamole to diagnose coronary artery disease. Coronary Artery Dis 1990;1:75–82.
46. Lam JY, Chaitman BR, Glaenzer M, et al. Safety and diagnostic accuracy of dipyridamole-thallium imaging in the elderly. J Am Coll Cardial 1988;11:585–9.
47. Homma S, Callahan RJ, Ameer B, McKusick KA, Strauss HW, Okada RD, et al. Usefulness of oral dipyridamole suspension for stress thallium imaging without exercise in the detection of coronary artery disease. Am J Cardiol 1986;57:503–8.
48. Nguyen T, Heo J, Ogilby JD, Iskandrian AS. Single photon emission computed tomography with thallium-201 during adenosine-induced coronary hyperemia: correlation with coronary arteriography, exercise thallium imaging and two-dimensional echocardiography. J Am Coll Cardiol 1990;16:1375–83.
49. O'Byrne GT, Rodrigues EA, Maddahi J, et al. Comparison of myocardial washout rate of thallium-201 between rest, dipyridamole with and without aminophylline, and exercise states in normal subjects. Am J Cardiol 1989;64:1022–8.
50. Ruddy TD, Gill JB, Finkelstein DM, et al. Myocardial uptake and clearance of thallium-201 in normal subjects: comparison of dipyridamole-induced hyperemia with exercise stress. J Am Coll Cardiol 1987;10:547–56.
51. Eichhorn EJ, Kosinski EJ, Lewis SM, Hill TC, Emond LH, Leland OS. Usefulness of dipyridamole-thallium-201 perfusion scanning for distinguishing ischemic from nonischemic cardiomyopathy. Am J Cardiol 1988;62:945–51.
52. Leppo JA, O'Brien J, Rothendler JA, Getchell JD, Lee VW. Dipyridamole-thallium-201 scintigraphy in the predictions of future cardiac events after acute myocardial infarction. N Engl J Med 1984;310:1014–8.
53. Younis LT, Byers S, Shaw L, Barth G, Goodgold H, Chaitman BR. Prognostic value of intravenous dipyridamole thallium scintigraphy after an acute myocardial ischemic event. Am J Cardiol 1989;64:161–6.

54. Younis LT, Byers S, Shaw L, Barth G, Goodgold H, Chaitman BR. Prognostic importance of silent myocardial ischemia detected by intravenous dipyridamole thallium myocardial imaging in asymptomatic patients with coronary artery disease. J Am Coll Cardiol 1989;14:1635–41.

55. Gimple LW, Hutter AM Jr, Guiney TE, Boucher CA. Prognostic utility predischarge dipyridamole-thallium imaging compared to predischarge submaximal exercise electrocardiography and maximal exercise thallium imaging after uncomplicated acute myocardial infarction. Am J Cardiol 1989;64:1243–8.

56. Brown KA, O'Meara J, Chambers CE, Plante DA. Ability of dipyridamole-thallium-201 imaging one to four days after acute myocardial infarction to predict in-hospital and late recurrent myocardial ischemic events. Am J Cardiol 1990;65:160–7.

57. Hendel RC, Layden JJ, Leppo JA. Prognostic value of dipyridamole thallium scintigraphy for evaluation of ischemic heart disease. J Am Coll Cardiol 1990;15:109–16.

58. Boucher CA, Brewster DC, Darling RC, Okada RD, Strauss HW, Pohost GM. Determination of cardiac risk by dipyridamole-thallium imaging before peripheral vascular surgery. N Engl J Med 1985;312:389–94.

59. Eagle KA, Singer DE, Brewster DC, Darling RC, Mulley AG, Boucher CA. Dipyridamole-thallium scanning in patients undergoing vascular surgery. Optimizing preoperative evaluation of cardiac risk. JAMA 1987;257:2185–9.

60. Eagle KA, Coley CM, Newell JB et al. Combining clinical and thallium data optimizes preoperative assessment of cardiac risk before major vascular surgery. Ann Intern Med 1989;859–66.

61. Cutler BS, Leppo JA. Dipyridamole thallium 201 scintigraphy to detect coronary artery disease before abdominal aortic surgery. J Vasc Surg 1987;5:91–100.

62. Lette J, Waters D, Lapointe J, et al. Usefulness of the severity and extent of reversible perfusion defects during thallium-dipyridamole imaging for cardiac risk assessment before noncardiac surgery. Am J Cardiol 1989;64:276–81.

63. Fletcher JP, Antico VF, Gruenewald S, Kershaw LZ. Dipyridamole thallium-scan for screening of coronary artery disease prior to vascular surgery. J Cardiovasc Surg (Torino) 1988;29:666–9.

64. Marwick TH, Underwood DA. Dipyridamole thallium imaging may not be a reliable screening test for coronary artery disease in patients undergoing vascular surgery. Clin Cardiol 1990;13:14–8.

65. Lane SE, Lewis SM, Pippin JJ, Kosinski EJ, Campbell D, Nesto RW, et al. Predictive value of quantitative dipyridamole-thallium scintigraphy in assessing cardiovascular risk after vascular surgery in diabetes mellitus. Am J Cardiol 1989;64:1275–9.

66. Brown KA, Rimmer J, Haisch C. Noninvasive cardiac risk stratification of diabetic and nondiabetic uremic renal allograft candidates using dipyridamole-thallium-201 imaging and radionuclide ventriculography. Am J Cardiol 1989;64:1017–21.

67. Villanueva FS, Kaul S, Smith WH, Watson DD, Varma SK, Beller GA. Prevalence and correlates of increased lung/heart ratio of thallim-201 during dipyridamole stress imaging for suspected coronary artery disease. Am J Cardiol 1990;66:1324–8.

68. Lette J, Lapointe J, Waters D, Cerino M, Picard M, Gagnon A. Transient left ventricular cavitary dilation during dipyridamole-thallium imaging as an indicator of severe coronary artery disease. Am J Cardiol 1990;66:1163–70.

69. Chouraqui P, Rodrigues EA, Berman DS, Maddahi J, Significance of dipyridamole-induced transient dilation of the left ventricle during thallium-201 scintigraphy in suspected coronary artery disease. Am J Cardiol 1990;66:689–94.

70. Iskandrian AS, Heo J, Nguyen T, Lyons E, Paugh E. Left ventricular dilation and pulmonary thallium uptake after single-photon emission computer tomography using thallium-201 during adenosine-induced coronary hyperemia. Am J Cardiol 1990;66:807–11.

71. Jain A, Mahmarian JJ, Borges-Neto S, et al. Clinical significance of perfusion defects by thallium-201 single photon emission tomography following oral dipyridamole early after coronary angioplasty. J Am Coll Cardiol 1988;970–6.

72. Homma S, Gilliland Y, Guiney TE, Strauss HW, Boucher CA. Safety of intravenous dipyridamole for stress testing with thallium imaging. Am J Cardiol 1987;59:152–4.

73. Lewen MK, Labovitz AJ, Kern MJ, Chaitman BR. Prolonged myocardial ischemia after intravenous dipyridamole thallium imaging. Chest 1987;92:1102–4.

74. Gerson MC, Moore EN, Ellis K. Systemic effects and safety of intravenous dipyridamole in elderly patients with suspected coronary artery disease. Am J Cardiol 1987;60:1399–401.

75. Pirelli S, Inglese E, Suppa M, Corrada E, Campolo L. Dipyridamole- thallium 201 scintigraphy in the early post-infarction period. (Safety and accuracy in predicting the extent of coronary disease and future recurrence of angina in patients suffering from their first myocardial infarction). Eur Heart J 1988;9:1324–31.

76. Bolognese L, Sarasso G, Aralda D, Bongo AS, Rossi L, Rossi P. High dose dipyridamole echocardiography early after uncomplicated acute myocardial infarction: correlation with exercise testing and coronary angiography. J Am Coll Cardiol 1989;14:357–63.

77. Laarman GJ, Niemeyer MG, van der Wall EE, et al. Dipyridamole thallium testing: noncardiac side effects, cardiac effects, electrocardiographic changes and hemodynamic changes after dipyridamole infusion with and without exercise. Int J Cardiol 1988; 20: 231–8.

78. Sylvén C, Beermann B, Jonzon B, Brandt R. Angina pectoris-like pain provoked by intravenous adenosine in healthy volunteers. Br Med J [Clin Res] 1986;293:227–30.

79. Pearlman JD, Boucher DA. Diagnostic value for coronary artery disease of chest pain during dipyridamole-thallium stress testing. Am J Cardiol 1988;61:43–5.

80. Chambers CE, Brown KA. Dipyridamole-induced ST segment depression during thallium-201 imaging in patients with coronary artery disease: angiographic and hemodynamic determinants. J Am Coll Cardiol 1988;12:37–41.

81. Lette J, Cerino M, Laverdiere M, Tremblay J, Prenovault J. Severe bronchospasm follewed by respiratory arrest during thallium- dipyridamole imaging. Chest 1989;95:1345–7.

82. Demer LL, Gould KL, Goldstein RA, et al. Assessment of coronary artery disease severity by positron emission tomography. Comparison with quantitative arteriography in 193 patients. Circulation 1989;79:825–35.

83. Gould KL, Goldstein RA, Mullani NA, et al. Noninvasive assessment of coronary stenoses by myocardial perfusion imaging during pharmacologic coronary vasodilation. VIII. Clinical feasibility of positron cardiac imaging without a cyclotron using generator-produced rubidium-82. J Am Coll Cardiol 1986;7:775–89.

18. Acute myocardial infarction: Evaluation by nuclear imaging techniques

ERNST E. VAN DER WALL, MENCO G. NIEMEYER,
ERNEST K.J. PAUWELS, PAUL R.M. VAN DIJKMAN,
JAKOBUS A.K. BLOKLAND, ALBERT DE ROOS and
ALBERT V.G. BRUSCHKE

Summary

In recent years, nuclear cardiology techniques have been successfully applied in patients with acute myocardial infarction. These scintigraphic measurements have provided important diagnostic, therapeutic and prognostic information based on the extent of myocardial damage and the functional reserve of the left ventricle. In particular in the thrombolytic era, myocardial perfusion imaging and radionuclide angiography proved to be valuable methods to study the effects of reperfusion on the extent of myocardial damage. Nuclear magnetic resonance imaging, preferably with contrast enhancement, is one of the newly developed nuclear imaging techniques that probably have the greatest potential in accurately delineating myocardial infarct size and in the evaluation of left ventricular function. Radionuclide procedures, on the other hand, employ more biologically oriented tracers and are therefore capable of monitoring biochemical changes in the course of acute myocardial infarction.

Introduction

Management of patients with infarction has become directed at strategies to salvage ischemic myocardium. Particularly in the thrombolytic era one wants to know the early and late benefits of reperfusion therapy. Myocardial infarction can be divided functionally into two phases: the acute phase of infarction when myocardial damage is evolving, and the recovery or convalescent phase, after the completed infarct. Acutely, one wishes know how much myocardium remains at risk, how much is permanently damaged, how much potentially reversibly damaged myocardium is present, the level of ventricular function, and the efficacy of any intervention employed in the early hours of the infarct. In the recovery phase, one wishes to define and determine myocardial functional reserve, the presence of ischemia, and the future risk and prognosis. In both phases, nuclear techniques can play an important role in providing the necessary data leading to an appropriate management strategy. The use of nuclear techniques in the recovery phase for functional

Johan H.C. Reiber & Ernst E. van der Wall (eds.), Cardiovascular Nuclear Medicine and MRI, 271–288.
© 1992 *Kluwer Academic Publishers.*

characterization and risk stratification has become routine; the value of newer nuclear techniques for acutely distinguishing reversibly from irreversibly damaged myocardium and assessing the efficacy of intervention is currently under active investigation. More than one nuclear imaging procedure is presently available and a relative newcomer for studying myocardial infarction is magnetic resonance imaging which offers promise in view of its high spatial resolution and nonionizing character. These features make magnetic resonance imaging potentially very suitable to evaluate patients with myocardial infarction.

Myocardial perfusion scintigraphy

Thallium-201 perfusion scintigraphy

Thallium-201 scintigraphy has been employed to detect and to localize acute myocardial infarction [1]. Wackers et al. [2] were the first to show that thallium-201 defects could be detected in nearly all patients who were evaluated within six hours of the onset of symptoms. However, when more than 24 hours have elapsed following the onset of symptoms, the sensitivity of thallium-201 decreases, presumably as a result of spontaneous reperfusion and development of collateral flow to the infarcted area. The potential for estimating prognosis by thallium-201 scintigraphy in acute infarct patients has been reported by Silverman et al. [3]. They attempted to quantify infarct size (Fig. 1), and observed that patients with a thallium-201 defect involving more than 40 % of the left ventricular circumference identified a patient group with 62 % mortality at 6 months, compared with a 6–month mortality of only 7 % in patients with lower thallium-201 defect scores.

In the era of thrombolytic therapy, thallium-201 scintigraphy has been used as a method of assessing efficacy of reperfusion. Schofer et al. [4] did find that patients who demonstrated improvement in regional wall motion in the infarct zone following successful thrombolysis had new thallium-201 uptake, and in patients with failed reperfusion, there was no change in either regional ejection fraction or thallium-201 uptake. However, immediate injection of the tracer after reperfusion overestimates the amount of viable tissue, whereas, when thallium is injected more than 48 hours after reperfusion, this phenomenon is not observed [5]. As a result, thallium-201 has no prominent role in the immediate assessment of reperfusion-related salvage but may be of use for follow-up studies. In this respect, Van der Wall et al. [6] demonstrated by thallium-201 exercise scintigraphy at 3 months after the acute event, that patients with reperfusion therapy showed a decrease in infarct size on thallium-201 images compared with those without reperfusion therapy, in particular in patients with an anterior infarction (Fig. 2).

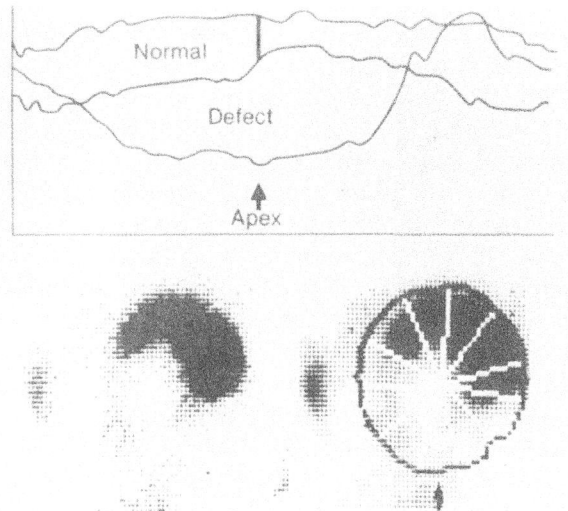

Figure 1. Scintigraphic (thallium-201) estimation of infarct size in a patient with a large antero-septal infarction based on circumferential profile analysis. (Reproduced with permission from Silverman et al., Ref. 3).

Predischarge Thallium-201 imaging

Predischarge thallium imaging combined with exercise or with pharmacologic-induced vasodilatation, has proven to be useful in predicting future cardiac events in patients recovering from acute myocardial infarction. The classic work on predischarge assessment was performed in 1983 by Gibson et al. [7], who assessed patients' prognosis before discharge by means of

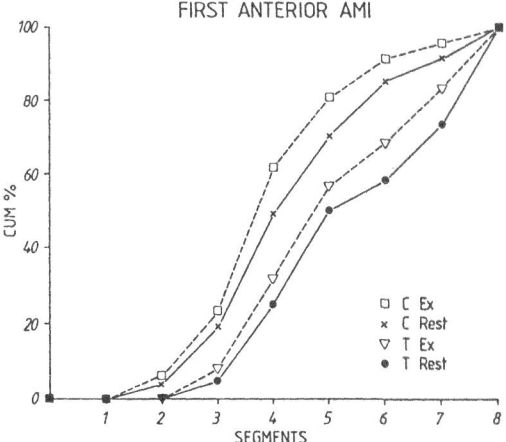

Figure 2. Cumulative percentage of normal thallium-201 segments in patients with a first anterior infarction. The number of normal segments is significantly higher in the patients with thrombolysis (T) compared to the control patients (C), both at rest and during exercise.

submaximal exercise testing, coronary angiography and thallium-201 scintigraphy. They then followed patients for 3 years to determine the subsequent event rate. A low- and high-risk pattern was defined for each of the 3 studies. Although the event rate in patients with a high-risk pattern was similar for exercise testing, coronary angiography and thallium-201 scintigraphy, the event rate in the low-risk group defined by thallium-201 (no redistribution, no defects in zones remote from the infarct zone and no lung uptake) was significantly lower (6 %) than that observed in the low-risk group defined by exercise electrocardiography (27 %), and coronary arteriography (22 %). Thus, in patients with uncomplicated acute myocardial infarction who are nearing discharge, low-level stress Tl-201 scintigraphy appears to be clinically useful in guiding management. A variation of this approach for patients who cannot exercise involves a 4–min intravenous infusion of dipyridamole followed by injection of thallium-201. Imaging then proceeds as it would after stress. The procedure can be used before discharge in patients with myocardial infarction and in patients with suspected coronary artery disease. Leppo et al. [8] were the first to report results of this technique in predicting new myocardial infarction or death in patients with acute myocardial infarction studied before discharge. The event rate within 1 year was only 6 % in patients whose scans showed no thallium-201 redistribution compared with 33 % in patients whose scans did show redistribution. The dipyridamole-thallium imaging technique thus identified a high-risk subset of patients and proved to be significantly more predictive of future events than submaximal exercise testing by electrocardiography alone. An extended variant of the dipyridamole approach is the combination with low-level exercise, as advocated by Laarman et al. [9]. The conjunction with low-level exercise significantly improves the image quality.

A major topic of interest at the current time is the value of 24–hr delayed imaging [10] and, in particular, reinjection of thallium-201 at rest following redistribution [11]. Conventional exercise/redistribution thallium-201 imaging may overestimate the extent of infarction because it has been shown that seemingly persistent defects may fill in on 24–hr delayed images or after reinjection, indicating residual myocardial viability in presumed necrotic areas [10,11]. This phenomenon is of major interest in patients after myocardial infarction, as in this group of patients one wishes to know whether the infarcted tissue is completely necrotic or still contains viable, potentially jeopardized, myocardial cells. This may have important implications for further patient management in terms of a more conservative approach in case of a definite necrotic area versus a more aggressive approach in case of remaining viable myocardial tissue.

Early predischarge Thallium-201 scintigraphy

A recently proposed different and more challenging approach is to perform thallium-201 exercise testing already in the subacute phase after myocardial infarction, i.e. within 3 days after the acute event. The rationale for this approach is early risk stratification of infarct patients and the potential early discharge of a subgroup of patients with negative findings, reducing health care costs. Topol et al. [12] studied 61 patients after reperfusion therapy for acute myocardial infarction who underwent a submaximal exercise test at 72 hours after the acute event. The exercise test was performed in conjunction with thallium-201 single photon emission computed tomography (SPECT). Of the 61 patients, 40 had no evidence of reversible ischemia by thallium-201 scintigraphy, and 17 patients showed reversible ischemic defects; 4 patients had equivocal results. At follow-up, 5 of 17 patients had an adverse clinical event vs none of 40 patients (P < 0.001). This trial documented the safety and feasibility of thallium-201 exercise testing 3 days after infarction, and presaged the safety of early hospital discharge following a negative thallium-201 SPECT test. Pirelli et al. [13] suggested that utilization of dipyridamole thallium stress in the very early post-infarct setting might be preferable to conventional exercise thallium-201 scintigraphy. With dipyridamole thallium-201 imaging, the hazard of early exercise in producing complications, such as sudden circulatory collapse or infarct extension, can be avoided.

Technetium-99m SestaMIBI scintigraphy

To circumvent the radiophysical limitations of thallium-201 (low gamma-emission of 80 keV, long half-life of 72 hr), technetium-99m labeled isonitrile complexes have been developed. Technetium-99m methoxy-isobutyl-isonitrile (technetium-99m SestaMIBI) exhibits the best biological properties for clinical implications. Due to the short half-life (6 hr), dosages up to 10 times as much as thallium-201 can be administered, resulting in better counting statistics. Similar to thallium-201, technetium-99m SestaMIBI accumulates in the myocardium predominantly according to myocardial blood flow. In contrast to thallium-201, it has a slow washout with minimal myocardial redistribution. These features make technetium-99m SestaMIBI more suitable for SPECT imaging and allow more flexibility in the time for starting the imaging procedure following tracer injection, according to findings by Verzijlbergen et al. [14]. The tracer is particularly useful for the immediate assessment of myocardial salvage in the reperfused regions without any delay in administration of thrombolytic therapy [15]. Performing subsequent comparative studies after repeat injections, e.g. 1 to 4 days later, the zone of hypoperfusion representing the final infarct can be identified and compared to the perfusion defect of the initial risk zone [16] (Fig. 3). Verani et al. [17] showed that a 30 % reduction of defect size was highly predictive of patency.

In the future, technetium-99m SestaMIBI may be more effective than thallium-201 for predischarge assessment because it will enable simultaneous assessments of exercise ejection fraction and exercise myocardial perfusion. The predischarge routine of the future may well incorporate a first-pass

MYOCARDIAL PERFUSION

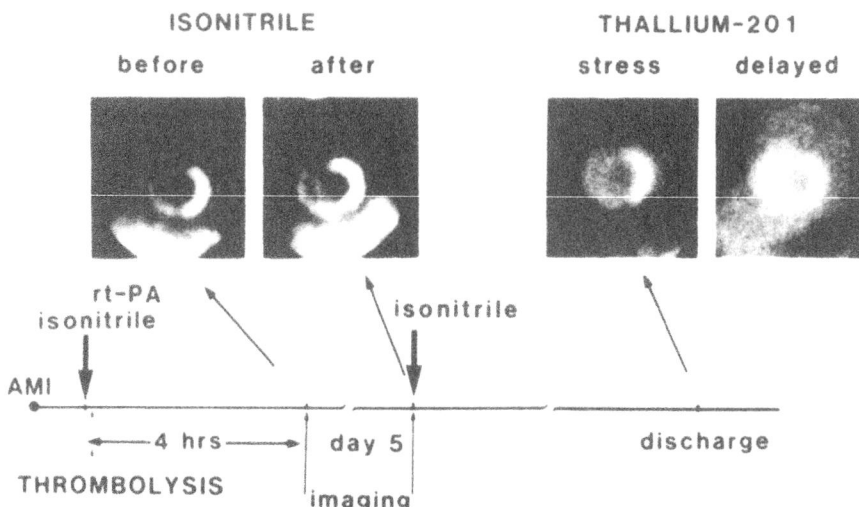

Figure 3. Images with technetium-99m SestaMibi (Tc-MIBI) injected before and after thrombolytic therapy. The images from Tc-MIBI injected before administration of tissue plasminogen activator (rt-PA) show a large septal defect. Images obtained after a second injection of Tc-MIBI (post-thrombolysis) show partial filling in of the defect. The predischarge low-level stress redistribution T1–201 study showed evidence of some viable myocardium in the previously jeopardized zone. AMI = acute myocardial infarction. (Reproduced with permission from Kayden et al., 1988, Ref. 16).

analysis of ventricular function at rest, a delayed gated tomographic assessment of the size of the perfusion defect, and the performance of the first-pass and gated tomographic procedures with exercise.

Rubidium-82 perfusion scintigraphy

Williams et al. [18] examined the use of the positron emitter rubidium-82 in the coronary care unit and clinical laboratory for detection of perfusion defects due to myocardial infarction. They studied 22 patients with myocardial infarction and the rubidium images showed similar sensitivity and specificity as for the thallium-201 and regional wall motion images. The positron emission tomographic technique, however, uses extremely expensive instrumentation and is unfortunately still limited to a small number of medical centres.

Myocardial infarct-avid scintigraphy

Imaging of acute myocardial infarction with infarct-avid imaging agents allows definition of the zone of acute myocardial necrosis as an area of increased radioactivity ('hot spot'). A number of agents have been used, such as technetium-99m pyrophosphate and more recently indium-111 labeled antimyosin.

Technetium-99m pyrophosphate

Technetium-99m pyrophosphate was first introduced as a means of diagnosing acute myocardial infarction in 1974, and proved to be highly sensitive for the clinical diagnosis of acute infarct [19]. Technetium-99m pyrophosphate forms a complex with calcium deposited in damaged myocardial cells. As myocardial uptake is flow dependent, the uptake is poor in the centre of low flow areas of a large infarct, where the uptake is predominantly epicardial. In experimental studies it was shown that technetium-99m pyrophosphate infarcts larger than 3 grams can be visualized by in vivo imaging [20]. Especially right ventricular infarction can be easily diagnosed as reported by Braat et al. [21]. The timing of the technetium-99m pyrophosphate study is of critical importance, and best results have been obtained 24–72 hours post-infarction by which ideally any intervention to salvage myocardium should have taken place [22]. However, Hashimoto et al. [23], who performed early technetium-99m pyrophosphate imaging with SPECT, showed that positive images were very adequate in sizing myocardial infarction soon after coronary reperfusion as early as eight hours after the onset of infarction. Although the sensitivity of pyrophosphate imaging is high, the specificity is rather low since a number of different disease processes show radioisotope accumulation by the myocardium. Positive images have been observed in patients with myocardial trauma, ventricular aneurysm, and after radiation therapy [24]. Additionally, the uptake of technetium-99m pyrophosphate in skeletal structures may restrict the proper interpretation of infarct size.

Indium-111 antimyosin

The development of easily applicable infarct-avid agents, that provide scintigrams which become abnormal within shorter periods with closer correlation between tissue uptake and severity of necrosis, is extremely important. Radiolabeled antimyosin (indium-111 antimyosin) is a monoclonal antibody that binds to cardiac myosin exposed upon cell death. Maximal uptake occurs in regions of lowest flow, and mostly in necrotic areas (Fig. 4). Infarct size in

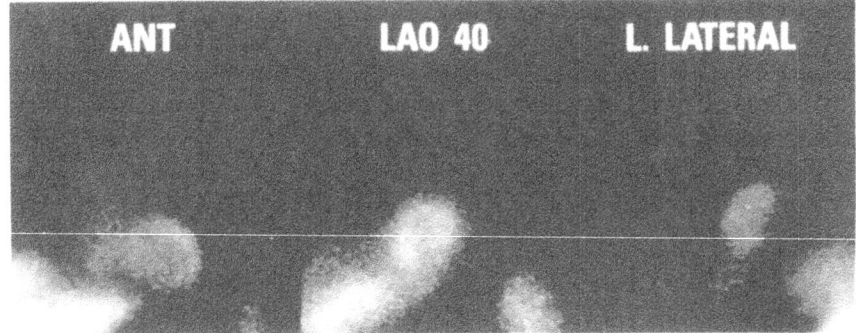

Figure 4. Indium-111 antimyosin scintigram of a patient with an anterior infarction. Uptake of the tracer is clearly visible in the anteriorly localized myocardial areas. (Image courtesy of W. van Prooyen, Centocor, Leiden).

grams can be calculated from transaxially reconstructed, normalized, and background corrected indium-111 antimyosin SPECT images [25]. By performing dual-isotope SPECT imaging with indium-111 monoclonal antibodies and thallium-201, infarct size and percentage of infarcted myocardium can be estimated accurately [26]. Furthermore, the antimyosin images can be then superimposed on the perfusion images to distinguish between viable and necrotic tissue.

Not only for detection of myocardial necrosis, but also for assessment of prognosis, indium-111 antimyosin has proven to be valuable. Follow-up for evaluation of major cardiac events was conducted in a large multicenter study to relate the extent of antimyosin uptake to the major event rate [27]. The incidence of cardiac events ranged from 5–8 % in patients with negative or minimally positive scans, up to an event rate of about 40 % in patients with extensive myocardial uptake of antimyosin. In a subsequent study, Johnson et al. [28] showed in 42 infarct patients that a mismatch pattern between thallium-201 defects and antimyosin uptake (i.e. regions with neither thallium-201 nor antimyosin uptake) identified patients at further ischemic risk. Van Vlies et al. [29], in patients following reperfusion therapy, showed that the level and extent of indium-111 antimyosin uptake could predict improvement of left ventricular wall motion. Drawbacks of indium-111 antimyosin are the blood pool contamination and interference from liver activity with indium-111, its suboptimal imaging characteristics (gamma-emission 170 and 247 keV, half-life 68 hr), and the late moment of reliable infarct definition at approximately 48 hours after infarction.

Biologically based scintigraphy

Radioactive tracers derived specifically for imaging on the basis of their known biological activity have been studied extensively. Scintigraphy with

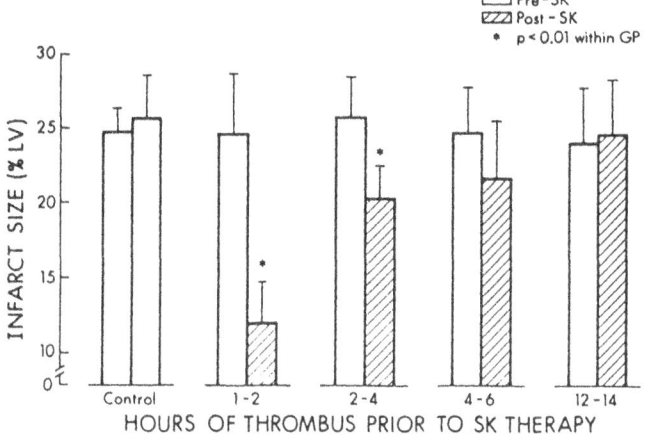

Figure 5. Histogram of tomographically estimated infarct size for control animals with sustained coronary occlusion (n = 6), and animals with 1–2 (n = 4), 2–4(n = 6), 4–6 (n = 4) and 12–14 hr of coronary occlusion prior to streptokinase (SK)(n = 3). Repeat tomography was performed 90 min after SK. Significant decreases of apparent infarct size (or increases in metabolic activity in jeopardized myocardium) occurred only in animals subjected to reperfusion within four hours of occlusion. The results illustrate the utility of positron emission tomography for sequential characterization of myocardium before and after reperfusion. (Reproduced with permission from Bergmann et al., 1982, Ref. 32).

radiolabeled metabolic substrates has become available for noninvasive studies of the normal and diseased myocardium. Metabolic imaging provodes insight into the in vivo myocardial biochemistry and may assist in guiding therapeutic interventions for acute ischemic states.

Carbon-11 palmitate, fluorine-18 deoxyglucose

Positron emitters as carbon-11 palmitate and fluorine-18 deoxyglucose, and the single photon agents, radioiodinated free fatty acids and their analogs, are suitable for assessing infarct size and viable myocardial tissue [30,31]. Positron emission tomography is valuable in delineating areas with reversible and irreversible injury, in assessing the feasibility of surgical revascularization, coronary angioplasty, or thrombolysis with respect to potentially salvageable tissue [32], (Fig. 5). The potential benefits of interventions could be evaluated more precisely in patients after myocardial infarction with advanced coronary disease and severely impaired ventricular function. Clinical studies in infarct patients showed that areas with persistent thallium-201 perfusion defects have evidence of remaining metabolic activity in 47 % of regions when studied with positron emission tomography, indicating overestimation of irreversible injury [33]. The implication, derived from this finding, is that in areas with perfusion defects, if glucose activity remains, the region is viable (mismatch pattern); conversely, if such activity is absent, the area is likely to be infarcted or necrotic (match pattern). In case of remaining viability, patients are more likely to benefit from therapeutical interventions than patients with definite necrotic myocardial areas. Although the assessment of a (mis)match pattern is unique to positron imaging, remaining myocardial viability can also be assessed by reinjection of thallium-201 immediately following the performance of the redistribution images, as stated before. Dilsizian et al. [11] demonstrated improved or normal thallium-201 uptake after reinjection in 49 % of apparently fixed defects, observed at redistribution.

Iodine-123 fatty acids

Metabolic imaging has also been performed with single-photon radiopharmaceuticals using radioiodinated free fatty acids. These can be imaged by both planar and tomographic techniques. Van der Wall et al. [34] demonstrated regionally decreased uptake of I-123 labeled heptadecanoic in patients with acute myocardial infarction. In addition, altered fatty acid metabolism was demonstrated in the infarcted regions. Visser et al. [35], in acute infarct patients, showed restored fatty acid metabolism in myocardial areas that were successfully reperfused.

The role of metabolic imaging in guiding and evaluating therapeutic interventions for acute ischemic states will hopefully expand.

Radionuclide angiography

In the setting of acute myocardial infarction, radionuclide angiography can be used for diagnosis and quantification of infarct size, evaluation of complications such as ventricular septum defect, (false) aneurysm and mitral regurgitation, assessment of the effects of interventions such as thrombolysis, and assessment of prognosis. Among clinical and angiographic variables, global left ventricular ejection fraction at rest, a direct measure of left ventricular function, is the most important predictor of mortality after acute myocardial infarction [36–38]. Analysis of regional left ventricular function may be a more direct means of assessing the efficacy of thrombolytic therapy than global ejection fraction, since global left ventricular ejection fraction obtained early in the course of acute myocardial infarction reflects the function of both viable and nonviable myocardium and thus may not necessarily predict whether reperfusion will improve function. Global ejection fraction determined at predischarge remains however the most important measurable prognostic endpoint following infarction [38]. A progressive increase in 1–year mortality rate occurs when left ventricular ejection fraction decreases below

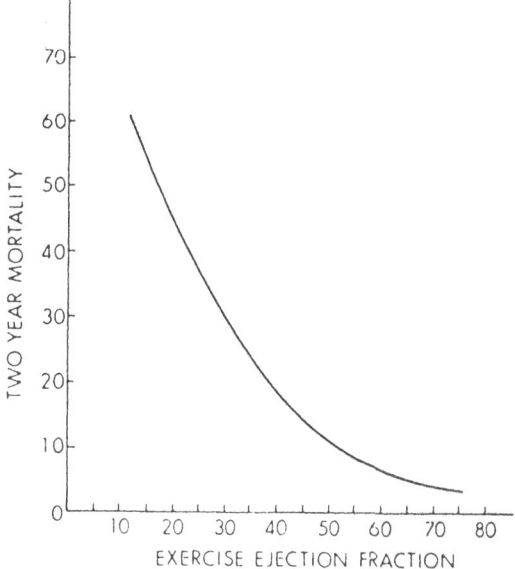

Figure 6. Relation of predischarge left ventricular ejection fraction to 1-year cardiac mortality in 799 patients with acute myocardial infarction. (Reproduced with permission from The Multicenter Post-infarction Research Group, 1983, Ref. 38)

40 % (Fig. 6). Combined rest and exercise radionuclide angiography at the time of hospital discharge, is an attractive procedure for risk assessment after acute infarction because its provides noninvasive measurements of both the severity of left ventricular dysfunction and the presence of potentially ischemic myocardium. Corbett et al. [39] studied 75 infarct patients with a mean resting ejection fraction of 55 % at predischarge. Failure to increase ejection fraction by 5 % or more was associated with a significantly increased rate of reinfarction. Similarly, Morris et al. [40] found a significant association between the time to death and ejection fraction at rest and during exercise in 106 consecutive survivors of acute myocardial infarction (Fig. 7). In a large study conducted by the Interuniversity Cardiology Institute of the Netherlands (ICIN), it was shown that patients with anterior infarction following reperfusion therapy – studied at 2 days, 2 weeks, and 3 months after the acute onset – had significantly improved left ventricular function compared to conventionally treated patients [41,42] (Fig. 8).

Nuclear magnetic resonance imaging

Magnetic resonance imaging has potential for quantifying and identifying areas of myocardial necrosis [43]. Magnetic resonance imaging is a nonionizing high resolution tomographic technique providing good soft tissue contrast, sharp delineation of the myocardium, and adequate characterization

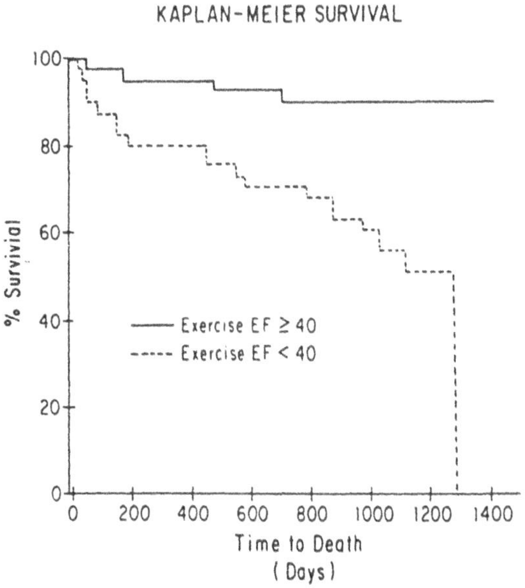

KAPLAN-MEIER SURVIVAL

Figure 7. Life-table survival of patient population by exercise ejection fraction (EF). (Reproduced with permission from Morris et al., 1985, Ref. 40)

of myocardial tissue. The area of acute myocardial infarction can be visualized as a high signal intensity area associated with prolonged T2 relaxation times. By using contrast enhancement with gadolinium-DTPA the infarct can be located more precisely [44] (Fig. 9). In our institution infarct size could be determined by nuclear magnetic resonance imaging using gadolinium-DTPA in patients receiving streptokinase for acute myocardial infarction [45]. Infarct size proved to be significantly smaller in patients with successful reperfusion in comparison with patients without reperfusion [46] (Fig. 10). Van Rossum et al. [47], in patients after thrombolysis, demonstrated that the dynamics of gadolinium-DTPA are useful for the noninvasive assessment of successful reperfusion.

Similar to positron emission tomography, drawbacks of magnetic resonance imaging are expenses and the limited availability of magnetic resonance facilities. Although promising, the clinical value in assessing infarct size and the extent of myocardial salvage after thrombolytic therapy remains to be settled.

Conclusion

In the assessment and management of the patient with acute myocardial infarction, nuclear studies have a role in both the acute and convalescent phase. In the acute phase, areas of decreased flow can be assessed by resting

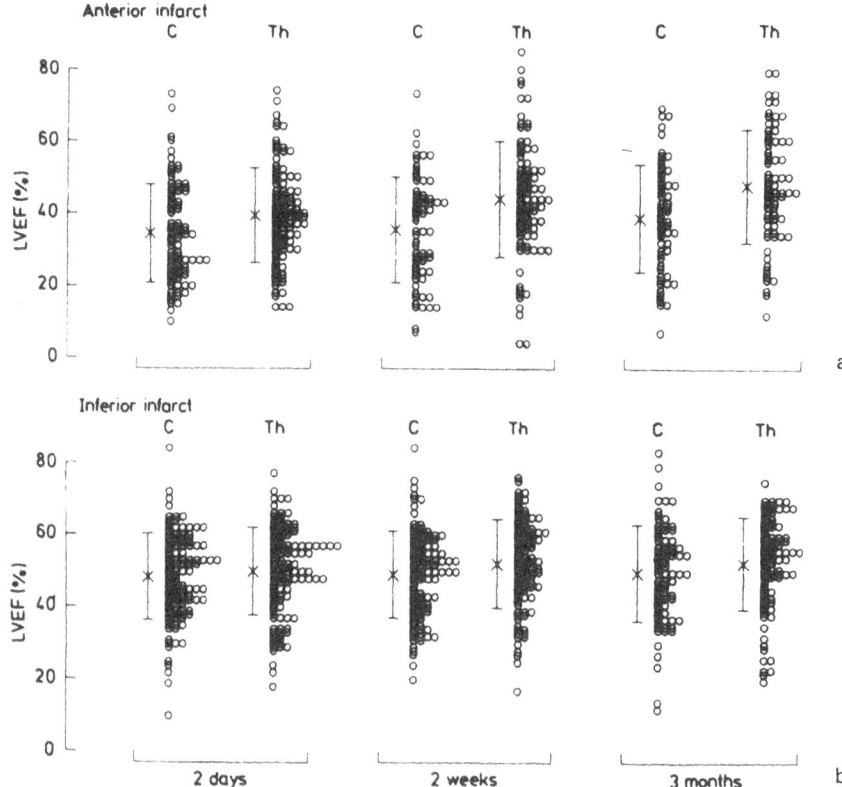

Figure 8. Distribution of left ventricular ejection fraction (LVEF) 2 days, 2 weeks and 3 months after admission, (a) in patients with anterior or anteroseptal infarction, and (b) in patients with inferior wall infarction. Means and standard deviations are indicated. C, conventional treatment; Th, patients allocated to thrombolytic treatment. In particular patients with anterior infarction showed significantly improved LVEF after reperfusion therapy. (Reproduced with permission from Res et al., 1986, Ref. 42)

perfusion imaging, and assessment of reperfusion and potential salvage of myocardium can be made qualitatively with delayed imaging. Thallium-201 and technetium-99m SestaMibi SPECT may provide additional quantification of infarct size, and possible quantitation of salvaged myocardium if serial studies are performed. Further studies are necessary to determine their role. Positron emission tomography is currently the only noninvasive technique that can identify and separate infarcted and ischemic myocardium on a metabolic basis. Whether the application of this expensive new technology to assessment of myocardial viability in patients with acute myocardial infarction will become practical for widespread use remains to be determined. In particular, reinjection of thallium-201 may circumvent the need for positron imaging in determining viability. In the convalescent phase, global and regional left ventricular function provide important prognostic information,

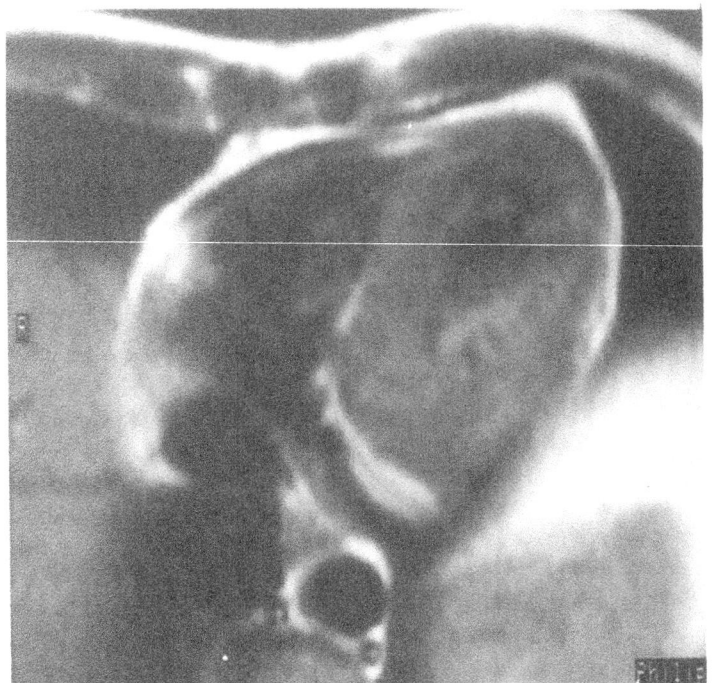

a

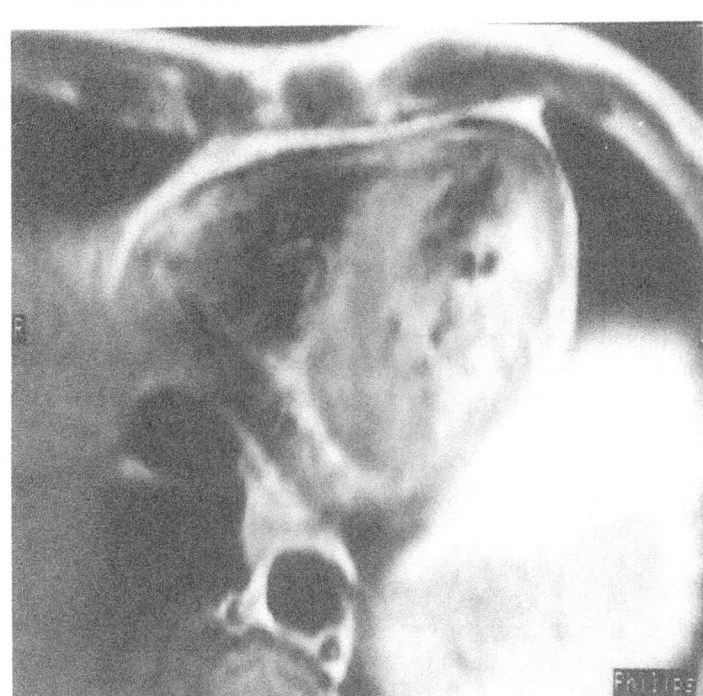

b

Anterior view

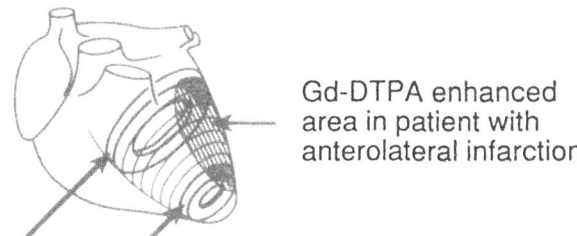

Gd-DTPA enhanced
area in patient with
anterolateral infarction

c   MRI slices (upper and lower)

Figure 9. Magnetic resonance images, (a) before, and (b) after administration of the contrast agent Gadolinium-DTPA from a patient with an acute anterolateral infarction. After administration of Gadolium-DTPA significant contrast enhancement is observed in the anteroseptal myocardial area. Summing up of the extent of contrast enhancement in the different tomographic slices covering the complete left ventricle, an estimate of infarct size can be obtained (c).

and the results of exercise testing combined with either thallium perfusion imaging or ventricular function studies to assess myocardial reserve can be used for risk stratification and to determine the most appropriate management strategies. Magnetic resonance imaging has shown to be useful in assessing infarct size and in following the sequelae after acute interventions. Although offering a great potential, the clinical utility of magnetic resonance imaging in patients with acute myocardial infarction has still to be settled.

Infarct size

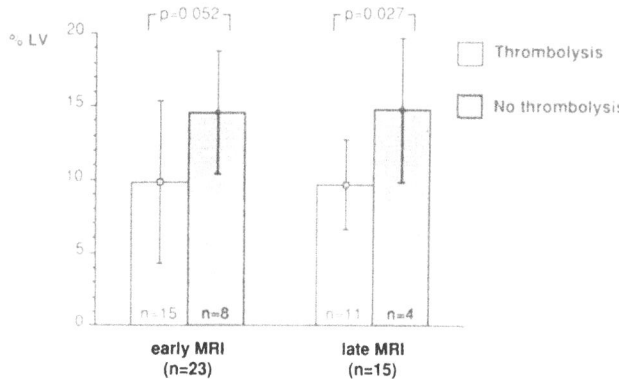

Figure 10. Following thrombolytic therapy a significant reduction of magnetic resonance imaging (MRI) determined infarct size is observed, in particular in patients with late MRI (5 weeks after the acute onset).

References

1. Niemeyer MG, Pauwels EKJ, Van der Wall EE, et al. Detection of multivessel disease in patients with sustained myocardial infarction by thallium 201 myocardial scintigraphy: No additional value of quantitative analysis. Am J Physiol Imaging 1989;4:105–114.
2. Wackers FJT, Busemann Sokole E, Samson G, et al. Value and limitations of thallium-201 scintigraphy in the acute phase of myocardial infarction. N Engl J Med 1976;295:1–5.
3. Silverman KJ, Becker LC, Bulkley BH, et al. Value of early thallium-201 scintigraphy for predicting mortality in patients with acute myocardial infarction. Circulation 1980;61:996–1003.
4. Schofer J, Mathey DG, Monty R, Bleifeld W, Strizke P. Use of dual intracoronary scintigraphy with thallium-201 and technetium-99m pyrophosphate to predict improvement in left ventricular wall motion immediately after intracoronary thrombolysis in acute myocardial infarction. J Am Coll Cardiol 1983;2:737–744.
5. De Coster PM, Melin JA, Detry J-M, Brasseur LA, Beckers C, Col J. Coronary artery reperfusion in acute myocardial infarction: assessment by pre- and post-intervention thallium-201 myocardial perfusion imaging. Am J Cardiol 1985;55:889–893.
6. Van der Wall EE, Res JCJ, Van den Pol R, et al. Improvement of myocardial perfusion after thrombolysis assessed by thallium-201 exercise scintigraphy. Eur Heart J 1988;9:828–835.
7. Gibson RS, Watson DD, Craddock GB, et al. Prediction of cardiac events after uncomplicated myocardial infarction; a prospective study comparing predischarge exercise thallium-201 scintigraphy and coronary angiography. Circulation 1983;68:321–336.
8. Leppo JA, O'Brien J, Rothendler JA, Getchell JD, Lee VW. Dipyridamole-thallium-201 scintigraphy in the prediction of future cardiac events after myocardial infarction. N Engl J Med 1984;310:1014–1018.
9. Laarman GJ, Bruschke AVG, Verzijlbergen FJ, Bal ET, Van der Wall EE, Ascoop CA. Efficacy of intravenous dipyridamole with exercise in thallium-201 myocardial perfusion scintigraphy. Eur Heart J 1988;9;1206–1214.
10. Kiat H, Berman DS, Maddahi J, et al. Late reversibility of tomographic myocardial thallium-201 defects: an accurate marker of myocardial viability. J Am Coll Cardiol 1988;12:1456–1463.
11. Dilsizian V, Rocco T, Freedman NMT, Leon MB, Bonow RO. Enhanced detection of ischemic but viable myocardium by the reinjection of thallium after stress-redistribution imaging. N Engl J Med 1990;323:141–146.
12. Topol EJ, Juni JE, O'Neil WW, et al. Exercise testing three days after onset of acute myocardial infarction. Am J Cardiol 1987;60:958–962.
13. Pirelli S, Inglese E, Suppa M, Corrada E, Campolo L. Dipyridamole-thallium scintigraphy in the early post-infarction period. Eur Heart J 1988;9:1324–1331.
14. Verzijlbergen JF, Cramer MJ, Niemeyer MG, Ascoop CA, Van der Wall EE, Pauwels EKJ. ECG-gated and static Technetium-99m-SestaMIBI planar myocardial perfusion imaging; a comparison with Thallium-201 and study of observer variabilities. Am J Physiol Imaging 1990;5:60–67.
15. Santoro GM, Bisi G, Sciagrà R, et al. Single photon emission computed tomography with technetium-99m hexakis 2–methoxyisobutyl isonitrile in acute myocardial infarction before and after thrombolytic treatment: assessment of salvaged myocardium and prediction of late functional recovery. J Am Coll Cardiol 1990;15:301–314.
16. Kayden DS, Mattera JA, Zaret BL, Wackers FJTh. Demonstration of reperfusion after thrombolysis with technetium-99m isonitrile myocardial imaging. J Nucl Med 1988;29:1865–1867.
17. Verani MS, Jeroudi MO, Mahmarian JJ, et al. Quantification of myocardial infarction during coronary occlusion and myocardial salvage after reperfusion using cardiac imaging

with technetium-99m 2-methoxyisobutyl isonitrile. J Am Coll Cardiol 1988;12:1573-1581.

18. Williams KA, Ryan JW, Resnekov L, et al. Planar positron imaging of rubidium-82 for myocardial infarction: a comparison with thallium-201 and regional wall motion. Am Heart J 1989;118: 601-610.

19. Willerson JT, Parkey RW, Stokely EM, et al. Infarct sizing with technetium-99m stannous pyrophosphate scintigraphy in dogs and man; relationship between scintigraphic and precordial mapping estimates of infarct size in patients. Cardiovasc Res 1977;11:291-296.

20. Stokely EM, Buja M, Lewis SE, et al. Measurement of acute myocardial infarcts in dogs with 99m-Tc-stannous pyrophosphate scintigrams. J Nucl Med 1976;17:1-5.

21. Braat SH, Brugada P, De Zwaan C, Coenegracht JM, Wellens HJJ. Value of electrocardiogram in diagnosing right ventricular involvement in patients with an acute inferior wall myocardial infarction. Br Heart J 1983;49:368-372.

22. Olson HG, Lyons KP, Butman S, et al. Validation of technetium-99m stannous pyrophosphate myocardial scintigraphy for diagnosing acute myocardial infarction more than 48 hours old when serum creatine kinase-MB has returned to normal. Am J Cardiol 1983;52:245-251.

23. Hashimoto T, Kambara H, Fudo T, et al. Early estimation of acute myocardial infarct size soon after coronary reperfusion using emission computed tomography with technetium-99m pyrophosphate. Am J Cardiol 1987;60:952-957.

24. Wynne J, Holman BL. Acute myocardial infarct scintigraphy with infarct-avid radiotracers. Med Clin North Am 1980;64:119-125.

25. Antunes ML, Seldin DW, Wall RM, Johnson LL. Measurement of acute Q-wave myocardial infarct size with single photon emission computed tomography imaging of indium-111 antimyosin. Am J Cardiol 1989;63:777-783.

26. Johnson LL, Lerrick KS, Coromilas J, et al. Measurement of infarct size and percentage myocardium infarcted in a dog preparation with single photon computed tomography, thallium-201 and indium 111–monoclonal antimyosin Fab. Circulation 1987;76:181-190.

27. Johnson LL, Seldin DW, Becker LC, et al. Antimyosin imaging in acute transmural myocardial infarctions: results of a multicenter clinical trial. J Am Coll Cardiol 1989;13:27-35.

28. Johnson LL, Seldin DW, Keller AM, et al. Dual isotope thallium and indium antimyosin SPECT imaging to identify acute infarct patients at further ischemic risk. Circulation 1990;81:37-45.

29. Van Vlies B, Baas J, Visser CA, et al. Dunning AJ. Predictive value of indium-111 antimyosin uptake for improvement of left ventricular wall motion after thrombolysis in acute myocardial infarction. Am J Cardiol 1989;64:167-171.

30. Ter-Pogossian MM, Klein MM, Markham J, Roberts R, Sobel BE. Regional assessment of myocardial metabolic integrity in vivo by positron-emission tomography with C-11–labelled palmitate. Circulation 1980;61:242-255.

31. Sochor H, Schwaiger M, Schelbert HR, et al. Relationship between Tl-201, Tc-99m (Sn) pyrophosphate and F-18 2-deoxyglucose uptake in ischemically injured dog myocardium. Am Heart J 1987;114:1066-1077.

32. Bergmann SR, Lerch RA, Fox KAA, et al. Temporal dependence of beneficial effects of coronary thrombolysis characterized by positron tomography. Am J Med 1982;73:573-581.

33. Brunken R, Schwaiger M, Grover-McKay M, Phelps ME, Tillisch J, Schelbert HR. Positron emission tomography detects tissue metabolic activity in myocardial segments with persistent thallium perfusion defects. J Am Coll Cardiol 1987;10:557-567.

34. Van der Wall EE, Den Hollander W, Heidendal GAK, Westera G, Majid PA, Roos JP. Dynamic scintigraphy with I-123 labelled free fatty acids in patients with myocardial infarction. Eur J Nucl Med 1981;6:383-389.

35. Visser FC, Westera G, Van Eenige MJ, Van der Wall EE, Heidendal GAK, Roos JP. Free fatty acid scintigraphy in patients with successful thrombolysis after myocardial infarction. Clin Nucl Med 1985;10:35-39.

36. Taylor GJ, Humphries JO, Mellits ED, et al. Predictors of clinical course, coronary anatomy and left ventricular function after recovery from acute myocardial infarction. Circulation 1980;62:960–970.
37. Sanz G, Castanar A, Betriu A, et al. Determinants of prognosis in survivors of myocardial infarction: a prospective clinical angiographic study. N Engl J Med 1982;306:1065–1070.
38. Multicenter Postinfarction Research Group. Risk stratification and survival after myocardial infarction. N Engl J Med 1983;309:331–336.
39. Corbett JR, Dehmer GJ, Lewis SE, et al. The prognostic value of submaximal exercise testing with radionuclide ventriculography before hospital discharge in patients with recent myocardial infarction. Circulation 1981;64:535–541.
40. Morris KG, Palmeri ST, Califf RM, et al. Value of radionuclide angiography for predicting specific cardiac events after acute myocardial infarction. Am J Cardiol 1985;55:318–324.
41. Van der Wall EE, Res JCJ, Van Eenige MJ, et al. Effects of intracoronary thrombolysis on global left ventricular function assessed by an automated edge detection technique. J Nucl Med 1986;27:478–483.
42. Res JC, Simoons ML, Van der Wall EE, et al. Long term improvement in global left ventricular function after early thrombolytic treatment in acute myocardial infarction. Br Heart J 1986;56:414–421.
43. Bouchard A, Reeves RC, Cranney G, Bishop SP, Pohost GM, Bischoff P. Assessment of myocardial infarct size by means of T2–weighted 1H nuclear magnetic resonance imaging. Am Heart J 1989;117:281–289.
44. Nishimura T, Yamade Y, Hayashi M, et al. Determination of infarct size of acute myocardial infarction in dogs by magnetic resonance imaging and gadolinium-DTPA: comparison with indium-111 antimyosin imaging. Am J Physiol Imaging 1989;4:83–88.
45. De Roos A, Matheijssen NAA, Doornbos J, Van Dijkman PRM, Van Voorthuisen AE, Van der Wall EE. Assessment of myocardial infarct size after reperfusion therapy using gadolinium-DTPA enhanced magnetic resonance imaging. Radiology 1990;176:517–521.
46. Van Dijkman PRM, Van der Wall EE, De Roos A, et al. Infarct size determined by gadolinium-DTPA enhanced magnetic resonance imaging in the evaluation of the efficacy of coronary thrombolysis. Neth J Cardiol 1990;3:95 (Abstract).
47. Van Rossum AC, Visser FC, Van Eenige MJ, et al. Value of gadolinium-diethylene-triamine pentaacetic acid dynamics in magnetic resonance imaging of acute myocardial infarction with occluded and reperfused coronary arteries after thrombolysis. Am J Cardiol 1990;65:845–851.

19. Prognostic assessment of coronary artery disease by exercise radionuclide ventriculography

RICHARD LIM and DUNCAN S. DYMOND

Summary

Exercise radionuclide angiography appears to contribute additional prognostic information to catheterisation and clinical data. Probably, the most important predictor of all-cause cardiovascular mortality is exercise radionuclide left ventricular ejection fraction. The prognostic value of exercise radionuclide ventriculography may be enhanced when performed *on* medical therapy, since an abnormal ejection fraction response to exercise despite anti-ischemic medications identifies the high-risk patient. For postthrombolytic patients the logistically optimum time for routine testing may be 6–8 weeks postinfarction and not much later to avoid missing the high-risk patient. In treated patients with silent ischemia, exercise radionuclide ventriculography may offer a simple means of individualizing and optimalizing such treatment.

Introduction

When revascularization is recommended for patients with limiting symptoms or prognostically significant coronary disease, it is hoped that this improves their quality of life and prolongs survival. By tradition, the assessment of prognosis in suspected or documented coronary disease has relied heavily on coronary arteriography and is influenced by three major randomized coronary surgery studies, supported by evidence of myocardial ischemia on exercise testing. Nonetheless, there remains a considerable patient residue with indeterminate (not necessarily intermediate) prognosis who defy stratification by arteriography or exercise electrocardiography. Furthermore, there are several reasons why the traditional approach may no longer be the best for an increasing number of patients.

Percutaneous coronary angioplasty has emerged as an attractive widely applicable treatment though its true place in the management of coronary disease is not yet established. The advent of thrombolysis as routine therapy in acute myocardial infarction has generated a large group of survivors who merit prognostic stratification. Aspirin has become routine treatment, newer and more anti-ischemic agents are now available to individualize medical

Johan H.C. Reiber & Ernst E. van der Wall (eds.), Cardiovascular Nuclear Medicine and MRI. 289–298.
© 1992 *Kluwer Academic Publishers.*

therapy, and control of angina has probably improved, though the importance of silent ischemia is increasingly recognized. Enthusiasm for applying high technology to the management of ischemic heart disease is being tempered by the need to contain the costs of assessment and treatment. Alternative noninvasive methods of prognostic testing have become available for refining the process of risk stratification in order to rationalize the allocation of invasive resources.

Exercise radionuclide ventriculography

Radionuclide ventriculography performed at rest and exercise is one such method that has been used increasingly to assess prognosis in coronary disease, whether suspected or documented by arteriography. The arteriogram, an invasive test of coronary anatomy, in clinical practice is often a crude visual assessment of luminal stenosis and cannot detect myocardial ischemia. The noninvasive radionuclide ventriculogram does not diagnose coronary artery disease, being a test of myocardial physiology, but provides a sensitive measurement of left ventricular function with a versatile ejection fraction range of 10–70 %.

Several workers have accordingly reported that the response to exercise during radionuclide ventriculography is of prognostic importance [1–7]. Jones et al. [1] found that patients with coronary disease and an abnormal exercise response had more favourable survival and pain relief if they underwent bypass surgery than if they were treated medically, suggesting that the test can be used to select patients who would or would not benefit from surgery. Bonow and colleagues [2] showed that in minimally symptomatic patients, the absolute exercise ejection fraction was significantly related to sudden death during medical therapy for three-vessel coronary disease, whilst a fall in ejection fraction from rest to exercise was associated with progressive angina requiring surgery. Conversely, patients with three-vessel disease but no evidence of exercise-induced ischemia appear to have a good outlook.

A preliminary study [3] by the Duke investigators followed by a fuller report [7] shared the major limitation that not all adverse cardiovascular events were primarily cardiac or necessarily ischemic and thus potentially amenable to preventive intervention. However, the same institution had separately reported that the change in ejection fraction with exercise was significantly associated with refractory angina requiring surgery [8]. Though the risk of *death* may be similar in two patients with an absolute exercise ejection fraction of 35 %, it is conceivable that the patient whose ejection fraction falls from 55 % is at greater risk of *ischemic* events than the patient whose ejection fraction rises from 30 %. This notwithstanding, possibly the most important predictor of all-cause cardiovascular mortality is exercise radionuclide ejection fraction [7]. Furthermore, the strength of the relationship between radionuclide variables and mortality matches that of prognostically important catheterisation variables, and radionuclide ventriculography appears to contribute additional prognostic information to catheterisation and clinical data.

On or off treatment?

One characteristic common to most reports of prognostic stress testing is that it has been performed with all or only some of the patients having stopped their regular anti-ischemic medications for a few hours to a few days, and several reports have omitted such treatment details altogether. Whilst diagnostic stress testing is better performed off medications to enhance its sensitivity for detecting disease, and whilst such testing may also yield prognostic information, it may be that the diagnostic usefulness of a stress test differs from its prognostic value in assessing patients with documented disease.

In some instances, it may be more appropriate to perform prognostic testing on medications, e.g. in the medically treated patient. The rationale for this is as follows. Firstly, when medical therapy rather than revascularization is recommended to patients with revascularizable coronary disease, we should offer some practicable means of testing the cardioprotective efficacy of that therapy. Secondly, since medical therapy which satisfactorily controls angina is the *raison d'être* for continuing with conservative management in non-critical coronary disease, should not prognostic testing be performed *on* rather than off such therapy?

We have therefore assessed the role of exercise radionuclide ventriculography performed *on* therapy in the evaluation of prognosis in 54 medically treated patients with significant but non-critical angiographic coronary disease [9]. Left ventricular ejection fraction was measured by the first-pass technique using technetium-99m pertechnetate and the Scinticor multicrystal gamma camera system (Scinticor Inc, Wisconsin, USA). Upright symptom-limited graded exercise was performed on a Fitron cycle.

At 6–month follow-up, we found that 10 of the 54 patients had experienced adverse events (Group I) comprising 1 cardiac death, 1 myocardial infarction, 3 cases of worsening angina requiring revascularization and 5 cases of unstable angina. Forty-four patients were event-free (Group II).

Univariate analysis (Table 1) showed that *off* treatment, there was an obvious but non-significant trend towards a greater fall in ejection fraction with exercise in Group I. However, on treatment, there was a highly significant difference in the ejection fraction response to exercise: a fall of 10 % in Group I vs a rise of 3 % in Group II. Expressed in another way (Fig. 1), the event-free group showed a rise in ejection fraction with exercise on treatment, whilst the adverse event group showed a persistent fall.

The study is ongoing to see what magnitude of fall in ejection fraction is most predictive of adverse outcome and whether long-term outcome worsens

Table 1. Grp I (adverse events) vs Grp 11 (event-free); values expressed as mean

	Grp 1	Grp 11	P value
Age	57	56	ns
Previous Ml	7	36	ns
+ve exECG	3	10	ns
No. diseased vessels	2	2	ns
3- vessel disease	0	9	ns
Ex LVEF off Rx %	37	43	ns
Ex LVEF on Rx %	43	43	ns
Change in LVEF off Rx	−8	−3	0.05[a]
Change in LVEF on Rx	−10	+3	0.0006[b]

[a]95% Cl= 6 to 19%.
[b]5% Cl = 0 to 11%.

if subsequent ejection fraction response to exercise deteriorates. The findings so far suggest that the prognostic value of exercise radionuclide ventriculography may be enhanced when performed *on* medical therapy, since an abnormal ejection fraction response to exercise *despite* clinically adequate medical therapy implies an adverse short-term outcome in medically treated coronary disease and suggests that early prognostic revascularization may need to be considered. The data appear to confirm what clinicians intuitively believe: that an exercise test which is abnormal despite anti-ischemic medications identifies the high-risk patient.

A trial is needed to compare outcome between patients with abnormal vs normal exercise radionuclide ventriculography performed on treatment and randomized to either revascularization or medical therapy. If such testing on clinically adequate medical therapy should become a routine method of

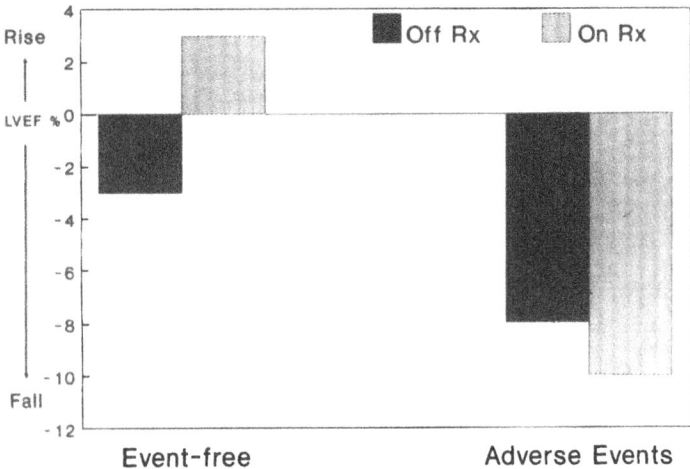

Figure 1. Change in LVEF with exercise. Exercise radionuclide ventriculography.

assessment in patients with suspected and known coronary disease, the clinical and resource implications will be far-reaching.

At the referral centre,

1. Can exercise radionuclide ventriculography performed on treatment improve patient selection for revascularization rather than medical therapy?
2. Can it help to 'triage' patients awaiting revascularization, especially where waiting lists are long?
3. Can invasive coronary angiography be reserved for patients who are potential candidates for revascularization because of limiting symptoms, or those with 'prognostically bad' exercise radionuclide ventriculography results? At the referring hospital where most patients originate, can exercise radionuclide ventriculography on treatment be performed reliably and serially to improve patient selection, and avoid referral for invasive angiography if test results are 'safe'?

Post-thrombolysis prognosis

Not only has effective thrombolytic treatment of acute myocardial infarction resulted in a large surviving population with residual coronary stenoses and the potential for myocardial jeopardy [10], it has also raised many questions concerning their post-reperfusion management and prognosis which are not properly addressed by data from the pre-thrombolytic era. For example, the traditional value of resting ejection fraction as a powerful marker of mortality has been questioned [11]. One possible explanation is that prompt reperfusion has resulted in fairly uniform preservation of ejection fraction so that its discriminatory power has diminished. Simoons et al. [12] found that ejection fraction as assessed by contrast ventriculography between 10–40 days post-infarction was better in patients who received thrombolysis than in those who did not and that this was the best predictor of long-term outcome. However the pooled evidence from other thrombolytic trials suggests that global resting ejection fraction may not be a useful surrogate endpoint in assessing thrombolytic efficacy (as opposed to prognostic importance post-infarction) [11]. This raises the hypothesis that it is the functional significance of residual anatomical lesions and not the irreversible aftermath of coronary thrombosis which is the crucial determinant of post-thrombolysis outcome.

So can the ventricular response to exercise now assume greater importance? Pre-thrombolytic data from exercise radionuclide ventriculography performed at roughly 3 weeks post-infarction showed that both the change in ejection fraction with exercise and the peak exercise ejection fraction were of prognostic value [8,13–15]. It is not known if these indices are applicable to present day assessment of prognosis following thrombolysis, but they probably still are relevant measures of risk.

That post-thrombolytic patients require some form of prognostic assessment is not in doubt. Many remain at risk of death, reocclusion, recurrent ischemia and need for revascularization. A recent report from the SWIFT (Should We Intervene Following Thrombolysis?) study group [16] is the latest in a series [17,18] supporting a conservative policy of post-thrombolysis intervention *only* for accepted clinical indications, amongst which is a positive test for inducible ischemia. However the predischarge exercise electrocardiogram does not seem to be able to predict reinfarction or death [12]. The outstanding issues are: which prognostic test is best for defining risk, and when should it be performed [19,20]. Moreover, given the progressive nature of coronary disease, how often should testing occur? If exercise radionuclide ventriculography is used, pre-discharge test interpretation may theoretically be confounded by myocardial stunning [21]. However the clinical data on recovery from stunning are conflicting [16,18,22–24]. In our own practice, a logistically optimum time for routine testing may be 6–8 weeks post-infarction and not much later to avoid missing the high-risk patient.

Subset analysis of the ongoing study at St Bartholomew's identified 31 medically treated stable patients (mean age 54) who had undergone exercise radionuclide ventriculography off anti-ischemic therapy between 6–8 weeks following thrombolysis for first myocardial infarction. The test was repeated within 4 weeks on therapy. At 1 year post-infarction, 5 patients had suffered significant recurrent symptoms (unstable angina in 1, non-fatal myocardial infarction in 1, worsening angina requiring revascularization in 3), but 26 remained well. Both groups were similar in mean number of diseased coronary arteries, exercise ejection fraction whether off (39 % vs 43 %) or on therapy (43 % vs 44 %), and change in ejection fraction with exercise off therapy (-11% vs -3%). However, on therapy, event-free patients showed an ejection fraction rise of 5 % with exercise whilst the group suffering recurrent symptoms showed a persistent fall of 11 % in ejection fraction ($P = 0.0008$, 95 % confidence interval = 7 to 23). These findings beg the question whether post-thrombolysis prognostic testing should be routinely and *only* performed *on* cardioprotective medication.

Silent myocardial ischemia

The need for accurate objective prognostic testing has been heightened by awareness that subjective symptoms are poor indicators of reversible myocardial ischemia and thus inadequate guides to management. Recent interest has focused on the prognostic implications of silent ischemia [25,26] and in particular whether its treatment improves prognosis (Fig. 2). Despite reported effects of anti-anginal medications on silent ischemia [27–30] data on how they affect patient outcome are still lacking.

We therefore examined whether the failure of anti-anginal therapy to abolish silent ischemia during exercise radionuclide ventriculography carried an adverse prognosis in medically treated coronary disease. We found that

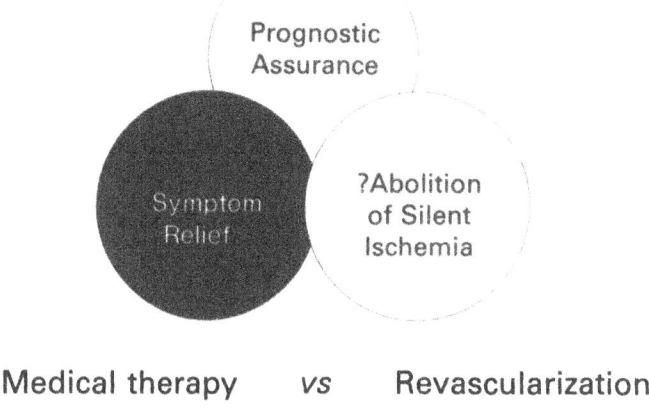

Medical therapy *vs* **Revascularization**

Figure 2. Treatment goals in coronary artery disease.

when such exercise-induced silent ischemia was not abolished by clinically adequate therapy, the relative risk of adverse cardiac events was increased nearly five-fold (Fig. 3).

These preliminary data suggest that persistent exercise-induced silent ischemia may be a marker of high-risk coronary disease and that, in medically treated coronary disease, the efficacy of medical therapy may need to be assessed by titration against ischemia and not just angina. If it is ultimately proved that silent ischemia requires treatment, then exercise radionuclide ventriculography may offer a simple means of individualizing and optimalizing such treatment.

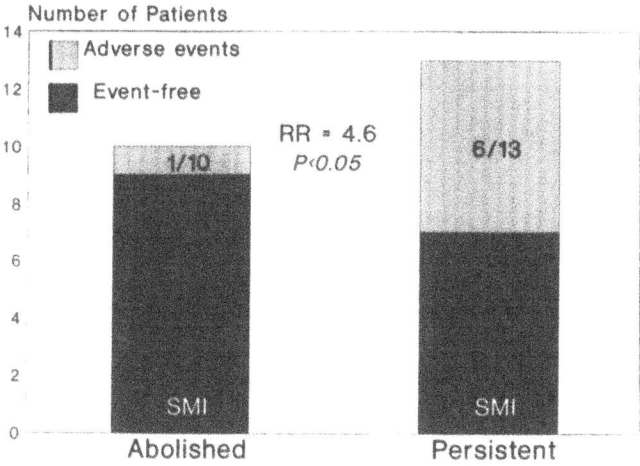

Figure 3. Adverse cardiac events. Effect of anti-ischemic therapy on silent ischemia.

Conclusions

Exercise radionuclide angiography appears to contribute additional prognostic information to catheterisation and clinical data. The strength of the relationship between radionuclide variables and mortality matches that of prognostically important catheterisation variables. Probably, the most important predictor of all-cause cardiovascular mortality is exercise radionuclide left ventricular ejection fraction. The prognostic value of exercise radionuclide ventriculography may be enhanced when performed *on* medical therapy, since an abnormal ejection fraction response to exercise despite medical therapy implies an adverse short-term outcome in medically treated coronary disease and suggests that early prognostic revascularization may need to be considered. The data appear to confirm what clinicians intuitively believe: that an exercise test which is abnormal despite anti-ischemic medications identifies the high-risk patient. For post-thrombolytic patients the logistically optimum time for routine radionuclide exercise testing may be 6–8 weeks post-infarction and not much later to avoid missing the high-risk patient. Pooled evidence from major thrombolytic trials suggests that global resting ejection fraction may not be a useful surrogate end-point in assessing thrombolytic efficacy (as opposed to prognostic importance post-infarction). This raises the hypothesis that it is the functional significance of residual anatomical lesions and not the irreversible aftermath of coronary thrombosis which is the crucial determinant of post-thrombolysis outcome. In addition, own data beg the question whether post-thrombolysis prognostic testing should be routinely and *only* performed *on* cardioprotective medication.

Recent interest has focused on the prognostic implications of silent ischemia and in particular whether its treatment improves prognosis. Despite reported effects of anti-anginal medications on silent ischemia, data on how they affect patient outcome are still lacking. If it is ultimately proved that patients with silent ischemia require treatment, exercise radionuclide ventriculography may offer a simple means of individualizing and optimalizing such treatment.

References

1. Jones RH, Floyd RD, Austin EH, Sabiston DC Jr. The role of radionuclide angiocardiography in the preoperative prediction of pain relief and prolonged survival following coronary artery bypass grafting. Ann Surg 1983;197:743–54.
2. Bonow RO, Kent KM, Rosing DR, et al. Exercise-induced ischemia in mildly symptomatic patients with coronary-artery disease and preserved left ventricular function. Identification of subgroups at risk of death during medical therapy. N Engl J Med 1984;311:1339–45.
3. Pryor DB, Harrell FE Jr, Lee KL, et al. Prognostic indicators from radionuclide angiography in medically treated patients with coronary artery disease. Am J Cardiol 1984;53:18–22.
4. Iskandrian AS, Hakki AH, Schwarz JS, Kay H, Mattleman S, Kane S. Prognostic impli-

cations of rest and exercise radionuclide ventriculography in patients with suspected or proven coronary heart disease. Int J Cardiol 1984;6:707–18.

5. Gibbons RJ, Fyke FE, Clements IP, Lapeyre AC, Zinsmeister AR, Brown ML. Noninvasive identification of severe coronary artery disease using exercise radionuclide angiography. J Am Coll Cardiol 1988;11:28–34.

6. Miller TD, Taliercio CP, Zinsmeister AR, Gibbons RJ. Risk stratification of single or double vessel coronary artery disease and impaired left ventricular function using exercise radionuclide angiography. Am J Cardiol 1990;65:1317–21.

7. Lee KL, Pryor DB, Pieper KS, et al. Prognostic value of radionuclide angiography in medically treated patients with coronary artery disease. A comparison with clinical and catheterization variables. Circulation 1990;82:1705–17.

8. Morris KG, Palmeri ST, Califf RM, et al. Value of radionuclide angiography for predicting specific cardiac events after acute myocardial infarction. Am J Cardiol 1985;55:318–24.

9. Lim R, Dyke L, Dymond DS. Prognostic importance of failure of medical therapy to normalise exercise ejection fraction response in coronary artery disease (abstract). J Am Coll Cardiol 1991;17 Suppl A:183A.

10. Schaer DH, Ross AM, Wasserman AG. Reinfarction, recurrent angina, and reocclusion after thrombolytic therapy. Circulation 1987;76 (2 Pt 2):II57–62.

11. Califf RM, Harrelson-Woodlief L, Topol EJ. Left ventricular ejection fraction may not be useful as an end point of thrombolytic therapy comparative trials. Circulation 1990;82:1847–53.

12. Simoons ML, Vos J, Tijssen JGP, et al. Long term benefit of early thrombolytic therapy in patients with acute myocardial infarction: 5 year follow-up of a trial conducted by the Interuniversity Cardiology Institute of The Netherlands. J Am Coll Cardiol 1989;14:1609–15.

13. Corbett JR, Dehmer GJ, Lewis SE, et al. The prognostic value of submaximal exercise testing with radionuclide ventriculography prior to hospital discharge in patients with recent myocardial infarction. Circulation 1981;64:535–44.

14. Hung J, Goris ML, Nash E, et al. Comparative value of maximal treadmill testing, exercise thallium myocardial perfusion scintigraphy and exercise radionuclide ventriculography for distinguishing high- and low-risk patients soon after acute myocardial infarction. Am J Cardiol 1984;53:1221–7.

15. DeBusk RF, Dennis CA. 'Submaximal' predischarge exercise testing after acute myocardial infarction: who needs it? Am J Cardiol 1985;55:498–500.

16. SWIFT trial of delayed elective intervention vs conservative treatment after thrombolysis with anistreplase in acute myocardial infarction. SWIFT (Should We Intervene Following Thrombolysis?). BMJ 1991;302:555–60.

17. Simoons ML, Arnold AE, Betriu A, et al. Thrombolysis with tissue plasminogen activator in acute myocardial infarction: no additional benefit from immediate percutaneous coronary angioplasty. Lancet 1988;i:197–203.

18. Rogers WJ, Baim DS, Gore JM, et al. Comparison of immediate invasive, delayed invasive, and conservative strategies after tissue-type plasminogen activator. Results of the Thrombolysis in Myocardial Infarction Trial (TIMI) Phase I-A trial. Circulation 1990;81:1457–76.

19. Ellis SG, Topol EJ, George BS, et al. Recurrent ischemia without warning. Analysis of risk factors for in-hospital ischemic events following successful thrombolysis with intravenous tissue plasminogen activator. Circulation 1989;80:1159–65.

20. ACC/AHA guidelines for the early management of patients with acute myocardial infarction. A report of the American College of Cardiology/American Heart Association Task Force on Assessment of Diagnostic and Therapeutic Cardiovascular Procedures. Circulation 1990;82:664–707.

21. Ellis SG, Henschke CI, Sandor T, Wynne J, Braunwald E, Kloner RA. Time course of functional and biochemical recovery of myocardium salvaged by reperfusion. J Am Coll Cardiol 1983;1:1047–55.

22. Sheehan FH, Doerr R, Schmidt WG, et al. Early recovery of left ventricular function after

thrombolytic therapy for acute myocardial infarction: an important determinant of survival. J Am Coll Cardiol 1988;12:289–300.

23. Pfisterer M, Zuber M, Wenzel R, Burkart F. Prolonged myocardial stunning after thrombolysis: can left ventricular function be assessed definitely at hospital discharge? Eur Heart J 1991;12:214–17.

24. Marzoll U, Kleiman NS, Dunn JK, et al. Factors determining improvement in left ventricular function after reperfusion therapy for acute myocardial infarction: primacy of baseline ejection fraction. J Am Coll Cardiol 1991;17:613–20.

25. Weiner DA, Ryan TJ, McCabe CH, et al. Comparison of coronary artery bypass surgery and medical therapy in patients with exercise-induced silent myocardial ischemia: a report from the Coronary Artery Surgery Study (CASS) registry. J Am Coll Cardiol 1988;12:595–9.

26. Breitenbucher A, Pfisterer M, Hoffmann A, Burckhardt D. Long-term follow-up of patients with silent ischemia during exercise radionuclide angiography. J Am Coll Cardiol 1990;15:999–1003.

27. Borer JS, Bacharach SL, Green MV, Kent KM, Johnston GS, Epstein SE. Effect of nitroglycerin on exercise-induced abnormalities of left ventricular regional function and ejection fraction in coronary artery disease. Assessment by radionuclide cineangiography in symptomatic and asymptomatic patients. Circulation 1978;57:314–20.

28. Imperi GA, Lambert CR, Coy K, Lopez L, Pepine CJ. Effects of titrated beta-blockade (metoprolol) on silent myocardial ischemia in ambulatory patients with coronary artery disease. Am J Cardiol 1987;60:519–24.

29. Mulcahy D, Keegan J, Cunningham D, et al. Circadian variation of total ischaemic burden and its alteration with anti- anginal agents. Lancet 1988;ii:755–9.

30. Van der Wall EE, Manger Cats V, Blokland JAK, et al. The effects of diltiazem on cardiac function in silent ischemia after myocardial infarction. Am Heart J 1989;118:655–61.

PART V

Cardiac magnetic resonance imaging

20. Magnetic resonance imaging of the cardiovascular system

RICHARD UNDERWOOD

Summary

Conventional magnetic resonance imaging offers excellent anatomical detail of the cardiovascular system, particularly in congenital heart disease and in diseases of the aorta, where invasive investigation can be avoided in selected cases. Global and regional ventricular function can be measured by cine imaging, valvular regurgitation and flow through shunts can be assessed, and filling defects such as thrombus and tumour are more readily recognised

Cine velocity mapping provides a display of velocity at each point wiᴛ in the heart, and offers flow measurements within the pulmonary and systeᴧ.ic circulations as well as in structures such as coronary bypass grafts. Velocity profiles through vessels can be used to demonstrate the functional significance of disease, and if it is possible to combine such measurements with three dimensional imaging of the coronary arteries, a completely noninvasive assessment of coronary artery disease may be possible.

An alternative approach to the assessment of vascular disease is the measurement of aortic compliance and we have demonstrated that compliance is low in patients with coronary artery disease and high in athletes. Aortic flow patterns are related to compliance and they are also disturbed in patients with disease. Atheroma can be imaged directly, and the ability to image fat and water separately indicates that it may be possible to direct treatment according to the chemical composition of the atheroma.

The wider application of these techniques will depend upon acceptance and understanding by cardiologists and the availability of resources for further development.

Introduction

Magnetic resonance is firmly established in imaging of the brain, the spinal cord and other static organs, because of the quality of the images produced and the natural contrast between different tissues. Over the last five years there has been increasing interest in cardiovascular magnetic resonance, because, despite the technical problems of imaging a moving organ, it is

Johan H.C. Reiber & Ernst E. van der Wall (eds.), Cardiovascular Nuclear Medicine and MRI, 301–309.
© 1992 *Kluwer Academic Publishers.*

possible to obtain both anatomical and functional information and to avoid invasive investigation in some cases.

Anatomy

The aorta

Many centres have reported the value of magnetic resonance in diseases of the aorta [1,2]. The aorta is particularly well seen because of its size and relative immobility, and because there is natural contrast between the wall and moving blood which usually gives no signal using conventional sequences.

Dissection is readily detected and its extent can be seen, including the involvement of other vessels. The entry and exit points are more difficult to localise, but there is no doubt that invasive investigation can be avoided with a combination of echocardiography and magnetic resonance [3]. The previous inability to detect involvement of the aortic valve is no longer a problem, since aortic regurgitation is now readily detected and quantified, and although an adequate assessment of the coronary arteries is not obtained, this is not always necessary preoperatively. Goldman et al. have compared the relative merits of echocardiography, magnetic resonance and X-ray computed tomography (CT) [4], and although the comparison with CT was only made in three patients, it seems likely that the two investigations are equivalent in their sensitivity for dissection. Magnetic resonance has the advantage of oblique planes and does not require contrast injection, but it is more difficult to image sick patients in the current generation of scanners. The investigation performed in most cases will depend upon practical problems such as whether magnetic resonance is available.

A virtue or a drawback of magnetic resonance, depending upon the circumstances, is the fact that slowly moving blood gives signal using conventional sequences. This can make the distinction of slowly moving blood in the false lumen from rapid flow in the true lumen very simple, but it can also make the distinction between thrombus and static blood in the false lumen difficult. Cine sequences that give high signal from blood and lower signal from thrombus are very helpful, and the ability to measure velocities in the two lumens [5,6] provides additional functional information, such as whether the false lumen is required to supply vital organs.

Other aortic abnormalities that are well seen by magnetic resonance are aneurysms [7] and stenoses, [8] and it is an ideal method for the long term follow-up of patients following coarctation repair [9] and patients with Marfan's syndrome [10,11].

Congenital heart disease

This is another area where invasive investigation can be avoided in selected cases. We are still at an early stage of the application of magnetic resonance in congenital heart disease and many of the reports are reviews of the findings in unselected cases [12,13], but the next stage is to establish the specific strengths and weaknesses of the technique.

One strength is in the detection of ventricular and atrial septal defects, [14] although specificity for the detection of atrial defects is a matter of debate. The very high figure reported by Diethelm et al. [15] disagrees with a previous report [16], and this is attributed to greater experience and superior image quality. Our own experience at Royal Brompton National Heart and Lung Hospitals is that specificity using conventional imaging in the transverse plane is not very good, but in practice, the debate will be eclipsed by different techniques such as the use of oblique planes, cine imaging and velocity mapping. The strength of magnetic resonance in the assessment of septal defects is not so much in detecting the lesion (which will usually have been found by echocardiography), but in assessing its functional significance by measurements of flow through the shunt.

Abnormalities of the atrioventricular valves are well seen [17], but again, magnetic resonance is of greatest value in assessing functional sequelae such as the patency of surgically created conduits [18], right ventricular function and pulmonary flow. In pulmonary atresia, the presence and state of the central pulmonary arteries and of systemic collaterals to the lungs is important, but this information can be very difficult to obtain, and magnetic resonance has reduced the number of invasive investigations that these patients endure [19]. Similarly, in transposition of the great arteries following the Mustard operation, right ventricular function and tricuspid competence are important determinants of long term morbidity and these are easily assessed by magnetic resonance imaging [20].

The role of magnetic resonance in assessing neonates and infants with congenital heart disease is unknown, and this, of course, is an area where echocardiography is particularly strong. Problems arise with magnetic resonance because high quality images are needed to see the anatomy of very small hearts but these are the least likely patients to stay still during acquisition. Rapid imaging techniques will help a great deal, but we may need to wait until real time acquisition is available before magnetic resonance can be widely applied in neonates [21].

Thrombus and tumours

A common reason for referral for magnetic resonance imaging is to adjudicate upon the presence of intracardiac filling defects. Tumours of the heart and surrounding structures are well demonstrated [22,23,24] but, with the possible exceptions of lipomata (high signal) and fibromata (low signal), it can be difficult to distinguish different tumours. This is not a problem restricted to cardiology, since it has not been possible to characterise cerebral or hepatic lesions by their relaxation times, and although the morphological appearances usually give clues, it is disappointing that it can sometimes be difficult to tell a cystic lesion from a solid one.

Thrombus is the commonest intracavitary filling defect and it is readily seen using a spin echo sequence. Confusion between thrombus and slowly moving blood can be avoided by using a cine sequence, where blood gives high signal and the thrombus appears as a filling defect.

The pericardium

The normal fibrous pericardium appears as a thin dark line around the heart using a short spin echo sequence, and it is usually most easily seen anteriorly [25]. Pericardial thickening and effusion can be seen although the appearances of both depend upon the pathology. Thickened pericardium usually has a low signal, although it may have an intermediate or high signal, presumably if there is active inflammation with cellular infiltration and oedema [26]. In contrast to X-ray computed tomography, pericardial calcification is not demonstrated. Pericardial fluid usually has a high signal although it may lose signal with motion. The result is that it can be difficult to distinguish pericardium from fluid, but cine imaging is helpful since the motion of the heart within the pericardial sac is seen. The functional difference between constriction and restriction cannot be appreciated but in the former, abnormal pericardium is invariably seen, and in the latter it is not [27].

Ventricular function

Because volumes can be measured accurately by summing areas in contiguous slices, there has been a rash of papers comparing volume measurements with other techniques. Muscle volume (hence mass) [28,29,30] is particularly interesting in patients with left ventricular hypertrophy and it has been possible to show regression of hypertrophy following only 3 months treatment of hypertension [31]. Wall thickness in hypertrophic cardiomyopathy is better demonstrated than by echocardiography because the three dimensional distribution is more easily seen [32]. It is not clear whether muscle that is hypertrophied secondary to increased afterload has different relaxation properties from myopathic muscle, but measurements of T2 of hypertrophied muscle in a magnetic resonance spectrometer have shown it to be different from normal myocardium [33]. Anecdotal experience is that the abnormal muscle in hypertrophic cardiomyopathy has even longer T2.

Muscle thinning is also readily recognised, and previous infarction can be detected and quantified by the presence and extent of thinning and wall motion abnormality [34,35]. Wall motion is usually measured from diastolic and systolic images by superimposition of endocardial contours, but this assumes that the time of end systole is known and that it is the same for all parts of the ventricle. These assumptions will be avoided by cine acquisition, which is described below.

Cavity volumes can be measured by a number of techniques. The most accurate is to sum areas in multiple contiguous slices, but a more rapid method is by area-length calculations on oblique images containing the long axis of the left ventricle [36,37,38]. For the right ventricle, the multislice method is needed since geometric assumptions are more difficult to make, but it is possible to calculate the regurgitant fraction in patients with valvular regurgitation from left and right ventricular stroke volumes [39]. This technique is only valid if a single valve is affected but it can be used in conjunction with cine imaging which gives a semiquantitative assessment of regurgitation through individual valves. Similarly, the pulmonary to systemic flow ratio can be calculated in patients with atrial or ventricular septal defects (although the latter is complicated in the presence of diastolic shunting).

Cine imaging and velocity mapping

It is difficult to repeat a spin echo sequence sufficiently rapidly to acquire images as a movie, but there has been considerable interest in variants of the gradient echo sequence, which can be repeated as rapidly as every 5 msec so that a multi-frame cine acquisition can be made in the same time as a single spin echo image (approximately 3 min). Moving blood does not lose signal but instead it gives a very high signal and appears white, except where there is turbulence when it loses signal and appears black.

There are several areas where cine acquisition can be helpful. Ventricular wall motion is more comprehensively defined because of the inclusion of a temporal component, although this has not yet been exploited. A second area is in the differentiation of thrombus and other filling defects from slowly moving blood. A third area makes use of the loss of signal from turbulent flow to detect and quantify valvular regurgitation and intracardiac shunts. The turbulent jets of mitral and aortic regurgitation are readily detected and their size provides a semiquantitative estimate of severity. Unfortunately, the same is not true of the turbulence distal to stenotic valves since abnormal valves, even if not stenosed, can lead to considerable turbulence.

A magnetic resonance image is a map of the amplitude of the magnetic resonance signal at each point within the imaging plane. The signal also has phase, however, and it is possible to encode velocity in the phase of the signal. A phase map then becomes a quantitative velocity map, and velocities of blood within the cardiac chambers and great vessels can be displayed [40,41,42]. If the velocity information is colour encoded and superimposed upon the grey scale anatomical image, then both anatomy and flow can be seen in a single display similar to that of colour Doppler cine velocity mapping [43]. The technique has become an important part of the assessment of congenital heart disease with measurements of flow through shunts and conduits [44], and the assessment of pressure gradients across stenoses from the peak velocity in the post-stenotic jet [45]. The measurement of velocity and flow in coronary artery bypass grafts has also been achieved [46].

Tissue characterisation

The longitudinal and transverse relaxation times, T1 and T2, are measures of how fast the magnetisation in a sample returns to equilibrium after it has been disturbed by a radiofrequency pulse, and they are in part determined by the chemical environment of the protons being imaged. One of the initial hopes of magnetic resonance imagers was that the relaxation times would uniquely define a tissue and that it would be possible to differentiate types of tumour. Unfortunately, this has not been possible because of the enormous overlap in the relaxation times of different tissues, and for the myocardium, if not for most other tissues, changes are mainly due to changes in water content or oedema. There are even greater problems for those wanting to characterise myocardium by its relaxation times: it is very difficult to measure the times accurately in imaging machines, and values obtained by one method may be very different from those obtained by another. In the brain, T2 is measured with an accuracy of 20 % at best [47], and there are added problems in a moving organ such as the heart. Motion artefact from blood often overlies the myocardium leading to spurious areas of high signal [48].

Notwithstanding the above, there has been an enormous interest in myocardial relaxation times in transplantation and infarction, because of the possibility of the early detection of rejection and of myocardium that is salvageable by reperfusion. When measured ex vivo after cardiac transplantation, T2 correlates well with the histological grade of rejection and with interstitial water content [49], although changes in T1 are less useful [50]. The problem is to apply these findings clinically where T2 measurements are inaccurate. It should be simplest in heterotopic transplantation, when there is the recipient's heart to act as a control [51], or in the monitoring of response to the treatment of established rejection.

The assessment of myocardial signal intensity in infarction is complicated by the different sequences used and by the alteration in signal with age of the infarct, but acute infarction can be detected by its altered signal [52], and the paramagnetic contrast agent gadolinium-DTPA aids detection acutely [53]. Following coronary occlusion and reperfusion, the myocardium has even higher signal than without reperfusion [54] and gadolinium-DTPA again increases the distinction [55,56]. The higher signal probably reflects oedema accompanying reperfusion. This is a shame because it means that we are not observing a property of the myocytes themselves, which might have led us to detect viable cells, but instead, we are observing nonspecific inflammatory changes.

Conclusion

Magnetic resonance of the cardiovascular system has progressed across a broad front in recent years, and it has now earned a place in the management of a variety of clinical problems. In those centres fortunate enough to have access to a machine, it contributes to patient management, and as this filters back to manufacturers and they produce machines tailored to examination of the cardiovascular system, its use can only increase. One area in which it has not yet contributed greatly is coronary artery disease. A combination of increased resolution with real time imaging may allow the coronary arteries to be imaged, and if it proves possible to measure velocity and flow in the coronaries, then there is hope for the future.

References

1. Dooms GC, Higgins CB. The potential of magnetic resonance imaging for the evaluation of thoracic arterial disease. J Thorac Cardiovasc Surg 1986;92:1088–95.
2. Mossard JM, Baruthio J, Germain P, et al. Apport de la résonance magnétique nucléaire dans le diagnostic des affections aortiques. Arch Mal Coeur 1986;79:456–61.
3. Goldman AP, Kotler MN, Scanlon MH, Ostrum BJ, Parameswaran R, Parry WR. Magnetic resonance imaging and two dimensional echocardiography. Alternative approach to aortography in diagnosis of aortic dissecting aneurysm. Am J Med 1986;80:1225–9.
4. Goldman AP, Kotler MN, Scanlon MH, Ostrum B, Parameswaran R, Parry WR. The complementary role of magnetic resonance imaging, Doppler echocardiography, and computed tomography in the diagnosis of dissecting thoracic aneurysms. Am Heart J 1986;111:970–81.
5. Dinsmore RE, Wedeen VJ, Miller SW, et al. MRI of dissection of the aorta: recognition of the intimal tear and differential flow velocities. Am J Roentgenol 1986;146:1286–8.
6. Bogren HG, Underwood SR, Firmin DN, et al. Magnetic resonance velocity mapping in aortic dissection. Br J Radiol 1988;61:456–62.
7. Winkler M, Higgins CB. MRI of perivalvular infectious pseudoaneurysms. Am J Roentgenol 1986;147:253–6.
8. Boxer RA, Fishman MC, LaCorte MA, Singh S, Parnell VA Jr. Diagnosis and postoperative evaluation of supravalvular aortic stenosis by magnetic resonance imaging. Am J Cardiol 1986;58:367–8.
9. Rees RSO, Somerville J, Ward C, et al. Magnetic resonance imaging in the late postoperative assessment of coarctation of the aorta. Radiology 1989;173:499–502.
10. Schaefer S, Peshock RM, Mallot CR, Katz J, Parkey RW, Willerson JT. Nuclear magnetic resonance imaging in Marfan's syndrome. J Am Coll Cardiol 1987;9:70–4.
11. Boxer RA, LaCorte MA, Singh S, Davis J, Goldman M, Stein HL. Evaluation of the aorta in the Marfan syndrome by magnetic resonance imaging. Am Heart J 1986;111:1001–2.
12. Boxer RA, Singh S, LaCorte MA, Goldman M, Stein HL. Cardiac magnetic resonance imaging in children with congenital heart disease. J Paediatr 1986;109:460–4.

13. Wolff F, Baruthio J, Wecker D, Brechenmacher C, Chambron J. Apport de l'imagerie par résonance magnétique dans les cardiopathies congénitales. Arch Mal Coeur 1986;79:1563–8.

14. Didier D, Higgins CB. Identification and localisation of ventricular septal defect by gated magnetic resonance imaging. Am J Cardiol 1986;57:1363–8.

15. Diethelm L, Déry R, Lipton MJ, Higgins CB. Atrial-level shunts: sensitivity and specificity of MR in diagnosis. Radiology 1987;162:181–6.

16. Lowell DG, Turner DA, Smith SM, et al. The detection of atrial and ventricular septal defects with electrocardiographically synchronised magnetic resonance imaging. Circulation 1986;73:89–94.

17. Fletcher BD, Jacobstein MD, Abramowsky CR, Anderson RH. Right atrioventricular valve atresia: anatomic evaluation with MR imaging. Am J Radiol 1987;148:671–4.

18. Sampson C, Martinez J, Rees S, Somerville J, Underwood R, Longmore D. Evaluation of Fontan's operation by magnetic resonance imaging. Am J Cardiol 1990;65:819–21.

19. Rees RSO, Somerville J, Underwood SR, et al. Magnetic resonance imaging of the pulmonary arteries and their systemic connections in pulmonary atresia: comparison with angiographic and surgical findings. Br Heart J 1987;58:621–6.

20. Rees RSO, Somerville J, Warnes CA, et al. Magnetic resonance imaging in the assessment of cardiac function and anatomy following Mustard's operation for transposition of the great vessels: a comparison with echocardiography and radionuclide angiography. Am J Cardiol 1988;61:1316–22.

21. Rzedzian R, Chapman B, Mansfield P, et al. Real-time nuclear magnetic resonance imaging in paediatrics. Lancet 1983;2:1281–2.

22. Applegate PM, Tajik AJ, Ehman RL, Julsrud PR, Miller FA Jr. Two-dimensional echocardiographic and magnetic resonance imaging observations in massive lipomatous hypertrophy of the atrial septum. Am J Cardiol 1987;59:489–91.

23. Conti VR, Saydjari R, Amparo EG. Paraganglioma of the heart. The value of magnetic resonance imaging in the preoperative evaluation. Chest 1986;90:604–6.

24. Grötz J, Steiner G, Josephs W, Sorge B, Wiechmann W, Beyer HK. Darstellung intra- und parakardialer raumfordernder Prozesse mit der magnetischen Resonanztomographie. Dtsch med Wochenschr 1986;111:1594–8.

25. Sechtem U, Tscholakoff D, Higgins CB. MRI of the normal pericardium. Am J Roentgenol 1986;147:239–44.

26. Sechtem U, Tscholakoff D, Higgins CB. MRI of the abnormal pericardium. Am J Roentgenol 1986;147:245–52.

27. Sechtem U, Higgins CB, Sommerhoff BA, Lipton MJ, Huycke EC. Magnetic resonance imaging of restrictive cardiomyopathy. Am J Cardiol 1987;59:480–2.

28. Florentine MS, Grosskreutz CL, Chang W, et al. Measurement of left ventricular mass in vivo using gated nuclear magnetic resonance imaging. J Am Coll Cardiol 1986;8:107–12.

29. Keller AM, Peshock RM, Malloy CR, et al. In vivo measurement of myocardial mass using nuclear magnetic resonance imaging. J Am Coll Cardiol 1986;8:113–7.

30. Caputo GR, Tscholakoff D, Sechtem U, Higgins CB. Measurement of canine left ventricular mass by using MR imaging. Am J Roentgenol 1987;148:33–8.

31. Eichstaedt HW, Felix R, Langer M, et al. Use of nuclear magnetic resonance imaging to show regression of hypertrophy with ramipril treatment. Am J Cardiol 1987;59:98D–103D.

32. Berghöfer G, Köhler D, Schmutzler H, Schneider R, Felix R. Die magnetresonanztomographische Darstellung bei hypertropher Kardiomyopathie im Vergleich zur Echokardiographie. Herz/Kreisl 1987;19:135–9.

33. Fried R, Boxt LM, Miller RH III, et al. Nuclear magnetic resonance spectroscopy of rat ventricles following supravalvar aortic banding. A model of left ventricular hypertrophy. Invest Radiol 1986;21:622–5.

34. Underwood SR, Rees RSO, Savage PE, et al. The assessment of regional left ventricular function by magnetic resonance. Br Heart J 1986;56:334–40.

35. Akins EW, Hill JA, Sievers KW, Conti CR. Assessment of left ventricular wall thickness

in healed myocardial infarction by magnetic resonance imaging. Am J Cardiol 1987;59:24–8.

36. Osbakken M, Yuschok T. Evaluation of ventricular function with gated cardiac magnetic resonance imaging. Cath Cardiovasc Diag 1986;12:156–60.
37. Buckwalter KA, Aisen AM, Dilworth LR, Mancini GBJ, Buda AJ. Gated cardiac MRI: ejection fraction determination using the right anterior oblique view. Am J Roentgenol 1986;147:33–7.
38. Underwood SR, Gill CR, Firmin DN, et al. Left ventricular volume measured rapidly by oblique magnetic resonance imaging. Br Heart J 1988;60:188–95.
39. Underwood SR, Klipstein RH, Firmin DN, et al. Magnetic resonance assessment of aortic and mitral regurgitation. Br Heart J 1986;56:455–62.
40. Nayler GL, Firmin DN, Longmore DB. Blood flow imaging by cine magnetic resonance. J Comput Assist Tomogr 1986;10:715–22.
41. Ridgway JP, Smith MA. A technique for velocity imaging using magnetic resonance imaging. Br J Radiol 1986;59:693–707.
42. Underwood SR, Firmin DN, Klipstein RH, Rees RSO, Longmore DB. Magnetic resonance velocity mapping: clinical application of a new technique. Br Heart J 1987;57:404–12.
43. Klipstein RH, Firmin DN, Underwood SR, Nayler GL, Rees RSO, Longmore DB. Colour display of quantitative blood flow and cardiac anatomy in a single magnetic resonance cine loop. Br J Radiol 1987;60:105–11.
44. Rees RSO, Firmin DN, Mohiaddin RH, Underwood SR, Longmore DB. Application of flow measurements by magnetic resonance velocity mapping to congenital heart disease. Am J Cardiol 1989;64:953–6.
45. Kilner PJ, Firmin DN, Rees RSO, et al. Valve and great vessel stenosis: assessment with magnetic resonance jet velocity mapping. Radiology 1991;178:229–35.
46. Underwood SR, Firmin DN, Klipstein RH, Rees RSO, Longmore DB. Magnetic resonance velocity mapping: clinical application of a new technique. Br Heart J 1987;57:404–12.
47. Johnson G, Ormerod IEC, Barnes D, Tofts PS, MacManus D. Accuracy and precision in the measurement of relaxation times from nuclear magnetic resonance images. Br J Radiol 1987;60:143–53.
48. Filpchuk NG, Peshock RM, Malloy CR, et al. Detection and localization of recent myocardial infarction by magnetic resonance imaging. Am J Cardiol 1986;58:214–9.
49. Sasaki H, Sada M, Nishimura T, et al. The expanded scope of effectiveness of nuclear magnetic resonance imaging to determine cardiac allograft rejection. Transplantation proceedings 1987;19:1062–4.
50. Lechat P, Eugene M, Hadjiisky P, Teillac A, Cabrol C, Grosgogeat Y. Détection du rejet de greffe cardiaque par résonance magnétique nucléaire du proton. Arch Mal Coeur 1986;79:1356–60.
51. Aherne T, Tscholakoff D, Finkbeiner W, et al. Magnetic resonance imaging of cardiac transplants:the evaluation of rejection of cardiac allografts with and without immunosuppression. Circulation 1986;74:145–56.
52. Johnston DL, Thompson RC, Liu P, et al. Magnetic resonance imaging during acute myocardial infarction. Am J Cardiol 1986;57:1059–65.
53. Eichstaedt HW, Felix R, Dougherty FC, Langer M, Rutsch W, Schmutzler H. Magnetic resonance imaging (MRI) in different stages of myocardial infarction using the contrast agent gadolinium-DTPA. Clin Cardiol 1986;9:527–35.
54. Johnston DL, Liu P, Rosen BR, et al. In vivo detection of reperfused myocardium by nuclear magnetic resonance imaging. J Am Coll Cardiol 1987;9:127–35.
55. Peshock RM, Malloy CR, Buja LM, Nunnally RL, Parkey RW, Willerson JT. Magnetic resonance imaging of acute myocardial infarction: gadolinium diethylenetriamine pentaacetic acid as a marker of reperfusion. Circulation 1986;74:1434–40.
56. Tscholakoff D, Higgins CB, Sechtem U, McNamara MT. Occlusive and reperfused myocardial infarcts: effect of Gd-DTPA on ECG-gated MR imaging. Radiology 1986;160:515–9.

21. Evaluation of cardiac function using MRI

UDO SECHTEM, PETER THEISSEN,
FRANK-MICHAEL BAER and HARALD SCHICHA

Summary

The clinical role of magnetic resonance imaging (MRI) is expanding in the evaluation of regional and global left ventricular function. Several unique features make MRI attractive for pharmacological studies of the left ventricle where reproducibility or three-dimensional imaging may be important, and for evaluation of the right heart. Apart from these specialized applications, evaluation of the various aspects of cardiac function by MRI will be clinically helpful if MRI is used as a second line technique in patients who cannot be adequately assessed by other noninvasive techniques such as echocardiography.

1. Introduction

The close relationship between cardiac anatomy and function defines the need for imaging techniques capable of providing detailed information of both aspects of organ integrity. MRI depicts cardiac anatomy with good spatial resolution and little motion artifact because of electrocardiographic gating and, after the recent introduction of faster gradient-echo sequences, has become an attractive modality for the assessment of cardiac function. Therefore, MRI is increasingly used to answer scientific and clinical questions in patients with cardiac disease. In this chapter, the technical requirements for the evaluation of cardiac function and the applications of functional MRI in three main groups of cardiac diseases – coronary artery disease, valvular disease, and congenital heart disease – are reviewed.

2. Technical considerations

2.1. *Spin-echo imaging*

A problem with a multisection spin-echo series of images is the fact that the time interval between the R-wave and data collection changes. Therefore,

Johan H.C. Reiber & Ernst E. van der Wall (eds.), Cardiovascular Nuclear Medicine and MRI, 311–331.
© 1992 *Kluwer Academic Publishers.*

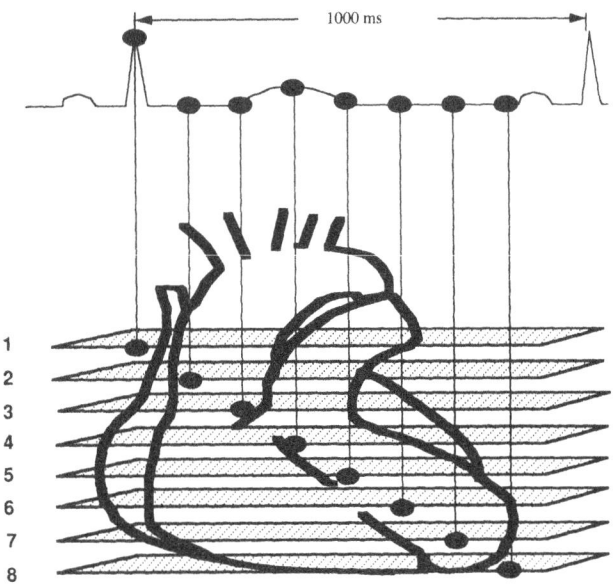

Figure 1. Schematic drawing of temporal order of sections obtained by routine spin-echo imaging of the heart.

the images of different tomographic planes are sampled at a different but fixed point in the cardiac cycle (Fig. 1). Consequently, analysis of cardiac function is not possible from such a set of images alone.

In order to overcome this limitation of spin-echo imaging and obtain a multisection and multiphase set of images, multislice imaging can be repeated with permutation of the initial slice order [1] (Fig. 2). With each repeated spin-echo sequence and permutation, slice one is imaged 50 msec later until 8 images of all are available evenly spaced in time by 50 msec. As result, a three-dimensional set of images of the heart is available for data analysis at eight different phases of the cardiac cycle (Fig. 3).

Another approach to functional spin-echo studies has been described which uses shorter echo-times in the order of 10 msec and shortens imaging times by taking advantage of the fact that cardiac volumes do not change during the approximately 60 msec of isovolumetric contraction and relaxation [2]. Up to four images at different anatomic levels are acquired during these periods, resulting in a set of enddiastolic and endsystolic images. However, to span the entire left ventricle, total imaging time is still in the order of 30 minutes although only two three-dimensional sets of images at enddiastole and endsystole are provided.

2.2. *Gradient-echo imaging*

To obtain a better temporal resolution than provided by spin-echo MRI, several MR imaging techniques have been developed which combine cardiac

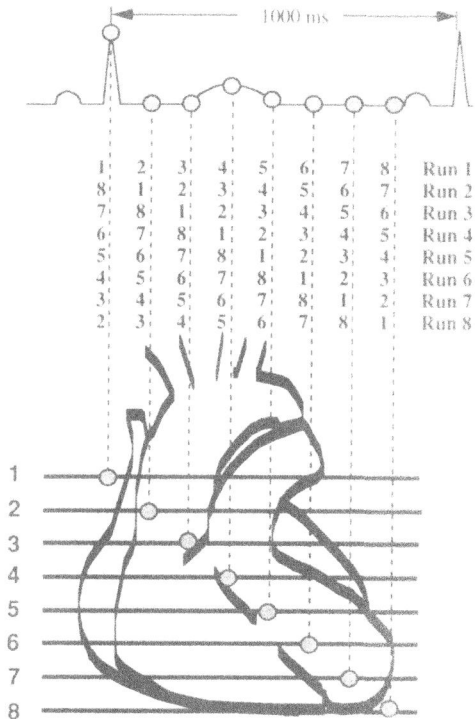

Figure 2. Temporal order of cardiac phases and sections for multisection-multiphase gated spin-echo sequence.

gating and depiction of an increased number of time frames per cardiac cycle within a somewhat shorter imaging time. These techniques are based on a combination of shortened pulse repetition times and reduced flip angles compared to conventional spin-echo MRI. These gradient-echo sequences apply only a single radiofrequency pulse and use reversal of the read gradient for echo formation [3–5]. Gradient-echo MRI of the heart also needs electrocardiographic gating which may be accomplished either by prospective or retrospective gating. For prospective gating, a minimum RR-interval must be chosen during which the pulse sequence can be applied. During longer RR-intervals, late diastole will not contribute to image formation. On the other hand, short RR-intervals will result in acquisition of early systolic contraction states of the next heart beat. Therefore, gradient images acquired with prospective gating have limitations for the exact depiction of late diastole. Retrospective gating requires additional hardware and software but has advantages for functional imaging because of its improved representation of the entire cardiac cycle. Imaging of late diastole may be important for analysis of atrial function [6].

Assuming a constant heart rate of 75 beats/min, a repetition time of 22 msec and an echo-time of 11 msec, 36 radiofrequency pulses with the appro-

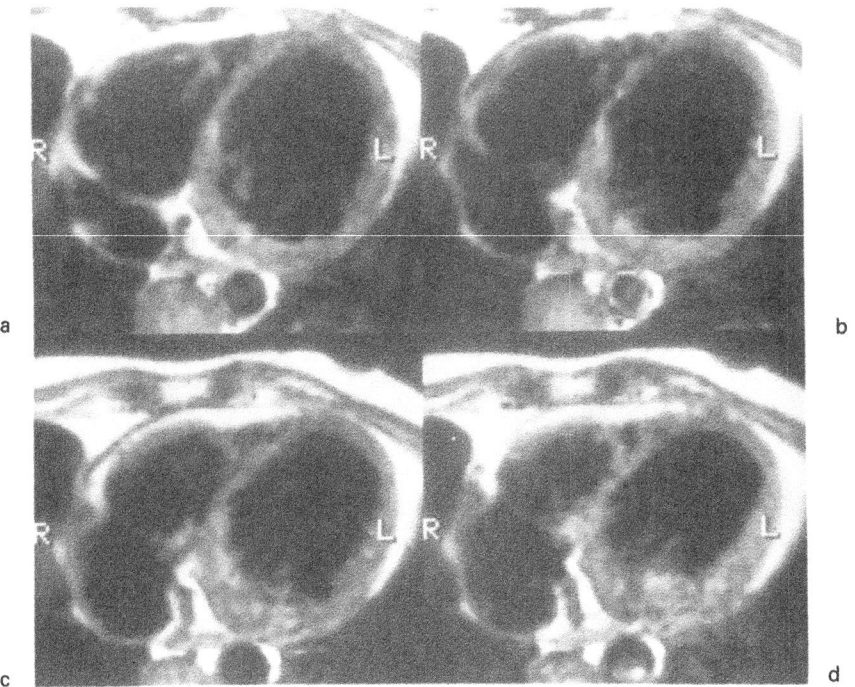

Figure 3. Four out of 8 phases of the same section of a multisection-multiphase spin-echo sequence (TE = 30 msec) in a patient with coronary artery disease and previous extensive infarction of the interventricular septum and the anterior wall. In the infarct regions, there is diastolic wall thinning and systolic wall thickening is virtually absent. (a) enddiastole; (b) 100 msec into systole; (c) midsystole; (d) endsystole.

priate gradient sequence can be applied during the RR-interval of 800 msec if retrospective gating is used (Fig. 4). After completion of the 128 phase steps commonly used in gradient-echo imaging, 36 images of the same plane can be reconstructed. Improvement of signal-to-noise ratio and image quality is achieved by repeating image acquisition two or four times amounting to a total imaging time of approximately: 800 msec × 128 × 2(4) = 3.5 (7) min. A multislice technique like described for spin-echo imaging can also be applied to gradient-echo sequences (Fig. 4). However, saving of imaging time results in lower temporal resolution.

In contrast to spin-echo images, gradient-echo images display flowing blood with higher signal intensity than myocardium. The blood pool in these images appears similar to contrast-enhanced computed tomography scans and cine-ventriculography. However, accelerated and especially turbulent blood flow is associated with signal loss [7]. Continuously replaying all time frames of one anatomic level of the heart yields a cinematic display of the

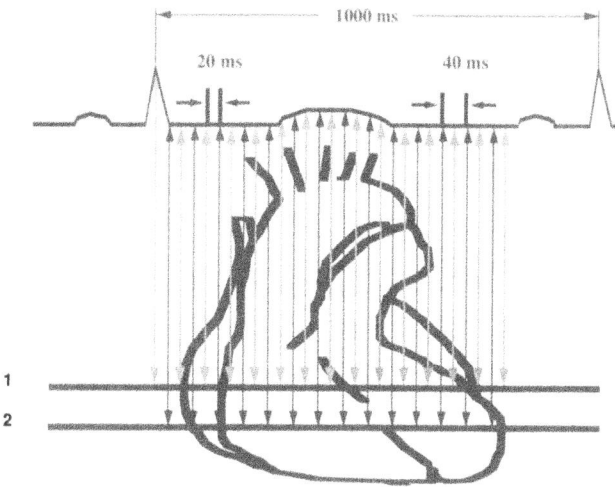

Figure 4. Temporal order of cardiac phases for gradient-echo sequence with 'simultaneous' acquisition of two anatomic sections. Repetition time of sequence is 20 msec but temporal resolution for one section is only 40 msec due to alternate excitation of sections. Imaging of section one occurs at the grey arrows, imaging of section two at the black arrows. Assumed heart rate 60 bpm.

entire cardiac cycle composed of information acquired over 256 or 512 cardiac cycles. Thus, it is possible to observe wall motion and wall thickening as well as blood flow phenomena.

2.3. *Ultrafast imaging techniques*

Despite the advances brought about by the introduction of gradient-echo imaging, imaging times are still in the order of several minutes, rendering image quality susceptible to subject motion. Significant reduction of motion artifacts in patients with arrhythmias and rapid breathing can be achieved if all the data required are obtained within one single cardiac cycle. By maximal shortening of the repetition time (3 msec) which requires a magnet with optimized hardware, a complete image of the heart can be acquired within 200 to 300 msec using a gradient-echo FLASH sequence [8]. With further hardware improvements, imaging times of 100 msec could be achieved in the near future. Even without cardiac gating, contraction of the heart can be appreciated from a series of these 'snapshot FLASH' images obtained from consecutive cardiac cycles [9,10]. The price for these impressively short imaging times is the low spatial resolution of an imaging matrix of 64 × 128 pixels. Further progress will be necessary before functional assessment will be possible using these so called snapshot images. However, the potential of

Table 1. Cardiac MR imaging sequences

	Permutation SE	Gradient-Echo	Snapshot	EPI
Imaging time/image	256 s*	256 s*	0.2 s	0.06
Imaging time LV**	34.1 min	17.1 min	3.3 min	0.13 min$^\circ$
Temporal resolution	100 msec	40 msec***	40 msec****	60 msec
Real time	no	no	almost	yes
Spatial resolution	+	+	–	–
SNR	+	(+)	(–)	(–)
Perfusion	limited	limited	possible	possible

* = for a heart rate of 60 bpm, 2 repetitions, 128 phase encoding steps; ** = imaging times assuming temporal resolution given below and 8 sections through left ventricular without computer reconstruction time; $^\circ$ = assuming continuous imaging through entire heart without interruption of sequence by changing sections; *** = simultaneous acquisition of 2 sections; **** = one image acquired per heart beat with subsequent initiation of imaging 40 msec later until section is imaged over the entire cardiac cycle after 25 heart beats; EPI = echo- planar imaging, LV = left ventricle; SE = spin-echo; SNR = signal-to-noise ratio; – = not good; (–) = acceptable but inferior to other sequences; (+) = better than (–); + = good.

this technique for assessment of left ventricular perfusion after application of contrast agents is considerable [11,12].

Another promising approach are echo-planar imaging techniques producing images with exposure times of 60 msec and less [13–15]. Similar to optimized snapshot FLASH techniques, major hardware alterations are necessary to implement echo-planar imaging on a magnet which could limit the widespread use of such technology. Functional imaging has not yet been reported with echo-planar imaging although the feature of real time imaging with artifact reduction and very short imaging times makes it very attractive for this purpose. Table 1 summarizes the various technical options for functional imaging of the heart.

3. Selection of imaging planes

Since MRI can be performed in any plane, considerable debate has arisen about the ideal imaging plane for evaluation of cardiac anatomy and global and regional cardiac function [16–19]. The transverse plane has the advantage of being perpendicular to the long axis of the body which makes orientation based on extracardiac landmarks easier. The transverse plane is oriented perpendicular to the anterior wall and the outflow tract and parallel to the diaphragmatic wall of the right ventricle which is useful for wall thickness measurements of the right ventricle. For the evaluation of right ventricular volumes, the transverse plane has mixed blessings because the large inferior section is prone to partial volume errors but a maximum of sections is available for three-dimensioned determination of volumes. Other useful features of the transverse plane include good visualization of the interventricular septum and the atrioventricular valves which may be advantageous for demonstration and measurement of valvular incompetence. Moreover, the extra time for exact determination of left ventricular axis angulation can be saved.

Sharp depiction of the left ventricular circumference is achieved by imaging in the short axis plane. Blood flow perpendicular to the imaging plane sometimes leads to somewhat higher signal intensity of flowing blood and improved delineation of the endocardial surface [20]. Although Dinsmore et al. expected less partial volume averaging problems [17], Buser et al. demonstrated that three-dimensional left ventricular volume measurements from transverse and short-axis images lead to identical results [18]. However, the short-axis plane is particularly well suited for assessment of left ventricular wall motion and wall thickening because artifactual thickening of lateral walls which is often observed on transverse images is avoided. An important advantage of the short-axis especially in patients with coronary artery disease is imaging of the diaphragmatic wall of the left ventricle. This is not possible from transverse sections which cut this region parallel and not perpendicular. Finally, the short-axis plane is used by echocardiography and scintigraphic techniques and is therefore useful for comparison of imaging modalities. However, a second imaging plane such as a long-axis plane parallel or perpendicular to the interventricular septum is necessary to assess the entire left ventricular because apex and mitral valve plane are not well seen in the short-axis plane.

For the sole purpose of left ventricular volume determination, two orthogonal planes intersecting along the intrinsic long axis of the heart (two chambers and four chambers) may be used. Instead of acquiring a three-dimensional stack of images as necessary for transverse and short-axis imaging of the left ventricular, only two sets of gradient-echo images are necessary. In addition, analysis times are considerably shortened from approximately 25 to 10 min [21]. However, assessment of regional wall motion from these images suffers the disadvantage that the left ventricular is only partially depicted and small abnormal areas may be missed.

Although fast and simple single oblique slice determinations of left ventricular volumes (area-length algorithm assuming an ellipsoidal shape of the left ventricle) have been described [22–25], the limitations of this approach especially in abnormally shaped ventricles are well known. If a single plane spin-echo technique is employed, flow signal in patients with regional or global wall motion abnormalities may obscure endocardial borders which is especially prominent with the use of short echo-times [22]. The single slice technique can therefore not be recommended for clinical application unless presaturation of adjacent sections diminishes flow signal and improves edge detection [26].

4. Cardiac function in coronary artery disease

4.1. *Ventricular volumes*

For the determination of left ventricular volumes, endocardial borders in enddiastolic and endsystolic images are outlined and volumes are calculated using Simpson's rule from a three-dimensional set of images or geometric formulas if mono- or biplane sections of the left ventricular are available. Stroke volume, cardiac output, and ejection fraction can be derived from these volumes.

The determination of left ventricular volume in a three-dimensional fashion from casts of canine and human hearts [28] yields an excellent correlation with the true volume determined by water displacement [27]. Ventricular volumes are calculated by outlining the endocardial borders in each section, multiplying the resulting area by slice thickness and using Simpson's formula or similar algorithms for endsystolic and enddiastolic volume determination. Although this method is considerable more time consuming than the single slice technique, it has the advantage of being independent of constraining geometric assumptions.

Van Rossum and coworkers [29] compared the single slice technique with a multiple slice technique for determination of ejection fraction. With monoplane left ventricular angiography as a gold standard, the correlation coefficient of the single slice technique was only 0.65, whereas an r value of 0.98 was found for the multislice technique.

Comparison of cardiac output measurements by spin-echo MRI, using the multiphasic imaging technique with a temporal resolution of 100 msec, and by thermodilution revealed a consistent underestimation of stroke volumes by MRI, which was possibly due to inaccurate determination of endsystole caused by the low sampling rate [27].

Using gradient-echo MRI, endocardial borders can be rapidly identified due to the high signal intensity of flowing blood. Normal values for ventricular volumes have been defined by gradient-echo MRI in a small cohort of volunteers [30]. Echocardiographic normal values correlate closely with the values found by gradient-echo MRI in the transverse and short-axis planes [18,30] despite the fact that echocardiography includes the papillary muscles in cavity volumes which would lead to overestimation of true volumes. This effect may be compensated for by systematic underestimation of volumes related to the exclusion of the true apex of the left ventricle [31]. In contrast, volumes measured from cine-angiography are larger than gradient-echo MRI volumes [21].

4.2. *Regional myocardial function*

Similar to echocardiography, regional left ventricular function may be assessed by describing wall motion and wall thickness or wall thickening abnormalities [32]. Because no agreement exists yet about the ideal MRI plane for depiction of the heart, segmental division varies between studies and the optimal approach for quantification of wall motion abnormalities has yet to be defined.

In general the semi-quantitative evaluation of segmental wall motion by two-dimensional echocardiography and MRI yields similar results for both imaging techniques [33]. However, imaging in the short-axis plane is mandatory for comprehensive wall motion analysis by MRI and comparison with echocardiography.

Regions of reduced wall thickness in patients with chronic myocardial infarction can easily be appreciated on transverse and short-axis spin-echo images [34,35]. The presence and location of reduced wall thickness correlates with wall motion abnormalities localized by ventriculography [35,36]. MRI also demonstrates utility for the diagnosis of left ventricular aneurysms identified by extremely thinned myocardium and a variable degree of regional bulging [37].

Due to its excellent definition of both the endo- and epicardial myocardial border MRI is well suited for analysis of regional myocardial function on the basis of wall thickening measurements. However, systolic wall thickening in healthy volunteers calculated from MR images varies considerably among various segments for individual patients [38,39]. Normal values may vary from one to another laboratory, depending on the ventricular sites at which the measurements are made and whether transverse or oblique (short-axis) imaging planes are used. Nevertheless, in most patients with previous transmural myocardial infarcts, regional wall thickening is reduced to less than 2 mm (Fig. 5) [39,40]. Relative values of percent wall thickening which is calculated as the difference in wall thickness at endsystole and enddiastole divided by wall thickness at enddiastole may be erroneously high in patients with diastolic myocardial thinning and little absolute thickening in systole. Therefore, absolute thickening values may more accurately reflect the difference in regional myocardial contractility.

Wall thickness and wall thickening as measured by gradient-echo MRI may be used to identify and quantify transmural myocardial scar. In patients with remote myocardial infarcts and angiographically documented severe wall motion abnormalities, segmental analysis of diastolic wall thickness and systolic wall thickening on gradient-echo images and segmental analysis of myocardial perfusion on corresponding 99mTc-methoxyisobutyl isonitrile (MIBI) tomographic (SPECT) images show an excellent agreement between normal and scarred regions with both techniques (Fig. 6) [41]. Three dimensional quantification of infarct size by MRI is possible by outlining the infarct area in each section and multiplying the resulting area by slice-thickness.

The clinical value of MRI in the assessment of coronary artery disease has been limited by the inability of imaging under exercise conditions. To overcome this limitation, dipyridamole can be used as a substitute for exercise

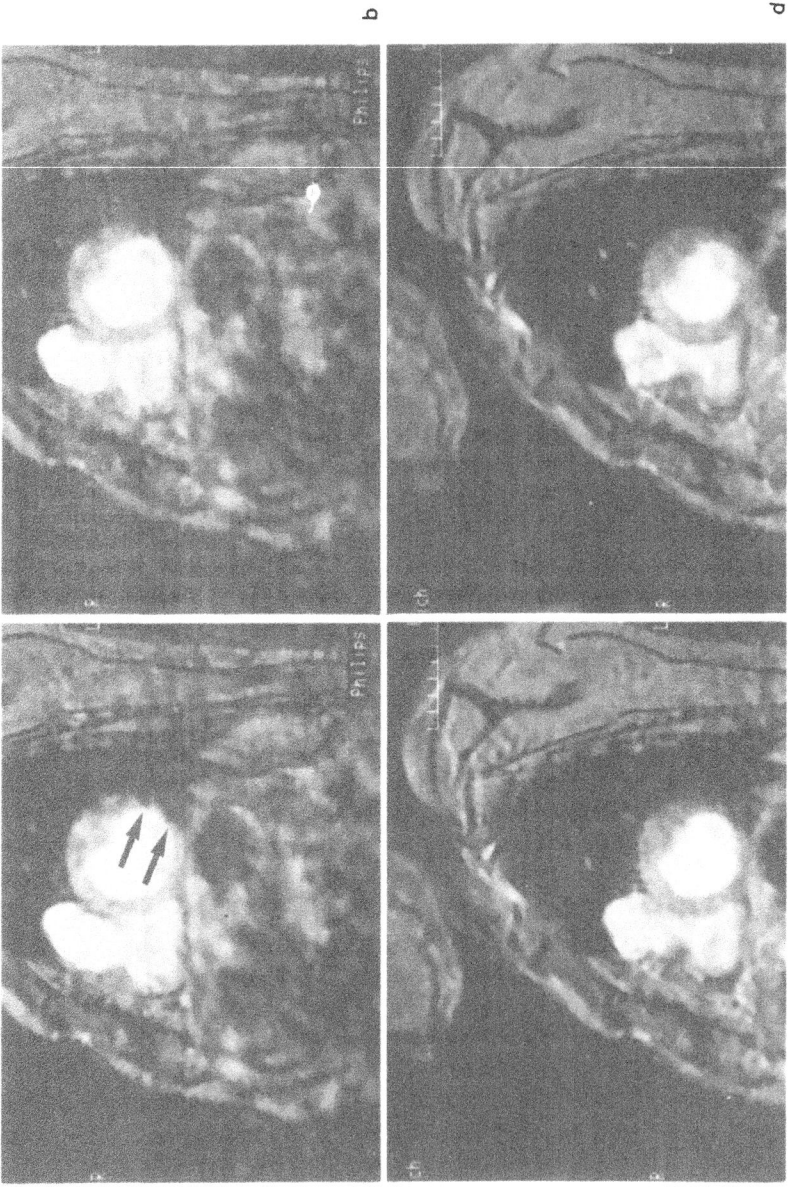

Figure 5. Short-axis gradient-echo images in a patient with posterolateral infarct. (a) Enddiastolic image. Wall thinning is evident posterolaterally (arrows). (b) Early systolic image. (c) Midsystolic image. (d) Endsystolic image. All regions except the posterolateral one show homogeneous wall thickening.

with gradient-echo MRI. Pennell et al. [42] were the first to report that gradient-echo MRI can demonstrate reversible myocardial wall thickening abnormalities induced by pharmacologic stress testing using dipyridamole. In our laboratory, the sensitivity of MRI in detecting significant coronary artery disease in patients with coronary stenoses of more than 70 % was 78 % [43]. However, imaging times are still rather long and complete scanning of the left ventricle poses considerable problems in patients suffering from dipyridamole induced angina within the magnet. Therefore, ultrafast MRI should be employed to improve the clinical feasibility of this kind of stress test.

5. Cardiac function in valvular lesions

5.1. *Qualitative assessment of valvular regurgitation*

As mentioned above, spin-echo MRI cannot demonstrate the presence of valvular regurgitation. In contrast, the jet of valvular regurgitation is clearly seen in its three-dimensional extent on a stack of gradient-echo images, for instance, encompassing the entire left atrium in a patient with mitral regurgitation (Fig. 7). The number of sections with a visible portion of the regurgitant jet correlates only loosely with the angiographic severity of the lesion.

Using maximal jet areas determined in a similar way as in color-coded Doppler echocardiography, significant differences exist between angiographic grades of severity although the overlap between groups is still considerable (Fig. 8A). The best means of discriminating among angiographic grades is by three-dimensional determination of maximal jet volumes: i.e. by planimetering jet areas in each section at the same phase of the cardiac cycle and addition of these areas (Fig. 8B). Nevertheless, there is no perfect agreement with angiography and some overlap remains which may to some extent be explained by the well known inaccuracies inherent to the qualitative angiographic grading [44,45].

5.2. *Quantitative assessment of valvular regurgitation*

The hemodynamic importance of valvular regurgitation may be more exactly measured by determination of regurgitant volumes. In patients with isolated or predominant regurgitation of one single cardiac valve, right and left ventricular stroke volumes can be derived from spin-echo and gradient-echo images and subsequently be subtracted to quantify regurgitant volumes [46,47]. MRI determined regurgitant volumes correlate closely with those measured at cardiac catheterization [48]. Comparison of MRI derived regurgitant fraction to angiographic estimation of lesion severity shows significant

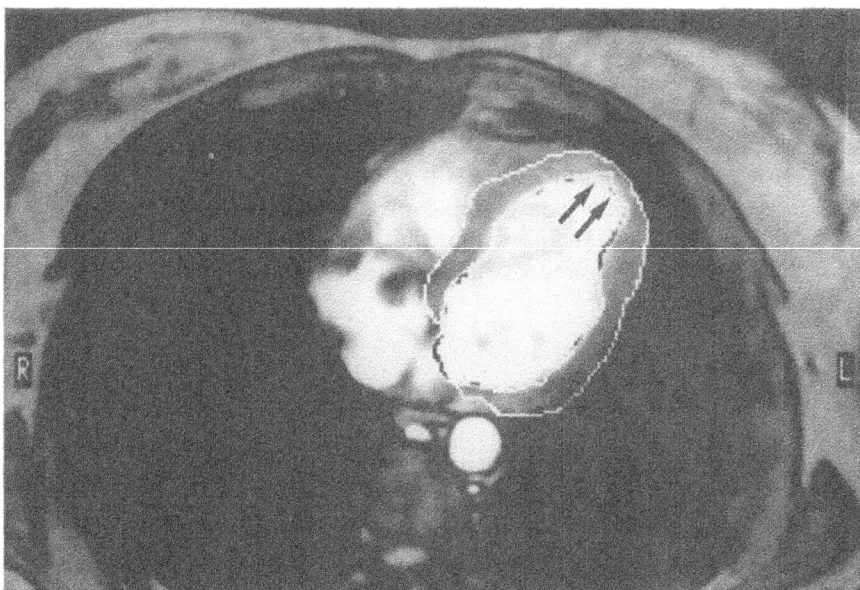

a

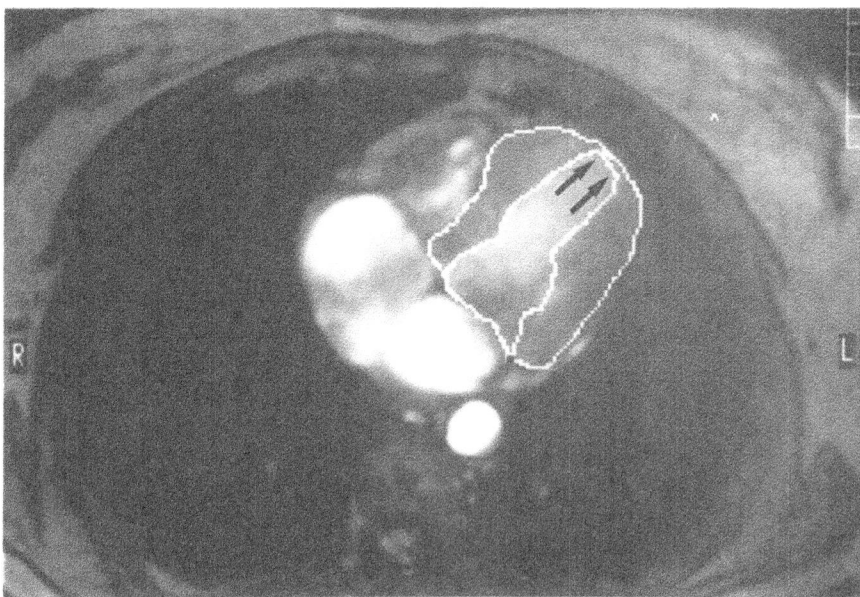

b

Figure 6. Congruity of regional diastolic wall thinning, absent systolic wall thickening on gradient-echo MR images and severe perfusion defect on MIBI SPECT image at rest in a patient with chronic myocardial infarction of the anterior wall of the left ventricle. (a) Diastolic MR image. Circumscript wall thinning is visible anteriorly (arrows). (b) Systolic MR image shows some wall thinning in the anterior region (arrows). (c) The corresponding MIBI SPECT image shows a severe perfusion defect of the same size at the same location. (See p. 323.)

differences between groups (Fig. 8C) [46,47]. Finally, a good correlation was found between gradient-echo MRI measurements of the volume of the signal void and the regurgitant volume [49].

5.3. *MRI and color-coded Doppler echocardiography*

Although the visualization of regurgitant jets by gradient-echo MRI and color coded Doppler echocardiography depends on entirely different physical principles, both techniques image the turbulent parts of the jet. It is therefore understandable that the maximal yellow-green core area of the reflux jet measured on the echo screen and the maximal dark core area planimetered on the MR screen correlate fairly well (r = 0.88) [50,51]. However, MR areas were systematically smaller than color Doppler areas. This may be due to the fact that MR sections are oriented to the body axes and not to maximize jet areas. In addition, it must be remembered that jet areas for both techniques depend on instrument settings [52] and hemodynamic factors [53].

Qualitative estimation of lesion severity by MRI seems to correspond better to angiographic grading than color Doppler estimations [54]. In our experience, jet volumes measured by MRI provide the best noninvasive grading of aortic and mitral regurgitation [51]. However, for daily clinical practice, color Doppler provides a much faster and in most patients sufficient

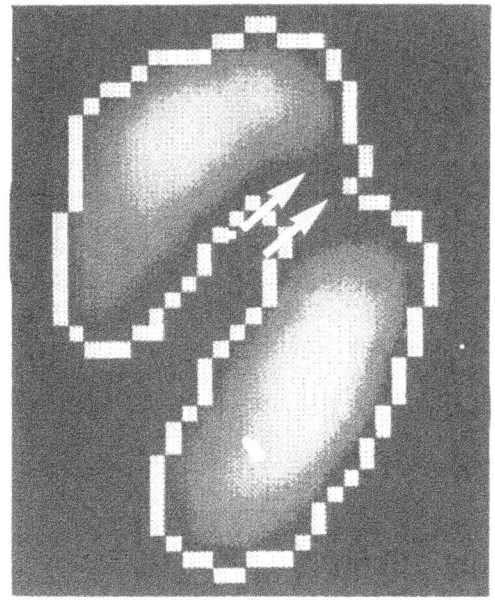

c

Figure 6c.

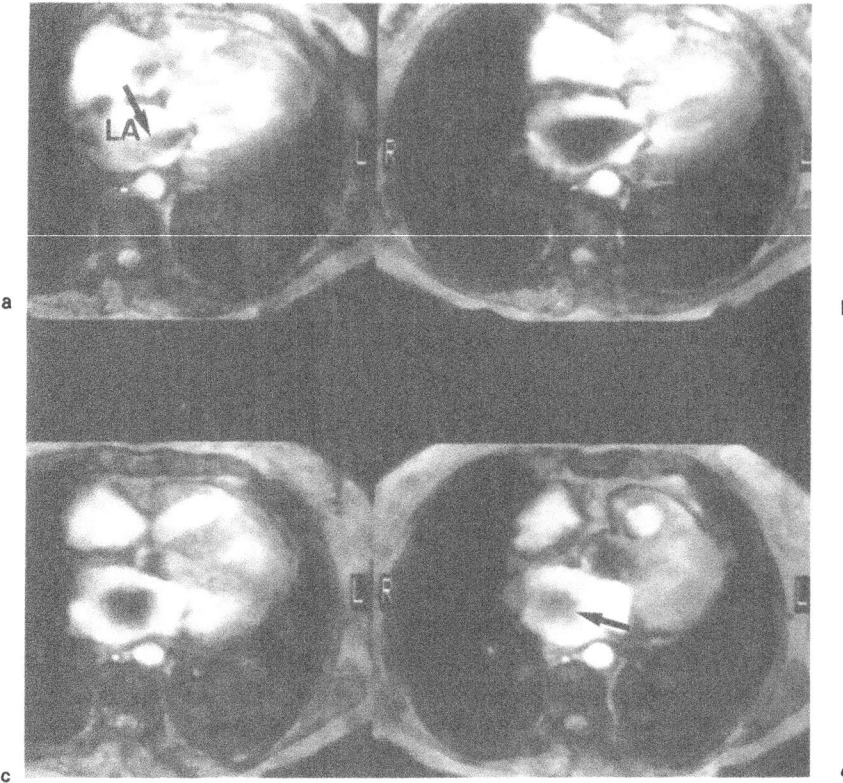

Figure 7. Four gradient-echo images at adjacent levels of the heart showing the same mid-systolic phase of the cardiac cycle in a patient with moderate mitral regurgitation. (a) Lowest level. Faint, narrow jet (arrow) in left atrium (LA). There is also a tiny jet within right atrium from insignificant tricuspid regurgitation; (b) One level more cranial. Jet larger, more distinct from surrounding high intensity blood within LA; (c) Another level further craniad. Jet smaller, still clear demarcation from normal blood. (d) Highest level. Faint rounded end portion of the jet (arrow).

orientation about valvular insufficiency. MRI which is much more expensive and time-consuming should be reserved for patients with discrepancies between clinical and echocardiographic estimation of lesion severity.

6. Cardiac function in congenital heart disease

Shunt flow and anatomical size of an atrial septal defect were previously reported to show a poor correlation [55]. Therefore, direct quantitation of shunt flow which is related to prognosis [56] seems to be better suited than measurement of the anatomical size of a defect to select patients for corrective surgery. This goal may be accomplished by measuring various parameters

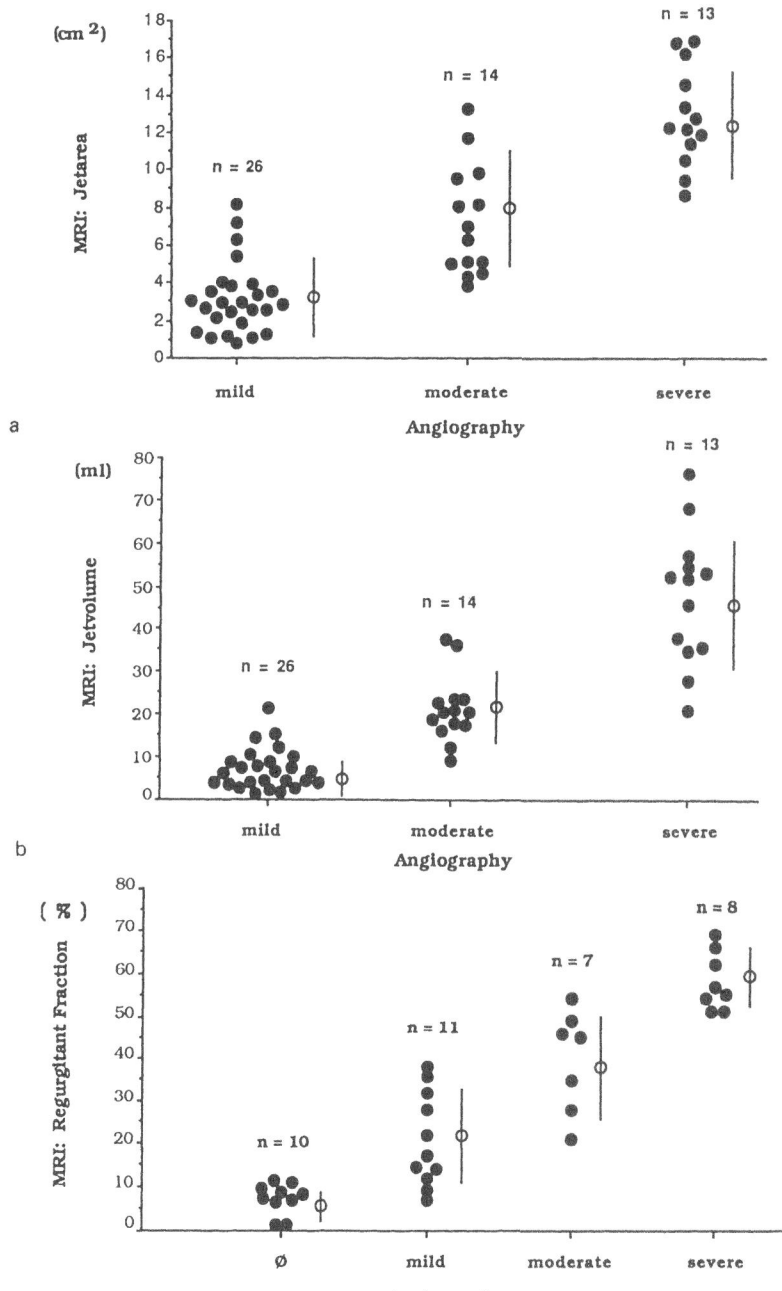

Figure 8. (a) MRI measured maximal jet areas in patients with aortic incompetence related to the angiographic estimation of severity; (b) MRI measured maximal jet volumes in patients with aortic incompetence related to the angiographic estimation of severity; (c) MRI derived regurgitant fractions in normals and patients with mild, moderate and severe aortic regurgitation.

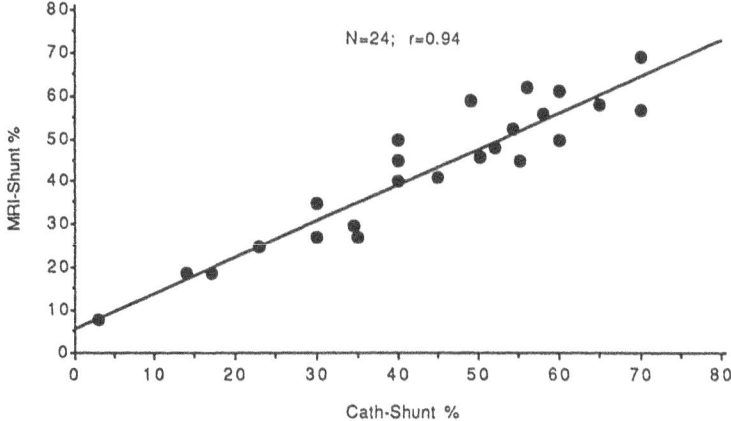

Figure 9. Comparison of atrial septal defect shunt fractions measured by MRI and cardiac catheterization.

of the jet like diameter, area, and volume. Alternatively, complete gradient-echo MRI examination of the right and left ventricle as described above provides the basis for three-dimensional determination of the difference between right and left ventricular stroke volumes which has been used to estimate the hemodynamic importance of the atrial septal defect in patients with left-to-right shunts [57]. In patients without associated valvular regurgitation or additional shunts, this method yielded a good correlation with shunt determinations obtained at cardiac catheterization (Fig. 9). Our preliminary results in patients with a ventricular septal defect demonstrate that the right ventricular stroke volume is also increased in left-to-right shunts depending on the location of the defect. Therefore, the stroke volume method does not seem to be applicable in patients with a ventricular septal defect.

Quantitation of shunt size can also be accomplished from phase analysis of gradient-echo images to measure volume flow in the pulmonary artery and aorta [58]. By measuring the velocity of blood from the phase shifts in each pixel of the cross-sectional area of the great vessels a velocity map is constructed which in conjunction with planimetry of the cross-sectional area permits calculation of blood flow through the pulmonary and systemic circulations. Recently, the velocity range which can be measured using this technique has been extended to 6m/s which is the upper limit encountered in patients with severe valvular stenosis [59].

In patients with surgically corrected congenital heart disease serial assessment of ventricular function is of great clinical importance [60]. Visualization and functional evaluation of the right ventricle may be difficult by noninvasive techniques such as echocardiography or radionuclide ventriculography. In contrast, MRI is not limited by the anatomic position of this ventricle or superposition of other anatomic structures and therefore is ideally suited for follow-up examinations in these patients. The degree of right ventricular

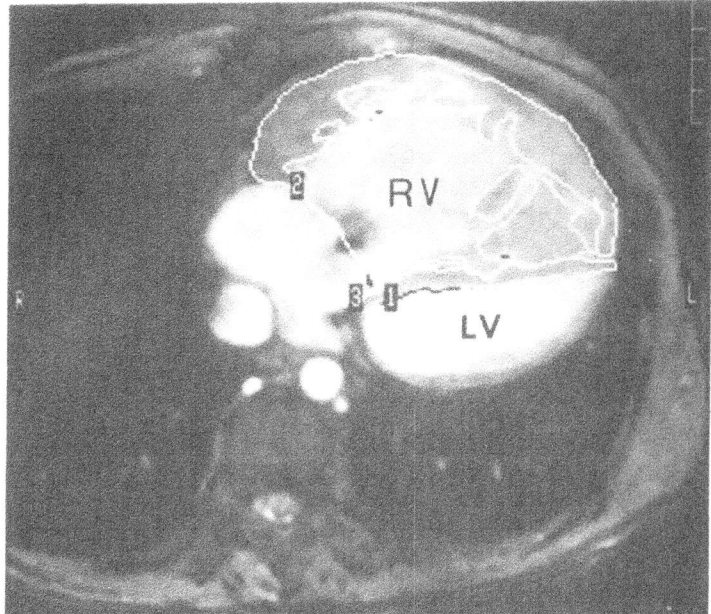

a

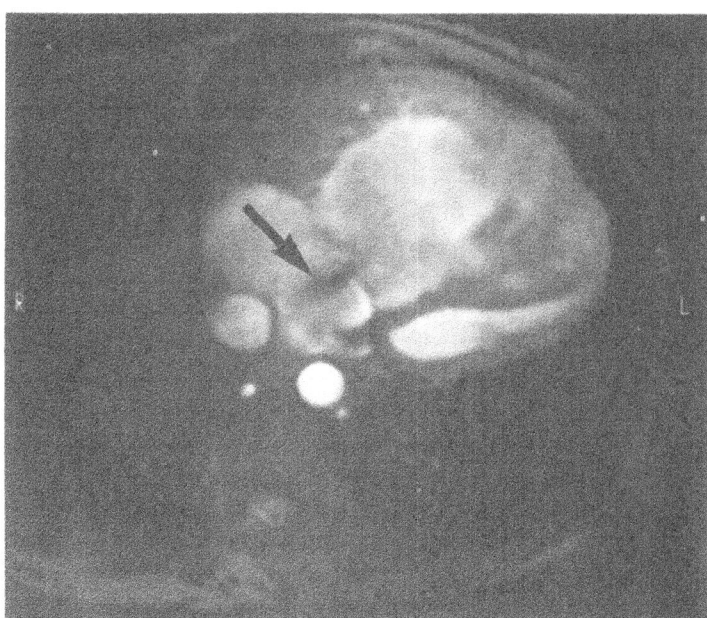

b

Figure 10. Transverse gradient-echo images in a patient with transposition of the great arteries 8 years after Mustard correction. (a) Diastolic image shows a dilated and hypertrophied right ventricle (RV) and a thin-walled small left ventricle (LV). Outlining indicates endocardial and epicardial borders used for determination of RV muscle mass. Numbers are related to quantitation software and should be disregarded. (b) Severely reduced contraction of the RV is evident on this systolic image. There is mild tricuspid regurgitation (arrow). The interventricular septum is shifted towards the normally contracting left ventricular posterior wall.

Table 2. Comparison of imaging techniques

	Echo	RNV	Cath	Cine-CT	MRI
Bedside technique	+	(+)	–	–	–
Noninvasive	+	+	–	+	+
Radiation exposure	–	(+)	+	(+)	–
Contrast media	–	–	+	+	–
Spatial resolution	(+)	–	+	+	+
Temporal resolution	+	+	+	+	+
Ease of quantitation	(+)	+	+	(+)	(+)
Pressures	(+)	–	+	–	(+?)
Reproducibility	(+)	+	+	+	+
Repeatibility	+	+	–	(+)	+
Three-dimensional	–	–	–	+	+
Right heart	–	(+)	(+)	+	+
Low cost	+	+	–	–	–

Cath = cardiac catheterization; echo = echocardiography including Doppler and transesophageal; RNV = radionuclide ventriculography; + = feature present and fully developed; (+) = feature present but some disadvantage compared to other techniques; (+?) = feature present at some centers, under development; – = feature not present or significant disadvantage to techniques with + sign.

hypertrophy and reduction of contractile function can be quantified by gradient-echo MRI in patients after atrial switch operation for transposition of the great arteries (Fig. 10) [61]. Significantly reduced mean right ventricular ejection fraction ($47.6 \pm 13.0\%$) was found in patients with additional closure of a ventricular septal defect whereas those without this associated lesion had a mean ejection fraction ($56.7 \pm 10.7\%$) which was not different from a normal population ($57.3 \pm 8.1\%$) [61].

7. Comparison with other imaging technique

Table 2 gives an overview of the strengths and weaknesses of the cardiac imaging techniques currently available for evaluation of cardiac function. At present, the clinical role of MRI is certainly not to replace established imaging techniques especially in the evaluation of regional and global left ventricular function (echocardiography, radionuclide ventriculography). However, some unique features make MRI attractive for pharmacologic studies of the left ventricle where reproducibility or three-dimensional imaging may be important and for evaluation of the right heart. Apart from these specialized applications, evaluation of the various aspects of cardiac function by MRI will be clinically helpful if MRI is used as a second line technique in patients who cannot be adequately assessed by other noninvasive techniques such as echocardiography.

Indications to perform MRI for diagnosis of anatomic abnormalities are discussed elsewhere in this book.

References

1. Crooks LE, Barker B, Chang H, et al. Magnetic resonance imaging strategies for heart studies. Radiology 1984;153:459–65.
2. Edelman RR, Thompson R, Kantor H, Brady TJ, Leavitt M, Dinsmore R. Cardiac function: evaluation with fast-echo MR imaging. Radiology 1987;162:611–5.
3. Van der Meulen P, Groen JP, Cuppen JJ. Very fast imaging by field echoes and small angle excitation. Magn Reson Imaging 1985;3:297–9.
4. Haase A, Frahm J, Matthaei D, Hanicke W, Merboldt KD. FLASH imaging. Rapid NMR imaging using low flip-angle pulses. J Magn Reson 1986;67:258–66.
5. Oppelt A, Graumann R, Barfuss H, Fischer H, Hartl W, Schajor W. FISP: A new fast MRI sequence. Electromedica 1986;54:15–8.
6. Glover GH, Pelc NJ. A rapid-gated cine MR technique. Magn Reson Annu 1988;4:299–333.
7. Sechtem U, Pflugfelder PW, White RD, et al. Cine MR imaging: potential for the evaluation of cardiovascular function. AJR Am J Roentgenol 1987;148:239–46.
8. Haase A. Snapshot FLASH MRI. Applications to T1, T2, and chemical-shift imaging. Magn Reson Med 1990;13:77–89.
9. Frahm J, Merboldt KB, Bruhn H, Gyngell ML, Hänicke W, Chien D. 0.3–second FLASH-MRI of the human heart. Magn Reson Med 1990;13:150–7.
10. Matthaei D, Haase A, Henrich D, Duhmke E. Cardiac and vascular imaging with a MR snapshot technique. Radiology 1990;177:527–32.
11. Atkinson DJ, Burstein D, Edelman RR. First-pass cardiac perfusion: evaluation with ultrafast MR imaging. Radiology 1990;174:757–62.
12. Wilke N, Machnig T, Engels G, et al. Ultraschnelle MR-Bildgebung für die dynamische Perfusionsuntersuchung: erste klinische Erfahrungen in der Kardiologie. Electromedica 1990;58:102–8.
13. Ordidge RJ, Mansfield P. Apid biomedical imaging by NMR. Br J Radiol 1981;54:850–5.
14. Rzedzian RR, Pykett IL. Instant images of the human heart using a new, whole-body imaging system. AJR Am J Roentgenol 1987;149:245–50.
15. Stehling MJ, Howseman AM, Ordidge RJ, et al. Whole-body echo-planar MR imaging at 0.5 T. Radiology 1989;170:257–63.
16. Dinsmore RE, Wismer GL, Levine RA, Okada RD, Brady TJ. Magnetic resonance imaging of the heart: positioning and gradient angle selection for optimal imaging planes. AJR Am J Roentgenol 1984;143:1135–42.
17. Dinsmore RE, Wismer GL, Miller SW, et al. Magnetic resonance imaging of the heart using image planes oriented to cardiac axes: experience with 100 cases. AJR Am J Roentgenol 1985;145:1177–83.
18. Buser PT, Auffermann W, Holt WW, et al. Noninvasive evaluation of global left ventricular function with use of cine nuclear magnetic resonance. J Am Coll Cardiol 1989;13:1294–300.
19. Lotan CS, Cranney CB, Bouchard A, Bittner V, Pohost GM. The value of cine nuclear magnetic resonance imaging for assessing regional ventricular function. J Am Coll Cardiol 1989;14:1721–29.
20. Pennell DJ, Underwood SR, Firmin DN, Longmore DB. Improved cine gradient echo imaging using gadolinium diethylenamine pentaacetic acid (abstract). 8th Annual Congress of the European Society of Magnetic Resonance in Medicine and Biology: book of abstracts. S.L.: European Society of Magnetic Resonance in Medicine and Biology, 1991:39.
21. Cranney GB, Lotan CS, Dean L, Baxley W, Bouchard A, Pohost GM. Left ventricular volume measurement using cardiac axis nuclear magnetic resonance imaging. Validation by calibrated ventricular angiography. Circulation 1990;82:154–63.
22. Van Rossum AC, Visser FC, van Eenige MJ, Valk J, Roos JP. Magnetic resonance imaging of the heart for determination of ejection fraction. Int J Cardiol 1988;18:53–63.
23. Stratemeier EJ, Thompson R, Brady TJ, et al. Ejection fraction determination by MR imaging: comparison with left ventricular angiography. Radiology 1986;158:775–7.

24. Buckwalter KA, Aisen AM, Dilworth LR, Mancini GB, Buda AJ. Gated cardiac MRI: ejection fraction determination using the right anterior oblique view. AJR Am J Roentgenol 1986;147:33–7.
25. Deutsch HJ, Smolorz J, Sechtem U, Hombach V, Schicha H, Hilger HH. Cardiac function by magnetic resonance imaging. Int J Card Imaging 1988;3:3–11.
26. Edelman RR, Wentz KU, Mattle H, et al. Projection arteriography and venography: initial clinical results with MR. Radiology 1989;172:351–7.
27. Markiewicz W, Sechtem U, Kirby R, Derugin N, Caputo GC, Higgins CB. Measurement of ventricular volumes in the dog using nuclear magnetic resonance imaging. J Am Coll Cardiol 1987;10:170–7.
28. Rehr RB, Malloy CR, Filipchuk NG, Peshock RM. Left ventricular volumes measured by MR imaging. Radiology 1985;156:717–9.
29. Van Rossum AC, Visser FC, Sprenger M, van Eenige MJ, Valk J, Roos JP. Evaluation of magnetic resonance imaging for determination of left ventricular ejection fraction and comparison with angiography. Am J Cardiol 1988;62:628–33.
30. Sechtem U, Pflugfelder PW, Gould RG, Cassidy MM, Higgins CB. Measurement of right and left ventricular volumes in healthy individuals with cine MR imaging. Radiology 1987;163:697–702.
31. Erbel R, Schweizer P, Henn G, Meyer J, Effert S. Apikale zweidimensionale Echokardiographie. Normalwerte für die monoplane und biplane Bestimmung der Volumina und der Ejektionsfraktion des linken Ventrikels. Dtsch Med Wochenschr 1982;107:1872–7.
32. Rackley CE. Quantitative evaluation of left ventricular function by radiographic techniques. Circulation 1976;54:862–79.
33. White RD, Cassidy MM, Cheitlin MD, et al. Segmental evaluation of left ventricular wall motion after myocardial infarction: magnetic resonance imaging vs echocardiography. Am Heart J 1988;115:166–75.
34. Higgins CB, Lanzer P, Stark D, et al. Imaging by nuclear magnetic resonance in patients with chronic ischemic heart disease. Circulation 1984;69:523–31.
35. Akins EW, Hill JA, Sievers KW, Conti CR. Assessment of left ventricular wall thickness in healed myocardial infarction by magnetic resonance imaging. Am J Cardiol 1987;59:24–8.
36. Underwood SR, Rees RS, Savage PE, et al. Assessment of regional left ventricular function by magnetic resonance. Br Heart J 1986;56:334–40.
37. McNamara MT, Higgins CB. Magnetic resonance imaging of chronic myocardial infarctions in man. AJR Am J Roentgenol 1986;146:315–20.
38. Fisher MR, von Schulthess GK, Higgins CB. Multiphasic cardiac magnetic resonance imaging: Normal regional left ventricular wall thickening. AJR Am J Roentgenol 1985;145:27–30.
39. Sechtem U, Sommerhoff BA, Markiewicz W, White RD, Cheitlin MD, Higgins CB. Regional left ventricular wall thickening by magnetic resonance imaging: evaluation of normal persons and patients with global and regional dysfunction. Am J Cardiol 1987;59:145–51.
40. Pflugfelder PW, Sechtem UP, White RD, Higgins CB. Quantification of regional myocardial function by rapid cine MR imaging. AJR Am J Roentgenol 1988;150:523–9.
41. Baer FM, Smolarz K, Sechtem U, et al. Viable and scarred myocardium: evaluation by gradient-echo magnetic resonance imaging and isonitrile SPECT (abstract). Circulation 1990;82(Suppl III):III-543.
42. Pennell DJ, Underwood SR, Ell PJ, Swanton RH, Walker JM, Longmore DB. Dipyridamole magnetic resonance imaging: a comparison with thallium-201 emission tomography. Br Heart J 1990;64:362–9.
43. Bacr FM, Smolarz K, Sechtem U, Jungehülsing M, Schicha H, Hilger HH. Feasibility of high dose dipyridamole MRI for the detection of coronary artery disease (abstract). 8th Annual Congress of the European Society for Magnetic Resonance in Medicine and Biology: book of abstracts. S.L.: European Society for Magnetic Resonance in Medicine and Biology, 1991:32.

44. Sellers RD, Levy MJ, Amplatz K, Lillehei CW. Left retrograde cardioangiography in acquired cardiac disease: technique, indications and interpretations in 700 cases. Am J Cardiol 1964;14:437–47.
45. Croft CH, Lipscomb K, Mathis K, et al. Limitations of qualitative angiographic grading in aortic or mitral regurgitation. Am J Cardiol 1984;53:1593–8.
46. Underwood SR, Klipstein RH, Firmin DN, et al. Magnetic resonance assessment of aortic and mitral regurgitation. Br Heart J 1986;56:455–61.
47. Sechtem U, Pflugfelder PW, Cassidy MM, et al. Mitral or aortic regurgitation: quantification of regurgitant volumes with cine MR imaging. Radiology 1988;167:425–30.
48. Globits S, Mayr H, Frank H, Neuhold A, Glogar D. Quantification of regurgitant lesions by MRI. Int J Cardiac Imaging 1990/91;6:109–16.
49. Wagner S, Auffermann W, Buser P, et al. Diagnostic accuracy and estimation of the severity of valvular regurgitation from the signal void on cine magnetic resonance images. Am Heart J 1989;118:760–7.
50. Welslau R, Sünger B, Sechtem U, et al. Comparison of colour coded Doppler and dynamic magnetic resonance imaging in semiquantitative estimation of aortic regurgitation (abstract). Eur Heart J 1989;10 (Abstract Suppl):403.
51. Welslau R, Kux R, Theissen P, Curtius JM, Sechtem U, Schicha H. Semiquantitative Schweregradabschätzung bei Mitralinsuffizienz: Vergleich Farbdopplerechokardiographie – Magnetresonanztomographie. Z Kardiol 1989;78 (Suppl 4):63.
52. Suzuki J, Caputo GR, Kondo C, Higgins CB. Cine MR imaging of valvular heart disease: display and imaging parameters affect the size of the signal void caused by valvular regurgitation. AJR Am J Roentgenol 1990;155:723–7.
53. Sahn DJ. Instrumentation and physical factors related to visualization of stenotic and regurgitant jets by Doppler color flow mapping. J Am Coll Cardiol 1988;12:1354–65.
54. Dulce MC, Friese K, Gast D, Albrecht A, Hamm B, Wolf KJ. Semiquantitative Beurteilung von Aortenklappeninsuffizienzen mittels Cine-MR im Vergleich zur Farb-Doppler-Echokardiographie und der Kardioangiographie. ROFO 1990;153:619–26.
55. Forfar JC, Godman MJ. Functional and anatomical correlates in atrial septal defect. An echocardiographic analysis. Br Heart J 1985;54:193–200.
56. Andersan M, Moller I, Lyngborg K, Wennevold A. The natural history of small atrial septal defects: long term follow-up with serial heart catheterizations. Am Heart J 1976;92:302–7.
57. Theissen P, Sechtem U, Linden A, Hilger HH, Schicha H. Noninvasive assessment of atrial septal defects and anomalous connection of pulmonary veins with MR (abstract). Radiology 1988;169 (Suppl P):270.
58. Nayler GL, Firmin DN, Longmore DB. Blood flow imaging by cine magnetic resonance. J Comput Assist Tomogr 1986;10:715–22.
59. Mohiaddin RH, Manzara CC, Kilner PJ, et al. Application of short echo time MR velocity mapping to characterization of blood flow through stenosed mitral valves (abstract). 8th Annual Congress of the European Society for Magnetic Resonance in Medicine and Biology: book of abstracts. S.L. European Society for Magnetic Resonance in Medicine and Biology, 1991:38.
60. Simpson IA, Chung KJ, Glass RF, Sahn DJ, Sherman FS, Hesselink J. Cine magnetic resonance imaging for evaluation of anatomy and flow relations in infants and children with coarctation of the aorta. Circulation 1988;78:142–8.
61. Theissen P, Kaemmerer H, Smolarz K, et al. Magnetic resonance imaging: functional and morphologic aspects of the heart in patients following Mustard procedure for transposition of the great arteries (abstract). Thorac Cardiovasc Surg 1991;39 (Suppl I):121.

22. Contrast-enhanced magnetic resonance imaging in myocardial disease

ALBERT DE ROOS, NIELS A.A. MATHEIJSSEN,
JOOST DOORNBOS, F. PAUL VAN RUGGE, PAUL R.M.
VAN DIJKMAN and ERNST E. VAN DER WALL

Summary

Magnetic resonance (MR) imaging with the aid of contrast agents may become a reliable noninvasive technique to assess myocardial perfusion. Dynamic MR imaging after administration of Gadolinium(Gd)-DTPA can differentiate reperfused from nonreperfused infarcts based on the early dynamics of contrast enhancement. Furthermore, Gd-DTPA enhanced MR imaging accurately delineates the infarcted region and can demonstrate infarct size reduction in patients with successful reperfusion. Ultrafast imaging methods in combination with MR contrast agents allow assessment of myocardial perfusion. The state-of-the-art developments in contrast-enhanced MR imaging in myocardial disease are reviewed.

Introduction

Magnetic resonance (MR) imaging and spectroscopy are able to provide high-resolution images of the heart, quantitative analysis of wall-motion abnormalities, evaluation of cardiac metabolism, and measurement of myocardial perfusion. MR imaging is essentially three-dimensional in nature and therefore well suited to evaluate the heart in any desired imaging plane. The MR images are acquired over many cardiac cycles and not real-time as with echocardiography. However, ultrafast and echo-planar techniques have recently become available for high-speed evaluation of dynamic cardiac events. Furthermore, critically ill patients with acute myocardial infarction can safely be studied with MR imaging, even in the early phase after infarct onset.

Several studies have shown that accurate quantification of regional myocardial first-pass perfusion by MR imaging in conjunction with MR contrast agents is feasible, indicating that MR imaging might become the preferred method for noninvasive screening of patients with ischemic heart disease [1]. High-speed MR scanning with paramagnetic and high-susceptibility MR contrast agents may allow assessment of regional myocardial perfusion, and evaluation of cardiac function and wall-motion both at rest and under pharm-

Johan H.C. Reiber & Ernst E. van der Wall (eds.), Cardiovascular Nuclear Medicine and MRI, 333–342.
© 1992 *Kluwer Academic Publishers.*

acologic stress [2]. This assessment may refine indications for surgery and angioplasty by providing distinction between reperfused-viable and reperfused-infarcted myocardium, evaluation of stunned myocardium and post-infarction prognostic factors such as infarct size, ejection fraction, end-systolic left ventricular volume and wall stress.

Pathophysiology of acute myocardial infarction

Thrombotic occlusion of an epicardial coronary artery is usually the cause of acute myocardial infarction [3,4]. After deprivation of arterial blood flow endocardial necrosis will occur within 20–40 minutes if coronary arterial flow is not reestablished. Following sudden and sustained coronary artery occlusion, the course of myocardial necrosis is rapid and will be completed within 3–6 hours after onset. The ischemic process is more severe in the inner, endocardial half of the myocardium than in the outer epicardial half. Acute myocardial infarction begins as subendocardial necrosis that spreads out as a 'wavefront' towards the epicardial layer as a function of time. The salutary effect of reperfusion therapy in acute myocardial infarction is due to salvage of reversibly damaged, ischemic myocardium. If reperfusion therapy is instituted at a time when viable ischemic myocytes are still present, the infarct size is limited.

Myocardial blood flow is provided by intramural coronary arteries which originate from the epicardial vessels. Under resting conditions, left ventricular flow is 70–85 ml per 100 g per min [4]. Left ventricular oxygen usage is 7–9 ml per 100 g per minute and most of this oxygen usage is expended during systole. About 80 % of total coronary flow occurs during diastole, when the perfusion pressure is reduced.

After the onset of acute myocardial ischemia, oxygen supply stops, ATP production ceases, and cardiac aerobic metabolism and energy production cannot continue. Since there is no glucose delivery during ischemia due to interruption of coronary arterial flow, increased glycogen breakdown becomes the major source for the increased anaerobic glycolysis which occurs during ischemia.

Phosphorus-31 MR spectroscopy can identify alterations in phosphocreatine (PCr), ATP, and inorganic phosphate (Pi) after coronary artery occlusion [5]. Within 5 minutes after coronary artery occlusion PCr levels drop significantly and a reciprocal rise in Pi levels occurs. The ATP levels decline over the first 45 minutes after initiation of ischemia. On reperfusion of the region with irreversible ischemia, there is incomplete recovery of PCr stores. In contrast, reversibly damaged myocardium demonstrates complete recovery of PCr stores and restoration of Pi to baseline values.

Importantly, it should be recognized that contrast-enhanced MR imaging is also able to distinguish reversibly and irreversibly damaged myocardium [6]. The occurrence of persistent and supernormal enhancement with albumin-Gd-DTPA is highly sensitive and specific for the presence of myocardial infarction. Reversible myocardial injury results in a uniform and equal enhancement of ischemic and normally perfused myocardium. Thus, both P-31 spectroscopy and contrast-enhanced MR imaging are able to separate reperfused-viable from reperfused-infarcted myocardium.

Contrast enhancement in myocardial infarction

The paramagnetic contrast agent Gd-DTPA can improve visualization of myocardial injury in both reperfused and nonreperfused infarcts [7]. Gd-DTPA shortens the T1 relaxation parameter in the infarcted zone, resulting in enhanced signal intensity of the infarct relative to normal myocardium using T1–weighted imaging techniques. Eichstaedt et al. examined 26 patients with acute myocardial infarction by MR imaging with the aid of 0.1 mmol/kg body weight Gd-DTPA [8]. MR imaging was performed in the acute phase (between 5–10 days), subacute (within 3 weeks), and chronic phase (after 3 weeks). Significant contrast enhancement was observed in the subgroup of acute infarcts. In the more chronic stages no differential contrast enhancement after Gd-DTPA was observed. This study suggested that injury of cell membranes and ingrowth of granulation tissue with capillary vessels were responsible for infarct enhancement between 5 and 10 days after infarct onset.

A preliminary study from our institution demonstrated the value of Gd-DTPA in the detection of acute myocardial infarction in five clinical patients at 2–17 days post-infarction [9]. It was concluded that MR imaging with the aid of Gd-DTPA improves detection and definition of acute myocardial infarction. These early results were confirmed in a larger series of 20 patients with acute myocardial infarction [10].

Infarct enhancement depending on the time after infarct onset

Nishimura et al. studied infarct enhancement after Gd-DTPA at different time intervals (average of 5, 12, 30 and 90 days post-infarction) [11]. Uptake of Gd-DTPA was a positive marker in acute myocardial infarction, but no significant uptake of Gd-DTPA occurred in chronic stages. Probably the absence of contrast enhancement in chronic infarcts is related to the development of poorly vascularized myocardial scar tissue. Van Dijkman et al. evaluated contrast enhancement of myocardial infarction in 84 patients at different points in time [12]. Gadolinium-DTPA improved visualization of acute myocardial infarction by MR imaging up to six weeks after onset of symptoms with a optimal effect within one week after the acute event.

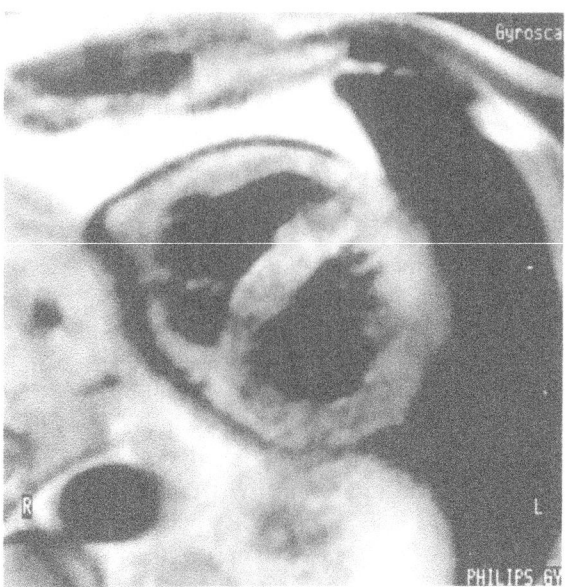

Figure 1. Homogeneous infarct enhancement in reperfused infarct. This pattern of contrast enhancement is indicative for reperfusion.

Assessment of infarct reperfusion by contrast enhancement

De Roos et al. assessed the diagnostic potential of Gd-DTPA-enhanced MR imaging to differentiate reperfused and nonreperfused infarcts [7]. Forty-five patients from two institutions were examined with MR imaging before and serially up to 30 minutes after intravenous administration of Gd-DTPA, 0.1 mmol/kg body weight. Coronary angiography after thrombolytic therapy was performed in all patients to assess reperfusion or coronary artery patency. Intensity ratios between both reperfused and nonreperfused infarcted areas and normal myocardium increased significantly up to 15–20 min after administration of Gd-DTPA and were still elevated 30 minutes after injection. In accordance with the findings in experimental studies, four distribution patterns of infarct enhancement were observed. With the use of Gd-DTPA as a marker for myocardial perfusion, we identified uniform, diffuse enhancement of the infarct in many reperfused infarcts (type 1 pattern; Fig. 1). In other reperfused infarcts we found predominantly subendocardial enhancement (type 2 pattern; Fig. 2). Dark areas of hemorrhage were particularly likely to be identified in patients with reperfused infarcts (type 3 pattern; Fig. 3). Variations in tissue edema and collateral circulation may affect the delivery of the amount of Gd-DTPA into the infarcted area. Hemorrhage and edema in the center of the infarct may prevent delivery of Gd-DTPA to the central core. This nonenhancing core may reflect the zone of no reflow within reperfused infarcts.

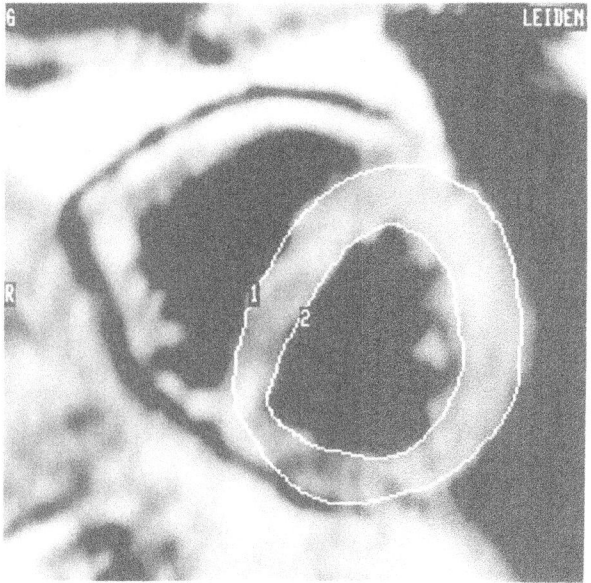

a

Figure 2a.

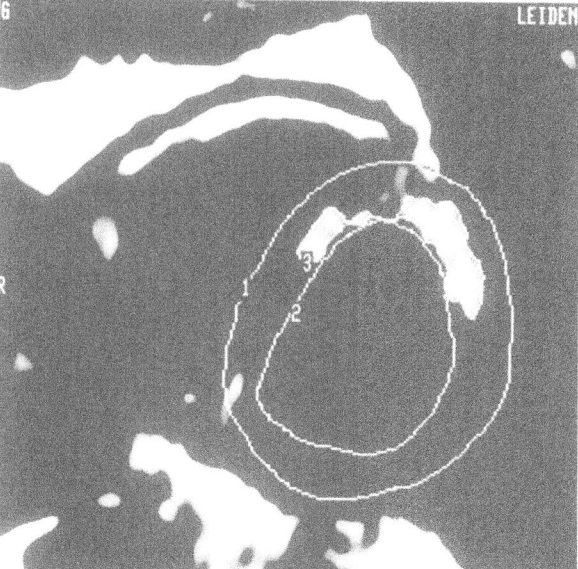

b

Figure 2. Post-gadolinium-DTPA MR image through the left ventricle in a patient with a recent anterior wall infarction. Note marked contrast enhancement in the anterior wall demarcating the subendocardial area of myocardial necrosis. Image is displayed before (a) and after (b) adjustment of window and level to visualize infarcted region. 1 = epicardial tracing; 2 = endocardial tracing; 3 = infarct tracing.

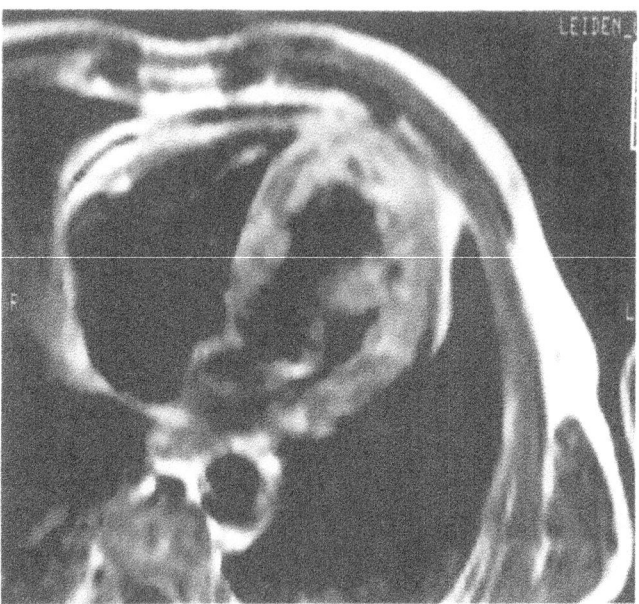

Figure 3. Inhomogeneous pattern of contrast enhancement. This pattern may be observed in reperfused infarct and is probably related to areas of hemorrhage in the infarcted region.

In nonreperfused infarcts we identified type 1,2, and 3 patterns of enhancement. The subendocardial (type 2) pattern was especially prevalent (61 %) in the group of nonreperfused infarcts. Partial enhancement with a doughnut pattern (type 4 enhancement) was found in one occlusive infarct. The overlap in enhancement patterns and similar maximal intensity ratios after Gd-DTPA administration for both reperfused and nonreperfused infarcts precluded a reliable differentiation on the basis of these factors alone. Significant enhancement of both reperfused and nonreperfused infarcts allowed adequate infarct imaging up to at least 30 minutes after administration of Gd-DTPA.

A separate analysis was performed in 27 patients who had a first acute myocardial infarction [13]. Intensity ratios were significantly higher in the 17 patients who underwent MR imaging more than 72 hours after onset of symptoms than in the 10 who underwent MR imaging earlier. When patients were compared considering the site and size of the infarcts, and the status of reperfusion or nonreperfusion, the intensity ratios both before and after Gd-DTPA were similar. However, there are indications that MR imaging early after Gd-DTPA injection may be clinically applicable to assess patency of the infarct-related coronary artery. Van Rossum et al. reported on the early dynamics of contrast enhancement using Gd-DTPA in 18 patients with myocardial infarction [14]. The patency of the infarct-related coronary artery was established by coronary angiography 36 ± 24 hr after infarct onset. A scoring system was used to quantify the severity of residual stenosis and to grade the collateral supply when total occlusion of the infarct-related coronary artery was found. Based on angiographic findings two groups of patients were distinguished. Group I included patients with occluded infarct-related coronary arteries without collateral filling. Group II patients had reperfused infarct vessels or occluded vessels with collateral supply. The maximum intensity ratio between infarcted and normal myocardium was not significantly different in group I and group II patients. Of note, a significant difference in intensity ratios was found between group I and II patients on images obtained early (i.e. 6–8 min) after injection of Gd-DTPA. This study indicates that assessment of the early dynamics of contrast enhancement with the aid of Gd-DTPA shows promise for the identification of coronary artery reperfusion after thrombolysis.

Assessment of the extent of myocardial necrosis by contrast enhancement

Recently, we assessed myocardial infarct size after reperfusion therapy using Gd-DTPA-enhanced MR imaging (Fig. 2) [15]. Twenty-one patients with proven acute myocardial infarction were studied. Early coronary angiography documented successful reperfusion after intravenous streptokinase therapy in a subset of 5 patients. In 4 patients early recanalization was established using acute percutaneous transluminal coronary angioplasty (PTCA) of the occluded infarct-related coronary artery. In 5 other patients coronary angiography documented absence of patency of the infarct-related coronary artery. Seven additional patients did not receive thrombolytic therapy for different reasons. Patients were divided into two groups. Group I includes patients with early reperfusion achieved by streptokinase therapy or PTCA (N = 9). Group II was comprised of patients with no reperfusion at coronary angiography and those without treatment by streptokinase administration or PTCA (N = 12). These group II patients were all considered to have no reperfusion. One group II patient was excluded from further analysis because of image degradation by motion artifacts. All patients underwent MR imaging at an average of 8 ± 4 days after infarct onset. Sixteen of 21 patients underwent a second MR examination at 26 ± 11 days after the acute event. MR imaging was started approximately 10 minutes after intravenous injection of 0.2 mmol/kg bodyweight Gd-DTPA. A control group of patients who were scheduled for enhanced MR imaging of the brain also underwent cardiac imaging. All MR images were evaluated by qualitative and quantitative analysis. All patients with acute myocardial infarction showed a myocardial region of contrast enhancement after Gd-DTPA injection in the distribution area of the proven or presumed infarct-related coronary artery. In the subjects without known cardiac disease, no abnormal myocardial regions of Gd-DTPA uptake were measured. Thus, Gd-DTPA appears to be a specific marker of myocardial necrosis in the setting of acute myocardial infarction in patients. The average MR-estimated infarct size in (reperfused) group I patients at the first MR study was $8 \pm 5\%$ compared to $15 \pm 4\%$ for (nonreperfused) group II patients ($p < 0.001$). No differences in infarct size were found between early and late scans or between group I and II patients at late time intervals. Thus, MR infarct sizing with the aid of Gd-DTPA is feasible in patients with or without successful reperfusion. This approach may be clinically useful to compare the effect of different reperfusion therapies aimed at the reduction of myocardial infarct size. Ovize et al. assessed myocardial infarct size by Gadolinium tetraazacyclododecanetetraacetic-acid (Gd-DOTA) after different time intervals of reperfusion [16]. Myocardial infarct size was accurately delineated on Gd-DOTA enhanced MR images, especially after a 6 hours delay after the onset of reperfusion [16].

Evaluation of myocardial perfusion with contrast agents

Assessment of the myocardial region at risk for ischemia may also be feasible using spin-echo MR imaging with the aid of continuous infusion of Gd-DTPA after vasodilation [17]. In that study regions at risk for ischemia were identified as perfusion defects during continuous infusion of Gd-DTPA after dipyridamole-induced vasodilation. Thus, contrast-enhanced MR imaging is useful to evaluate both the infarcted myocardial region and the area at risk for ischemia.

Recently the availability of subsecond, ultrafast MR techniques has provided new avenues for assessing myocardial perfusion by MR imaging in conjunction with contrast agents [1]. Van Rugge et al. evaluated first-pass through the ventricular cavities and myocardial perfusion using subsecond MR imaging and a bolus injection of Gadolinium-DTPA on a commercially available Philips ACS system operating at 1.5 Tesla (Fig. 4) [18]. The addition of wide area prepulses of 120–150 degrees resulted in T1–weighting of the image contrast and presaturation of the inflowing blood into the imaging plane. The subsecond MR technique was performed with a short repetition time of 7.8 msec and a reduced echo delay time of 4 msec. The imaging sequence was timed as follows: R-wave trigger-trigger delay-spatial presaturation pulse-prepulse delay-64 phase encoding steps.

Significant myocardial enhancement was demonstrated over time. Gadolinium-DTPA enhanced subsecond MR imaging may offer clinical useful information on the early dynamics of myocardial perfusion in patients with coronary artery disease.

Conclusions

MR imaging provides clinically useful information in patients with ischemic heart disease which is not available from other imaging modalities. High-speed MR imaging with the aid of contrast agents may become a valuable

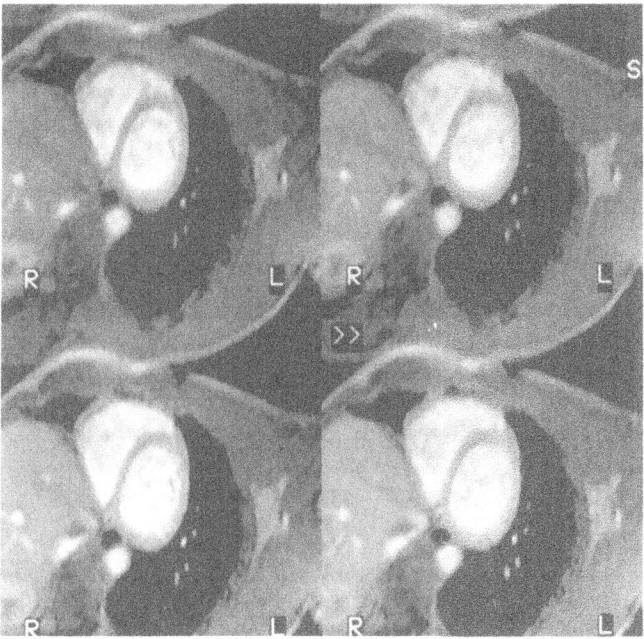

Figure 4. Subsecond MR images through the left ventricle after bolus injection of Gadolinium-DTPA. Note marked enhancement of ventricular cavities and normal myocardium evolving over time (courtesy of F.P. van Rugge, Ref. 18).

tool for assessing myocardial perfusion in patients with ischemic heart disease. The current applications of contrast-enhanced MR imaging include: 1. improved visualization and detection of acute myocardial infarction, especially in the first week after infarct onset, 2. quantification of myocardial infarct size in the setting of reperfusion therapy, 3. evaluation of regional myocardial perfusion in ischemic heart disease.

References

1. Atkinson DJ, Burstein D, Edelman RR. First-pass cardiac perfusion: evaluation with ultrafast MR imaging. Radiology 1990;174:757–62
2. Pettigrew RI. Four-dimensional cardiac MR imaging: diagnostic procedure of the future. Radiology 1989;173 (Suppl):50 (abstract)
3. Braunwald E. Myocardial reperfusion, limitation of infarct size, reduction of left ventricular dysfunction, and improved survival. Should the paradigm be expanded? Circulation 1989;79:441–4
4. Bianco JA, Alpert JS. Current and future role of noninvasive studies in acute myocardial ischemia and infarction. Am J Physiol Imaging 1986;1:142–53
5. Higgins CB. Malcolm Hanson memorial lecture. MR of the heart: anatomy, physiology, and metabolism. Am J Roentgenol 1988;151:239–48
6. Wolfe CL, Moseley ME, Wikstrom MG, Sievers RE, Wendland MF, Dupon JW, et al.

Assessment of myocardial salvage after ischemia and reperfusion using magnetic resonance imaging and spectroscopy. Circulation 1989;80:969–82

7. De Roos A, Van Rossum AC, Van der Wall EE, Postema S, Doornbos J, Matheijssen N, et al. Reperfused and nonreperfused myocardial infarction: diagnostic potential of Gd-DTPA enhanced MR imaging. Radiology 1989;172:717–20

8. Eichstaedt HW, Felix R, Dougherty FC, Langer M, Rutsch W, Schmutzler H. Magnetic resonance imaging (MRI) in different stages of myocardial infarction using the contrast agent gadolinium-DTPA. Clin Cardiol 1986;9:527–35

9. De Roos A, Doornbos J, Van der Wall EE, Van Voorthuisen AE,. MR imaging of acute myocardial infarction: value of Gd-DTPA. Year Book Medicine 1989;323–5

10. Van Dijkman PR, Doornbos J, De Roos A, Van der Laarse A, Postema S, Matheijssen NA, et al. Improved detection of acute myocardial infarction by magnetic resonance imaging using gadolinium-DTPA. Int J Card Imaging 1989;5:1–8

11. Nishimura T, Kobayashi H. Ohara Y, Yamada N, Haze K, Takamiya M, et al. Serial assessment of myocardial infarction by using gated MR imaging and Gd-DTPA. Am J Roentgenol 1989;153:715–20

12. Van Dijkman PRM, Van der Wall EE, De Roos A, et al. Quantitative analysis of acute, subacute and chronic myocardial infarction by Gadolinium-DTPA enhanced magnetic resonance imaging. Radiology. In press.

13. Van der Wall EE, Van Dijkman PR, De Roos A, Doornbos J, Van der Laarse A, Manger Cats V, et al. Diagnostic significance of Gadolinium-diethylenetriamine penta-acetic acid enhanced magnetic resonance imaging in thrombolytic treatment for acute myocardial infarction: its potential in assessing reperfusion. Br Heart J 1990;63:12–7

14. Van Rossum AC, Visser FC, Van Eenige MJ, Sprenger M, Valk J, Verheugt FN, et al. Value of gadolinium-diethylene-triamine-pentaacetic acid dynamics in magnetic resonance imaging of acute myocardial infarction with occluded and reperfused coronary arteries after thrombolysis. Am J Cardiol 1990;65:845–51

15. De Roos A, Matheijssen NA, Doornbos J, Van Dijkman PR, Van Voorthuisen AE, Van der Wall EE. Myocardial infarct size after reperfusion therapy: assessment by Gd-DTPA-enhanced MR imaging. Radiology 1990;176:517–21

16. Ovize M, Pichard JB, de Lorgeril M, Dandis G, Revel D, Renaud S, et al. Accurate quantitation of infarct size by gadolinium-DOTA enhanced magnetic resonance imaging in the dog. J Am Coll Cardiol 1991;17: Suppl A: 242 A (abstract)

17. Galjee MA, Van Rossum AC, Visser FC, Valk J, Roos JP. MRI of myocardial ischaemia using continuous infusion of Gd-DTPA after dipyridamole (abstract). In: 2nd International Symposium on Computer Applications in Nuclear Medicine and Cardiac Magnetic Resonance Imaging. Book of Abstracts. 1991:208

18. Van Rugge FP, Boreel JJ, Van der Wall EE, et al. Assessment of cardiac first-pass and myocardial perfusion in normal subjects using Gadolinium-DTPA enhanced subsecond magnetic resonance imaging. J Comput Assist Tomogr 1991. In press

23. Assessment of hypertrophy and regression in arterial hypertension: Value of magnetic resonance imaging

HERMANN EICHSTAEDT

Summary

Increasing interest has been paid to the effects of antihypertensive treatment on the myocardium. In particular regression of left ventricular hypertrophy (LVH) has been the focus of recent studies. Regression of LVH can be decisive in improving oxygen consumption of the myocardium and may prevent serious long-term cardiac complications of hypertension, such as dilatation of tissue structures and heart failure. Regression of hypertrophy under antihypertensive treatment was first demonstrated in rats. Marked regression was observed after alpha-methyldopa, beta-blocking agents, and angiotensin converting enzyme (ACE) inhibitors. Effects of diuretics and direct vasodilators like hydralazine and minoxidil were less impressive.

In patients with hypertension, cardiologists first made use of echocardiography for the direct in vivo demonstration of regression of hypertrophy. Previous to echocardiography, only indirect electrocardiographic methods were available. With echocardiography, antihypertensive drugs such as alpha-methyldopa, beta-blocking agents, and ACE-inhibitors showed similar effects on LVH as observed in rats.

Thallium-201 perfusion imaging for quantification of hypertrophy has been shown useful for demonstration of LVH, but the radionuclide technique lacks the spatial resolution to accurately determine regression of LVH.

Magnetic resonance imaging (MRI) has emerged as a new imaging modality the heart since 1983. Due to its high spatial resolution, MRI is an excellent technique for assessing cardiac dimensions, volumes and myocardial mass. MRI is therefore very suitable to determine changes in these myocardial parameters before and after antihypertensive treatment.

1. Introduction

Corresponding interdependency has been demonstrated across many animal species between the mass of the heart and external work of the ventricle [1]. Thus, within any single species of animals, any prolonged augmentation in the hemodynamic overload imposed on the ventricle will result in hypertrophy of

Johan H.C. Reiber & Ernst E. van der Wall (eds.), Cardiovascular Nuclear Medicine and MRI, 343–367.
© 1992 *Kluwer Academic Publishers.*

that cavity sustaining the overload. Systemic arterial hypertension is the most common condition leading to left ventricular hypertrophy since the left ventricle is the chamber that should provide the augmented energy needed to overcome the chronic obligation of the pressure overload.

Already in 1868, it was G. Johnson who utilized sphygmographic evidence of increased arterial pressure to make the true association between arterial hypertension and left ventricular hypertrophy, as described by Pickering [2]. In 1933, Chanutin and Barksdale actually demonstrated that LVH could be produced by inducing experimental hypertension [3]. These investigators used a renoprival model of arterial hypertension and showed that left ventricular mass increased with the development of experimental hypertension. This pioneering work indicated clearly that the increased mass of the left ventricle could be attributed to ventricular hypertrophy since it was demonstrated that left ventricular myocyte fiber diameter was increased in direct proportion to the height of arterial pressure [4].

2. Incidence of left ventricular hypertrophy

2.1. *Animal hypertension*

Left ventricular hypertrophy is caused entirely by enlargement of individual cells in adult animals. In contrast, when hypertrophy develops immediately after birth and for a number of weeks thereafter, it is due to an increase in cell number and in cell size [5].

Time of onset of the rise in blood pressure is much more clearly defined in animal models of secondary hypertension than in human hypertension and can be accurately related to the time course of development of LVH. Increased protein synthesis occurs within an hour after rising in blood pressure in a range of hypertrophy models [6–8]. In rats with experimental renovascular hypertension a gross increase in left ventricular mass can be detected within 2–3 days and the process of hypertrophy is complete within about 3 weeks after elevation of blood pressure [9]. Similarly in renal hypertensive dogs, rabbits and rats, the ratio of left ventricular weight to bodyweight is increased by about 50–100 % after 4–6 weeks of hypertension [10–13]. As expected, the increased ratio affects virtually all the animals.

In spontaneously hypertensive rats, a significant increase in left ventricular weight has been found by several investigators soon after birth [14,15], when there is only little elevation in blood pressure. In studies on the time course of the development of LVH, in rats from 4 to 50 weeks of age, there were little differences in left ventricular mass/body weight ratio at 4 weeks between carefully age- and weight-matched spontaneously hypertensive rats and Wistar-Kyoto normotensive control rats [16]. In these series no obvious differences were observed in systolic or in mean arterial blood pressure between the strains at 4 weeks. The left ventricular mass/bodyweight ratio was only about 6–8 % higher (P = NS) in spontaneously hypertensive rats than in Wistar-Kyoto normotensive control rats. The main increase in left ventricular mass occurred between 4 and 14 weeks and was associated with the main rise in blood pressure during the rapid growth phase. At the end of this time, left ventricular mass/bodyweight ratio in spontaneously hypertensive rats exceeded that of Wistar-Kyoto normotensive control rats by about 25 %, and rose by a further 10 % by 20 weeks to the final difference between the strains [17].

2.2. *Human hypertension*

Assessment of LVH was based largely on X-Ray and electrocardiographic (ECG) findings in the early literature. Both these methods are relatively insensitive to minor changes in left ventricular mass. So it is likely that many patients diagnosed as having left ventricular *hypertrophy*, may have had some degree of left ventricular *dilatation*. The latter may have contributed to the strikingly poor prognosis of LVH in the earlier epidemiological surveys, such as the Framingham study [18].

Since the midseventies, M-mode echocardiography followed by development of two-dimensional echocardiography with associated Color-Doppler methods, have allowed more precise assessment of human left ventricular dimensions and function with a range of about 1–2 mm. There are now validated formulae for assessing left ventricular mass from measurements of wall thickness and other dimensions, which permit diagnosis of milder degrees of LVH [19]. However, despite these more sensitive techniques, the reported prevalence of human LVH is still surprisingly low when compared to the almost 100 % prevalence in animal models [20,21].

Estimates of the prevalence range from 20–60 % in patients with established hypertension, with the findings of most series closer to the lower end of this range [22]. Possible reasons for the discrepancy between human and experimental hypertension include: (1) a greater severity of hypertension in experimental models, (2) prior treatment with antihypertensive drugs in many studies in human hypertension, which could reduce the apparent prevalence by causing regression of LVH, and (3) use of genetic traits in animal experiments with a smaller normal range of variation of left ventricular mass than in the human population. The latter is genetically more heterogenous with respect to the factors likely to influence left ventricular mass. For example, there is a much greater variation in body build in the human population than in Wistar-Kyoto normotensive controls and spontaneously hypertensive rats.

In the normal population there is a high variance of left ventricular mass which makes it more difficult to establish realistic criteria that take adequately into account the numerous biological factors that influence the normal variation. The conventional standard is to define as abnormal a value that is more than two standard deviations above the mean of the normal population. This criterion is rather severe with a variable like left ventricular mass where the range of normal variation is large, and will define as abnormal only those with gross degrees of LVH. With other criteria of congruence, such as matching individuals for the same body build or lean body mass, we could probably detect hypertensive individuals with smaller degrees of LVH. Such an approach for providing the best index of left ventricular mass has been suggested [22]. An alternative way is to use anatomical variables with a smaller range of variation in the normal population that provided similar information about LVH. With a low variance, the categorization of 'abnormality' will be less ambiguous when considering, as our standard, values that are two standard deviations above the mean of the normal population.

It seems to be the high variance of left ventricular mass index in the normal human population that contributes to the low estimate of prevalence of LVH in hypertension [23]. The study population of Laufer et al. [23] included normal subjects and hypertensive patients with mild (borderline) and established hypertension. None of the patients had previously received antihypertensive drug treatment. However, despite this, only 30 % of the patients with established hypertension, and only 12 % of those with mild hypertension, had values of left ventricular mass index that were at least two standard deviations above the mean of the normal group. This corresponds exactly with the low level of prevalence reported in the earlier literature and suggests that prior drug treatment was not the major determinant of the estimated low prevalence of LVH in some of the earlier series. With anatomical variables, including wall thickness corrected for body surface area and the ratio of wall thickness/internal radius in which the variance in the normal population was lower, a greater proportion of hypertensives was categorized as having LVH. With either of the latter variables about 60–65 % of patients with established hypertension and about 30 % with mild hypertension were classified as having 'abnormal' left ventricular structure on the basis of values two standard deviations above the mean of the normal group.

Multivariate discriminant function analysis is another approach, that allows maximum separation between hypertensive and normotensive individuals [24]. In the study of Laufer et al. [23], where two predictor variables were used to categorize the groups, left ventricular mass index, or wall thickness and left ventricular internal diameter, were classified correctly in 72 % of normal subjects and 70 % of patients with long-lasting hypertension. For those patients classified as having only mild hypertension, the above-mentioned parameters were not significantly different from normals. With the multivariate technique of the estimates, the prevalence of LVH in hypertension was identical whether left ventricular mass index or wall thickness was used, suggesting that the multivariate technique makes some allowance for more congruent matching of individuals in the two populations.

When in addition to anatomical variables, functional predictor variables were added to the discriminant function, one could obtain still greater improvement in discriminating capacity. The most important variable was the ratio of transmitral flow velocities in early (E) and late (A wave-related) diastole (E/A velocity ratio). In mild and established hypertension, the E/A ratio falls progressively when compared with corresponding normal values. The E/A ratio deals with diastolic events which, in the context of hypertension, are largely a reflection of decreased left ventricular compliance. The latter is an early abnormality in hypertension, so that the E/A ratio can be regarded as a pseudo-anatomical variable. Fractional systolic shortening (ratio of end-systolic/end-diastolic left ventricular diameter) was also used in the analysis. Fractional shortening was slightly elevated in mild hypertension, but in established hypertension there was an almost complete overlap with the normal range. In the multivariate analysis, the use of fractional shortening greatly helped in the correct classification of patients with *mild* hypertension. Using three predictor variables (wall thickness, E/A velocity ratio, and fractional shortening), there was correct classification of 81 % of normal male subjects, 72 % of those with established hypertension and 60 % of those with mild hypertension [25].

Left ventricular mass index turns out to be one of the least discriminating anatomical variables, and the criterion of abnormality of more than two standard deviations above the mean of the normal population appears to be too severe. Of the univariate variables that Korner et al. [25] have studied the estimated prevalence of LVH is greatest with wall thickness or wall thickness/internal radius. But the use of multivariate analysis with combined anatomical and functional variables provides the highest estimate of prevalence of LVH.

With the technique of the multivariate analysis, the prevalence of LVH is very high and is not very far from the almost universal prevalence in animal models of hypertension. The results of Laufer et al. [23] suggest that, if some allowance is made for problems of matching of hypertensive and normal individuals, LVH in stable hypertension occurs in virtually all patients. In mild human hypertension, the prevalence of LVH appears to be lower. Slightly more than half of this group has characteristics distinctive from the normal population. This is in accordance with early epidemiological studies, in which about half the subjects with borderline hypertension went on to develop chronic hypertension, whereas the blood pressure returned to normal in the others [18].

3. Cellular changes in smooth muscle and vessels

3.1. *Hypertrophy and hyperplasia*

In arterial hypertension the hypertrophy of vessel walls is the result of multiple cellular events including smooth muscle proliferation (hyperplasia and polyploidy) [26–29], cell hypertrophy [30], fibrous proteins synthesis and deposit in the extracellular matrix [31,32]. With exception of malignant forms leading rapidly to the disruption of the arteriolar architecture, the early phases of hypertension usually respect the normal appearance of the arterial wall. All the cellular components participate in the process of hypertrophy, which appears relatively homogenous. In chronic hypertension, collagen and glycosaminoglycans synthesis predominates and leads to a progressive arterial fibrosis [33]. One of the goals for hypertension treatment is a return to normal of the smooth muscle cell activity. Assuming that this objective is achieved, the return to a normal arterial trophicity will then depend on the turnover rate of the major structural proteins.

Wolinsky et al. [34] produced the first evidence of dissociated responses of the arterial components following an antihypertensive treatment. Unclipping renovascular hypertensive rats made it possible to lower the aortic alcali-soluble proteins to normal values, indicating the reversal of the cellular hypertrophy. However, the collagen content remained unchanged or even increased in males after several months of normotension.

Smooth muscle cell hypertrophy is most rapidly and completely reversed among the arterial structural changes [35–38]. Extracellular deposition of fibrous proteins, mainly of collagen, seems considerably more difficult to heal. A number of studies did not detect any change in arterial collagen content induced by treatment [30,39–41]. It was reported that collagen turnover remained high in arteries during antihypertensive treatment allowing a progressive decrease in collagen content [42]. Long-lasting inhibition of collagen deposition in spontaneously hypertensive rat arteries can be induced by an early and prolonged antihypertensive therapy [43,44]. The intensity of this effect is directly related to blood pressure control during the treatment period and is normally not facilitated by any of the different antihypertensive medications.

The most difficult parameter to control seems to be cell hyperplasia of smooth muscle. In the arteries of adult rats, muscle cell DNA metabolism is inactive, as indicated by the very low labeling index after tritiated thymidine injections [28]. Arterial mitotic activity is high in two cases: during the first hours and day of acute blood pressure rise in secondary hypertension [26,28] and at the prehypertensive phase of genetic hypertension in particular in the spontaneously hypertensive rats [33,38]. In both cases, the intense DNA synthesis activity is a transient phenomenon. The nucleic acid metabolism returns to normal or near normal values in chronic hypertension and appears to be only slightly affected by antihypertensive treatment [17,37]. Arterial smooth muscle hyperplasia is normally impossible to reverse. Experiments in renovascular hypertensive rats illustrated the complete dissociation of cell hypertrophy and cell hyperplasia following a 12–week unclipping period [45]. The aortic wet weight and the aortic alkali-soluble proteins content of the unclipped resumed normotensive values. By contrast, the aortic DNA content as well as the residual tritiated thymidine radioactivity injected after 4 days of hypertension, an estimate for early DNA synthesis, was not different in the treated animals compared to the hypertensive controls [38].

Preventive administration of antihypertensive agents in prehypertensive spontaneously hypertensive rats has oftenly no effect on the smooth muscle cell hyperplasia that develops very early in the middle-sized arteries of these animals [43]. Only alpha-methyldopa is able to prevent the early increase in DNA content, but calcium-antagonists, ACE-inhibitors and alpha-blockers failed to show this effect despite significant inhibition of hypertension development.

3.2. *Genetic factors of hypertrophy*

Myocardial hypertrophy has been shown to be associated with a gradual decline in the maximum velocity of cardiac muscle shortening that usually correlates with the decreased calcium ATP-ase activity of myosin [46]. Recently, it has been demonstrated that during persistent cardiac hypertrophy, cardiac myosin isoforms shift from type V_1, a faster migrating type, to type V_3, a form that migrates more slowly [47–49]. It has been demonstrated that the change in myosin isozymes during the development of hypertrophy is a result of cellular regulation of myosin biosynthesis depending on two separate genes that code for two types of heavy chains. V_1 and V_3 are the two homodimer phenotypes of the genes, whereas V_2 is the mixed heterodimer phenotype involving both genes [50–52]. Recently, Sen and Young [53] have shown that in renal hypertensive rats there is a significant shift of myosin isoforms from type V_1 to type V_3, which can be corrected or reversed by either antihypertensive therapy with captopril or sodium deprivation from V_3 to V_1. On the other hand, treatment with the beta-blocker atenolol increases V_3 myosin phenotypes. This observation was confirmed by Dussaule et al. [54]; they demonstrated in two-kidney, one-clip hypertensive rats that treatment with captopril induced regression of hypertrophy. They also showed that upregulation of myosin isoform from V_3 to V_1 occurred. Sen and Young [55] continued this study and confirmed the similar shifting of myosin isoform in spontaneously hypertensive rats. It was demonstrated that the type of myosin isozyme distribution pattern can be corrected by either captopril therapy or by sodium deprivation. Dussaule et al. [54] concluded that the cardiac effect most probably relates to normalization of blood pressure in the absence of any stimulation of the sympathetic nervous system. However, Sen and Young [55] showed that the changes in myosin isozyme distribution can occur independent of muscle mass and heart rate, blood pressure and sympathetic outflow. Therefore, the factor responsible for signaling of myosin V_1 or V_3 biosynthesis is still not clear.

3.3. *Proportions of collagen and muscle*

During development of hypertrophy in hypertension an alteration in collagen component of the myocardium takes place. Sen [56] showed that an increase in rate of collagen synthesis parallelled an increase in content of myocardial collagen in spontaneously hypertensive rats. Not only did the total collagen change, but also the collagen phenotypes of type III and type V changed during development of hypertension and hypertrophy. These changes can be corrected by normalization of blood pressure. Recently, Weber et al. [57] demonstrated that in pressure-overloaded hypertrophied myocardium, clinical and experimental evidence indicates that the proportion of collagen relative to muscle is increased. Factors that appear to influence collagen growth during the hypertrophy process include age, species, rapidity with which the overload occurs, the nature of lesion leading to pressure overload and the severity and duration of overload. Morphologically the collagen matrix of myocardium consists of a complex weave with tendinous insertions that surround myocytes, grouping them into myofibers, strands of collagen that connect adjoining myofibers, and collagenase struts that join myocytes to other myocytes and capillaries. In a primate preparation of perinephritis with systemic hypertension, it was observed that the tendinous elements of the weave and the strands of collagen lying between the myofibers were increased in number and physical dimension [57]. The functional consequences of remodeling of collagen matrix that accompanies myocardial hypertrophy remain to be elucidated. A better understanding of the dynamic behavior of collagen matrix may offer new insights into the pathogenesis of ventricular dysfunction that accompanies chronic pressure-overloaded state.

4. Hypertrophy regression

4.1. *Animal models*

Different antihypertensive drugs produce different degrees of regression of LVH, a phenomenon which Sen et al. [58] first showed in spontaneously hypertensive rats. For example, with alpha-methyldopa there was substantial lowering of left ventricular mass, but similar lowering of blood pressure produced by minoxidil did not cause regression of LVH. In addition, propranolol produced substantial reversal of LVH in doses that did not lower blood pressure. In contrast, Motz et al. [59] found that the vasodilator agent hydralazine induced regression of LVH. However, further reduction in left ventricular mass occurred when metoprolol was added to hydralazine, with only slight additional lowering of blood pressure. There was substantial reduction in left ventricular mass/volume ratio, indicating structural remodeling similar to the findings in humans. In spontaneously hypertensive rats, lowering mean arterial pressure is associated with substantial reduction in left ventricular mass, though the values reached remain usually somewhat above the levels of Wistar-Kyoto normotensive controls [59,60]. This was also observed by Fletcher [61] after normalizing blood pressure following reversing renal cellophane wrap hypertension in rabbit by removal of the fibrous capsule encasing the kidney: in untreated renal hypertensive rabbits, left ventricular mass/bodyweight was 2 g/kg, compared with a mean value of 1.3 g/kg in normal rabbits. Six weeks after unwrapping the kidneys, left ventricular mass/bodyweight was 1.5 g/kg, indicating substantial regression of LVH.

Development of LVH parallels the rise of blood pressure from 4–20 weeks in spontaneously hypertensive rats [16]. Korner et al. [25] studied three groups of spontaneously hypertensive rats with the ACE-inhibitor enalapril, using a dose that normalized blood pressure. Treatment was given from (a) 4 to 10 weeks, (b) 4–14 weeks – which corresponds to the major phase of development of hypertension –, and (c) 14–20 weeks, when adult levels of blood pressure have been reached [24]. In all three groups, LVH reversed completely by the end of treatment, and the left ventricular mass/bodyweight ratios were the same as those for Wistar-Kyoto normotensive controls. When treatment was discontinued, blood pressure remained stable and at significantly lower values than in untreated spontaneously hypertensive rats. In spontaneously hypertensive rats treated for 4–14 weeks, blood pressure rose by only a small amount till the end of study, when the rats were 3–40 weeks of age. This was associated with a corresponding slight redevelopment of LVH. In the other two groups, 15–20 weeks after treatment, blood pressure had stabilized about half-way between the levels obtained in untreated spontaneously hypertensive rats and Wistar-Kyoto normotensive controls. This went along with corresponding redevelopment of a modest degree of LVH, which was somewhat greater than in spontaneously hypertensive rats treated for 4–14 weeks.

During antihypertensive therapy, LVH can be completely reversed in young animals, as shown by the above-mentioned studies. Its subsequent redevelopment is in proportion to the elevation in blood pressure. In older animals, regression of LVH, though substantial, appears to be less complete. This may relate to the development of irreversible structural changes, such as the deposition of collagen, owing to damage associated with poor perfusion of the hypertrophied muscle fibres.

4.2. Methods for measurement in patients

4.2.1. Electrocardiographic methods

Diagnosis of LVH was confirmed mainly by electrocardiographic criteria of LVH (ECG-LVH) until recently. These various criteria of ECG-LVH were based upon increased electromotive precardial voltage forces plus repolariz-

Table 1. Left ventricular hypertrophy: amplitude criteria in electrocardiography

1) R_I
2) $R_I + S_{III}$ (Gubner/Ungerleider
3) R_{aVL}
4) max.S_{V1-V3}
5) max.R_{V4-V6}
6) $S_{V1} + R_{V5/V6}$ (Sokolow/Lyon)
7) max.S_{V1-V3} + max.R_{V4-V6}
8) max.$S_{V1/V2}$ + max.$R_{V5/V6}$
9) max.S_{V1-V3} od.max.R_{V4-V6}
10) $\Sigma S_{V1-V3} + \Sigma R_{V4-V6}$
11) Total amplitude aVF + V2 + V6 (Manning/Smiley)

Note: In our hypertrophy studies left ventricular hypertrophy was calculated comparing the 11 most often cited hypertrophy-criteria from the ECG-literature.

ation changes on the standard electrocardiogram. There are more than 30 different criteria that have been developed by various investigators to relate electrocardiographic measurements to more direct evidence of increased anatomic ventricular mass (Table 1). In general, these electrocardiographic criteria of LVH are rather consistently insensitive, but they are fairly specific for detecting increased left ventricular mass [62]. These electrocardiographic criteria by definition provide only a categorial variable for the continuous variable of left ventricular mass. Therefore, the direct correlation of the actual LVH mass with ECG findings has been disappointing [63]. It follows that the clinical premorbid diagnosis of LVH has generally referred to the ECG pattern rather than actual mass of the left ventricle.

The relative risk for the patient to develop an adverse cardiovascular event or death is markedly increased when LVH in the ECG is preexistent [64]. In the prospectively conducted Framingham study, development of ECG-LVH was documented in individuals having had previously normal ECGs. Thirty-five percent of all men that first manifested ECG-LVH died within five years of the appearance of this adverse marker. Furthermore, men and women between 35 and 64 years of age had a 10 to 19–fold increased risk of cardiovascular mortality when ECG-LVH was present when compared to age- and gendermatched individuals without ECG-LVH [65]. Moreover, risk of sudden death is particularly increased in patients with ECG-LVH [66]. Left ventricular ectopy appears to be more prevalent on ambulatory monitoring in individuals with ECG-LVH [67,68].

Prognostic implications of ECG-LVH are also observed in other forms of adverse cardiovascular events. Risk of later development of angina pectoris, myocardial infarction, stroke, symptomatic peripheral vascular disease, and overt congestive heart failure are all significantly increased in patients with ECG-LVH [65]. Indeed, the greatest risk of developing overt congestive heart failure could be predicted from the presence of ECG-LVH. In the Framingham study, asymptomatic men and women with ECG-LVH had

Table 2. Left ventricular hypertrophy: amplitude criteria in vectorcardiography

Scalar vectors	Planar maximal vectors
Rx	H
Ry resp. Sy	F
Rz	S
max. R $_{x/y/z}$	max. H, F or S
Rx + Ry (resp.Sy)	H + F
Rx + Rz	H + S
Rz + Ry (resp.Sy)	F + S
Rx + Rz + Ry (resp.Sy)	H + F + S
MVr = $\sqrt{R^2_x + R^2_y + R^2_z}$	rMV = $\sqrt{(H^2 + F^2 + S^2)/2}$

MV = maximal vector; H = horizontal; F = fontal; S = sagittal
Note: The most often cited amplitude criteria in vectorcardiography were used for identification of left ventricular hypertrophy.

more than a 17–fold chance of ultimately developing congestive heart failure than age- and gendermatched cohorts without evidence of ECG-LVH [65].

With vectorcardiography similar criteria for quantification have been developed and show a comparable value for diagnosis and prognosis of arterial hypertension (Table 2).

4.2.2. *Echocardiography*

Anatomical evidence of LVH can certainly be present without being detected by the ECG. It has become apparent that echocardiography provides an excellent noninvasive means for more accurately assessing the presence of increased left ventricular mass. In expert hands, pre-mortem echocardiographic measurements of left ventricular mass has correlated very closely with actual anatomic measurements performed in patients with a wide range of ventricular weights who died as a result of a wide variety of cardiovascular disorders [69]. Conversely, correlations with ECG and vectorcardiography are relatively poor (Tables 3,4).

Echocardiographic techniques provide a reliable measure of left ventricular mass, but since mass is a continuous variable, it follows that for this noninvasive diagnostic measurement to be applied to general populations it must address more directly the question of the true prevalence of increased left ventricular mass. Levine and coworkers [19] performed echocardiographic evaluations in almost 5000 participants of the Framingham Heart Study. This important study demonstrated that LVH by echocardiographic criteria was not uncommon in the general population, being present in 16 % of the men and 19 % of the women evaluated. Moreover, an important age affect was demonstrated as well as a significant association between blood pressure levels and the presence of echocardiographic evidence of LVH. Another finding of this population based study was the influence of exogenous obesity as an independent risk for the occurrence of echocardiographic

Table 3. Left ventricular hypertrophy: correlation between electrocardiography and echocardiography

	Cross-sectional plane		Volume of muscle in in diastole		Total ventricular volume in diastole	
	Concentric	Eccentric	Concentric	Eccentric	Concentric	Eccentric
R_I	0.17	0.36	0.15	0.38	0.15	0.35
$R_I + S_{III}$	0.19	0.41	0.22	0.43	0.21	0.40
R_{aVL}	0.18	0.34	0.23	0.38	0.22	0.39
max.S_{V1-V3}	0.45	0.23	0.40	0.34	0.39	0.44
max.S_{V1-V3} + max.R_{V4-V6}	0.35	0.28	0.31	0.38	0.36	0.46
$S_{V1} + R_{V5/V6}$	0.21	0.23	0.19	0.32	0.21	0.40
$\Sigma S_{V1-V3} + \Sigma R_{V4-V6}$	0.36	0.33	0.31	0.41	0.31	0.46
aVF + V2 + V6	0.35	0.34	0.29	0.42	0.28	0.47

concentric n = 45; eccentric n = 30
Note: Nearly all correlations between electrocardiography and echocardiography were rather poor.

LVH. The importance of both age and the level of systolic arterial pressure on the prevalence of echocardiographically demonstrable LVH support the concept that the height of arterial pressure, as well as duration of hypertension, are important determinants of actual LVH. We also investigated different types and locations of LVH in patients with hypertension compared to aortic stenosis [70].

4.2.3. *Magnetic resonance studies*

Magnetic resonance imaging (MRI) has emerged as a method for visualization of the heart and has been available in our institution for cardiac imaging since the end of 1983. Because MRI displays the blood pool as very low or no signal intensity with the spin-echo technique, the cardiac chambers are visualized without contrast medium. This method is excellent for determining the cardiac axis, layer depth, dimensions and volumes, and the time of triggering in the cardiac cycle. Therefore, MRI is a very suitable method for determination of myocardial parameters before and after drug treatment

Table 4. Left ventricular hypertrophy: correlation between vectorcardiography and echocardiography

	Cross-sectional plane		Volume of muscle in diastole		Total ventricular volume in diastole	
	Concentric	Eccentric	Concentric	Eccentric	Concentric	Eccentric
R_x	0.18	0.30	0.21	0.42	0.22	0.51
R_z	0.49	0.14	0.46	0.25	0.43	0.34
max.$R_{x/y/z}$	0.47	0.26	0.47	0.38	0.45	0.49
MV_r	0.39	0.24	0.40	0.36	0.36	0.47
MV – H	0.40	0.05	0.44	0.24	0.47	0.44
MV – H + MV – S	0.43	0.04	0.46	0.21	0.47	0.39

concentric n = 24; eccentric n = 16
MV = maximal vector; H = horizontal; S = sagittal

[71]. Until now there have been very few studies on hypertrophy regression with magnetic resonance [72–76]. The main reason seems to be that normally the treating cardiologist is the same person who performs the echocardiographic study, but the radiologist performs the MRI study. We have the rare chance to work with MRI as cardiologists. In the last eight years we undertook a lot of LVH regression studies to assess the effects of diuretics, alpha-blockers, calcium-antagonists, beta-blockers, Clonidine, and different ACE-inhibitors on LVH. In the following we will, as an example, describe the study with the ACE-inhibitor Ramipril, which was the first MRI-regression study published in the literature [71,73].

The study population comprised 32 patients (23 men and 9 women) aged 41–63 years with arterial hypertension. Diastolic blood pressure was measured noninvasively and ranged from 95 to 120 mmHg. Ten untreated control subjects were also included in our study protocol. Patients with myocardial failure controlled by drugs, dysrhythmias, coronary heart disease, stenosis of the renal artery, or endocrine hypertension were excluded from the study. The study protocol consisted of a 2 week washout phase followed by a treatment phase of 5 mg ramipril per day over a period of 3 months.

Prior to ramipril treatment, blood pressure, plasma calcium, potassium, magnesium, sodium, creatinine, and ACE levels (Hoechst AG, Frankfurt, Germany) were measured and the baseline values for ventricular parameters were determined by electrocardiography, echocardiography, and MRI. Four hours after the first oral dose of 5 mg ramipril, a MRI scan was obtained and the serum samples for ACE levels were taken.

After 2 weeks of treatment, blood pressure was measured, blood samples taken for ACE levels, and MRI scans obtained before intake of ramipril and 4 hours after intake of 5 mg ramipril. Final measurements of blood pressure, MRI scans, echocardiograms and electrocardiograms were performed after 3 months of ramipril treatment. Serum calcium, potassium, magnesium, sodium, and creatinine were measured against at this time.

Blood pressure was measured noninvasively using a mercury sphygmomanometer in patients and normal controls. Electrocardiograms at rest were also recorded with quantification of the left precordial R-waves. Measurements of left ventricular wall thickness were made in three planes and the mean of three readings calculated for each. M-mode echocardiograms were performed using standard techniques with a Diasonics DRF-400 (digital radio frequency). Measurements of interventricular septal thickness had to amount to more than 15 mm at endsystole and 12 mm at enddiastole. Baseline values for posterior wall thickness were allowed to be 1 mm less. The left ventricular enddiastolic diameter had to be <50 mm and the left ventricular endsystolic diameter had to be 30 mm in keeping with concentric hypertrophy.

The magnetic resonance tomograph (Siemens Magnetom) used a superconducting magnet operating at a field strength of 0.5 T (Table 5). The Sirecust 404 ECG system with ultrathin copper leads assured exact end-

Table 5. Specification of technical parameters of the MR imaging system at the University Hospital Berlin-Charlottenburg

Diameter of the magnet	50 cm
Magnetic field strength	0.5 T
High-frequency field strength	8 to 10 kW
Duration of excitation impulse	0.5 to 1.0 sec
Spin-echo sequence	35 and 70 msec
Trigger delay time	≈ 360 msec
Slice thickness	≤ 10 mm
Imaging matrix	256 × 256 matrix points
Resolution between 2 lines (735 matrix lines and 31–cm diagonal screen)	< 2 mm
Recording in three planes	Frontal, axial, sagittal
Recording time (depending on measure sequence)	≤ 6 min + ≥ 10 min

systolic and end-diastolic triggering. The repetition rate, or interval between sets of radiofrequency pulses, was determined by the heart rate of each subject heart rate and ranged from 400 to 1000 msec. MRI scans were recorded in four slices and three planes (frontal, transverse, and sagittal) with multiple angulations (Figs. 1,2,3). The imaging sequence was spin-echo with echo delay time of 35, 70 and 105 msec and a proton resonance frequency of 15 MHz. The selection gradient was 3 mT/m. A 256 × 256 reconstruction matrix was used. Angulation was started in the frontal plane to define the correct angle in the transversal plane (Figs. 4,5). Signal intensity was determined at three points as a mean from three measurements and expressed in arbitrary units (a.U.) ranging from 0 (for air) to 2000 a.U. (for

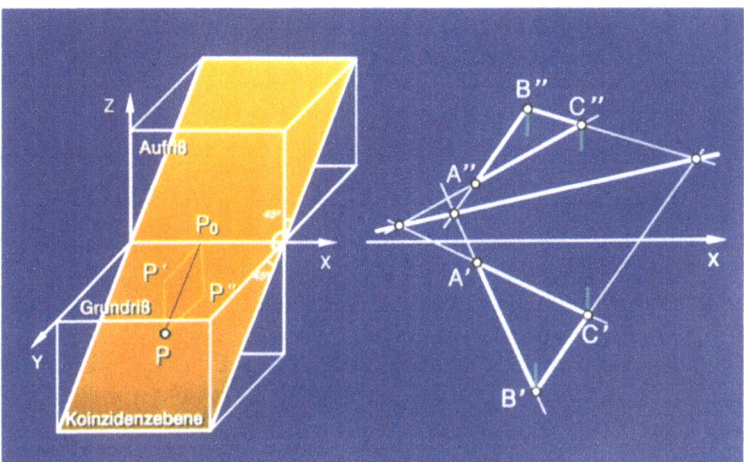

Figure 1. Angulation is the most important process in the algorithm for quantification in magnetic resonance measurements. The real distance between the points P and Po is only represented in the plane of coincidence (yellow). In the case of wrong angulation we will measure the wrong distances between P' and Po or P'' and Po. Aufriss = vertical projection; Grundriss = horizontal projection; Koinzidenzebene = coincidence level or plane.

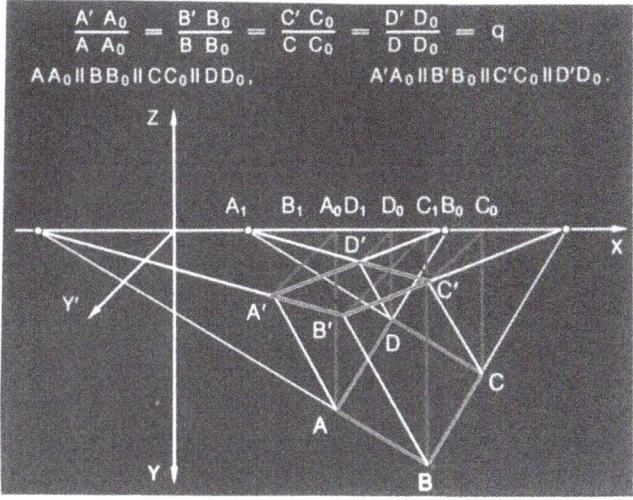

$$\frac{A'\,A_0}{A\,A_0} = \frac{B'\,B_0}{B\,B_0} = \frac{C'\,C_0}{C\,C_0} = \frac{D'\,D_0}{D\,D_0} = q$$

$$A A_0 \parallel B B_0 \parallel C C_0 \parallel D D_0. \qquad A'A_0 \parallel B'B_0 \parallel C'C_0 \parallel D'D_0.$$

Figure 2. When imaging a square (A, B, C, D), a completely wrong presentation and quantification will be received in case of incorrect angulation (A', B', C', D').

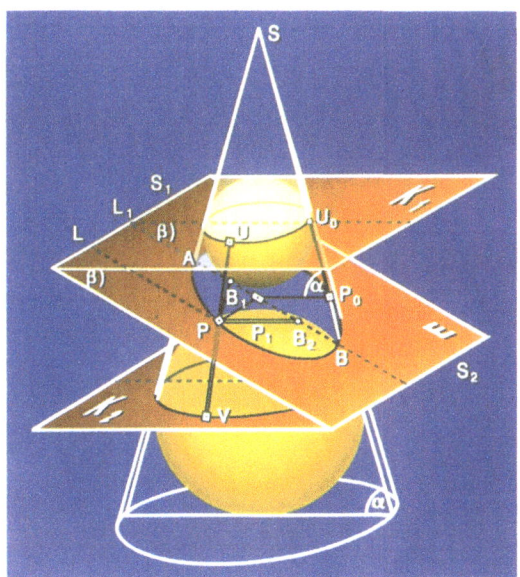

Figure 3. The most complicated mistakes can be done with wrong projections of volumes. The upper sphere (U) in the plane K_1 is symbolizing a small heart. In the case of wrong angulation we can have a projection of this sphere in the plane of K_2, where it appears as a very large organ.

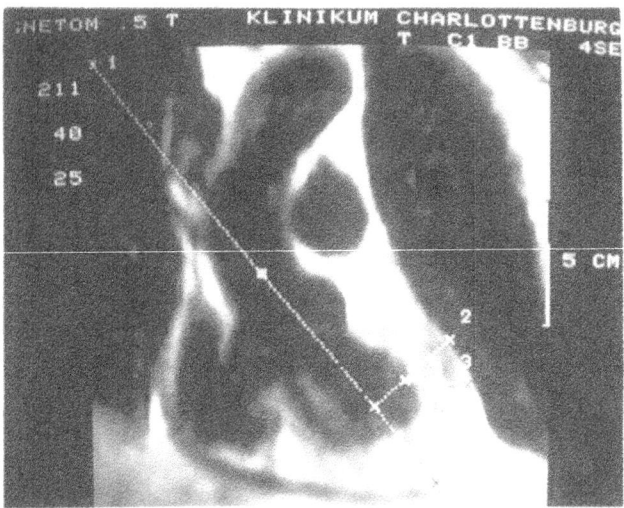

Figure 4. After definition of the long axis of the left ventricle in the frontal plane, the transversal plane rectangular to this axis can be reconstructed.

fatty tissue). The inclusion criteria for hypertrophy were the same as for echocardiography and in addition myocardial signal intensity had to amount to more than 600 a.U. at each measuring point.

Measurements obtained by MRI and by echocardiography were validated

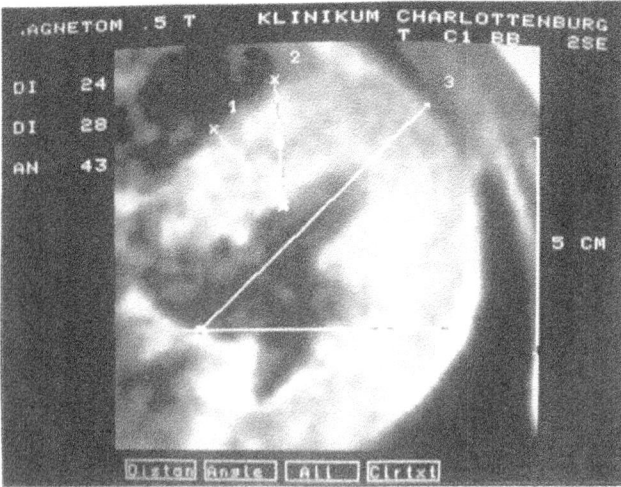

Figure 5. After angulation the transversal plane represents the real distances in the long axes of the left ventricle. Now the direction of the apex has to be angulated in an anterior-posterior direction.

by calculating the correlation. The mean value of interventricular septal thickness on MRI scans was 19.57 ± 5.24 mm, whereas echocardiography produced a value of 18.78 ± 6.23 to the correlation coefficient of $r = 0.911$ for corresponding measurements. The values for posterior wall thickness measured by MRI and echocardiography also correlated well ($r = 0.892$). The mean MRI value for the three measuring points was 20.03 ± 3.96 mm with a corresponding echocardiographic value of 18.42 ± 4.02 mm.

The internal diameter of the left ventricle at enddiastole is a very sensitive index of the degree of concentric LVH. Transversal MRI scans encompassing the left ventricle at the level of the lateral papillary muscle showed a mean diameter of 31.72 ± 4.05 mm. The corresponding echocardiographic measurements resulted in somewhat lower values of 29.68 ± 3.97 mm. In addition to morphological parameters, functional parameters were measured to establish whether ventricular function deteriorates as a result of regression of myocardial mass. Earlier studies on regression of hypertrophy have suggested measurement of ejection fraction, and this was determined by both echocardiography and MRI. These measurements showed high values of ventricular ejection fraction: a mean of 75.42 ± 11.21 % measured by MRI and 73.61 ± 13.68 measured by echocardiography.

The first series of investigations up to 2 weeks after administration of ramipril showed no significant regression of hypertrophy. After 3 months, however, considerable decrease of wall thickness was found. MRI demonstrated a decrease of interventricular septal thickness from 19.57 to 15.20 mm with a corresponding decrease in echocardiographic values from 18.78 to 14.57 mm. An impressive decrease of posterior wall thickness from 20.73 to 15.96 mm on MRI scans and from 18.42 to 14.21 mm on echocardiography was noted and found to be reproducible in serial measurements (Fig. 6). Analyses of left ventricular function showed that the ejection fraction remained largely unchanged with ramipril, despite the striking reduction of wall thickness. This can probably be attributed to a considerable decrease in afterload. Ejection fraction changed from 75.42 to 73.18 % measured by MRI and from 73.61 to 70.92 % by echocardiography. The changes in ejection fraction were statistically not significant.

During 4 hours after intake of the first dose of ramipril, the angiotensin converting enzyme activity was inhibited to less than 10 % of the pretreatment activity. Values remained at this level or even decreased throughout the study.

In keeping with the marked decrease of hypertrophy measured by imaging methods, the R-wave amplitudes in lead V5 of the ECG decreased from 1.9 to 1.1 mV, which may be related mainly to the change of the electrical axis. MRI measurements of myocardial signal intensity decreased from 839 to 778 a.U., indicating change in density of the hypertrophic myocardium. Diastolic blood pressure levels were reduced below 90 mmHg or 15 % below baseline and remained at this level throughout the treatment period. Ramipril was well tolerated by all patients throughout the study.

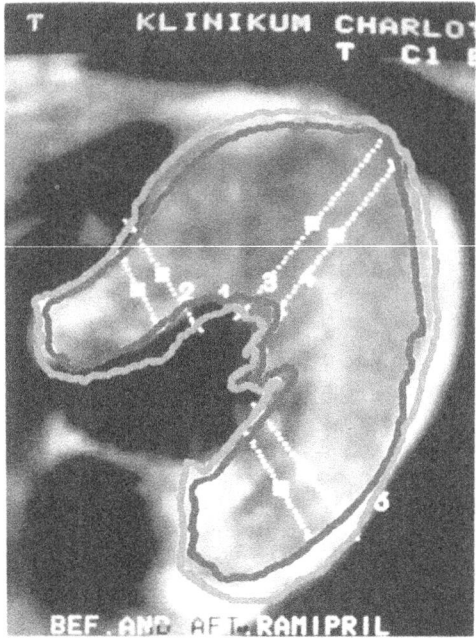

Figure 6. In a point-by-point-measurement the contour of the left ventricle is outlined before and after therapy. The subtraction image shows the dimension of hypertrophy regression after three months of treatment with the ACE-inhibitor ramipril.

5. Discussion

There is increasing interest in the effect of antihypertensive treatment on myocardial hypertrophy. Myocardial hypertrophy results in impairment of oxygen supply to the left ventricle even if the physiologic coronary reserve is completely exploited. Antihypertensive drugs may reduce left ventricular wall stress by lowering left ventricular afterload, leading to regression of LVH.

On a cytochemical basis, regression is paralleled by a decrease of intracellular RNA content related to myocardial muscle fibers. Interstitial components such as collagen, structural proteins, or hydroxyproline once formed appear irreversible and therefore determine the absolute limits of any regression of hypertrophy. Thus, for example, if hypertensive left ventricular failure has occurred with the formation of fiber-rich connective tissue in the hypertrophic ventricle, then impaired ventricular function can no longer be improved by regression of myocardial hypertrophy with reduction of afterload.

Methods: Earlier studies showed regression of LVH using simple measurements of R-waves on the chest wall-electrocardiogram [62,63]. More recent investigations made use of echocardiography and levocardiography

[19,69,70,77]. However, with the latter method, reliable interpretation of myocardial dimensions is only possible if levels of contrast medium in the myocardium are sufficiently high.

Thallium-201 scintigraphy also allows quantification of myocardial hypertrophy. The larger cell surface areas found in hypertrophic myocardium permit a more intense exchange of isotopes, resulting in higher impulse rates. We feel that this remains one of the most sensitive methods available for imaging hypertrophy. However, the quantification of impulse density is an elaborate procedure [78–80] and cannot be compared directly with echocardiography, the most widespread imaging method used for measuring wall thickness.

We have used multislice gated multiplanar magnetic resonance images as an alternative method to measure cardiac hypertrophy [71]. Gated magnetic resonance imaging can generate cardiac images with excellent morphological contrast and permits easy reproduction of cardiac phases measured, depth of the level, and angle of determination. In comparison to echocardiography, MRI provides superior images and also permits superior accuracy of measurements.

Substances: Adrenergic inhibiting agents [15,78,81], calcium channel blockers [74,82,83] and ACE-inhibitors [71–73,84,85] tend to reverse LVH, whereas diuretics [81] and direct vasodilators like hydralazine [15] or minoxidil [40,82] do not, even though blood pressure is well-controlled. These findings suggest that hypertrophy cannot be explained solely on a hemodynamic basis [86]. There are exceptions, however. Beta-blockers do not prevent or reverse hypertension or LVH in spontaneously hypertensive rats [87] or in renal hypertensive rats [88], but the non-ISA beta-blockers do reverse LVH in hypertensive patients [89–91]. Methyldopa has consistently reversed LVH in rats and man [15,81]. Yet clonidine, a drug with similar action on the adrenergic nervous system does not influence LVH, unless doses large enough to exert a peripheral adrenergic agonist effect were used [92,93]. Furthermore, diuretics have not been shown to reverse LVH [81], but they reduce vascular reactivity to norepinephrine infusions [94,95].

In our studies in hypertensive patients receiving treatment with ACE-inhibitors (ramipril, spirapril, lisinopril, trandolapril,captopril), severe LVH was present in all patients prior to treatment. After 3 months of treatment with the ACE inhibitors, left ventricular wall thickness decreased by almost 5 mm (ramipril). Follow-up examinations after this time showed no evidence of further regression, indicating that maximum reduction of hypertrophy occurs before 3 months [71–73].

Various other antihypertensive agents, as diverse in their pharmacological actions as beta-blockers and calcium-antagonists, have shown abated degrees of regression of cardiac hypertrophy (Table 6).

Many studies have shown that reduction of blood pressure, irrespective of the drugs that were prescribed, can reverse LVH to a certain degree [96–

Table 6. Studies with antihypertensive drugs on preventing or reversing evidence of LVH

Drug	Rats	Humans
Methyldopa	yes [58,92,93]	yes [81]
Methyldopa + diuretic		yes [81]
Methyldopa + minoxidil	yes [15,58]	
Diuretic	no [58]	no [81]
Minoxidil	no [55,82]	
Hydralazine	no [55]	
Penbutolol		yes [78]
Metoprolol		yes [89]
Propranolol	yes/no [55], no [87]	
Atenolol	no [88]	yes [90]
Timolol	no [87]	yes [91]
Propranolol + minoxidil	no [55]	
Calcium channel blockers	yes [82]	yes [74,83]
Clonidine	no [92,93]	
Clonidine (high dose)	yes [92]	
Moxonidine		yes [75]
ACE-inhibitors	yes [84]	yes [85,71–73,76]
ACE inhibitors + diuretic	yes [84]	

yes = regression of LVH demonstrated.
no = no regression of LVH demonstrated.
Numbers denote References.

99], even when hypertension is suboptimally controlled [100]. Whether this improves prognosis is not known, but it is unlikely to reduce the risk to the level of uncomplicated but treated hypertension [101].

6. Conclusion

Regression of LVH may prevent serious long-term cardiac complications of hypertension, such as dilatation of tissue structures and heart failure. Regression of hypertrophy under antihypertensive treatment was first demonstrated in rats, and marked regression was observed after alpha-methyldopa, beta-blocking agents, and ACE-inhibitors. Effects of diuretics and direct vasodilators like hydralazine and minoxidil were less impressive. In patients with hypertension, many (mostly echocardiographic) studies have shown that reduction of blood pressure, irrespective of the drugs that were prescribed, can reverse LVH to a certain degree, even when hypertension is suboptimally controlled. Antihypertensive drugs such as alpha-methyldopa, beta-blocking agents, and ACE-inhibitors showed marked regression of LVH. Whether this improves prognosis is not known, but it is unlikely to reduce the risk to the level of uncomplicated but treated hypertension. MRI proves to be an excellent technique for assessing cardiac dimensions, volumes and myocardial mass, and appears to be very suitable to determine changes in these myocardial parameters before and after antihypertensive treatment.

References

1. Holt JP, Rhode EA, Kines H. Ventricular volumes and body weight in mammals. Am J Physiol 1968;215:704–15.
2. Pickering G. Systemic arterial hypertension. In: Fishman AP, Richards DW, editors. Circulation of the blood: men and ideas. Bethesda: American Physiological Society 1982;487–541.
3. Chanutin A, Barksdale EE. Experimental renal insufficiency produced by partial nephrectomy: relationship of left ventricular hypertrophy, width of cardiac muscle fiber and hypertension in rat. Arch Intern Med 1933;52:739–51.
4. Frohlich ED, Pfeffer MA. Heart and hypertension: the magnitude of the problem. In: Safar ME, Fouad-Tarazi FM, editors. The heart in hypertension: a tribute to Robert Tarazi (1925–1986). Dordrecht: Kluwer Academic Publishers 1989;169–79.
5. Bugaisky L, Zak R. Biological mechanism of hypertrophy. In: Fozzard HA, Jennings RB, Haber H, Katz AM, editors. The heart and cardiovascular system: scientific foundations. New York, Raven Press 1986;1491–506.
6. Wikman-Coffelt J, Parmley WW, Mason DT. The cardiac hypertrophy process. Analyses of factors determining pathological vs physiological development. Circ Res 1979;45:697–707.
7. Tarazi RC, Sen S. Catecholamines and cardiac hypertrophy. In: Mezey KC, Caldwell ADS, editors. Catecholamines and the heart. The Royal Society of Medicine 1979.
8. Schreiber SS, Evans CD, Oratz M, Rothschild MA. Protein synthesis and degradation in cardiac stress. Circ Res 1981;48:601–11.
9. Lundgren Y, Hallbäck M, Weiss L, Folkow B. Rate and extent of adaptive cardiovascular changes in rats during experimental renal hypertension. Acta Physiol Scand 1974;91:103–15.
10. Fletcher PJ, Korner PI, Angus JA, Oliver JR. Changes in cardiac output and total peripheral resistance during development of renal hypertension in the rabbit: lack of conformity with the autoregulation theory. Circ Res 1976;39:633–9.
11. Folkow BU, Hallbäck MI. Physiopathology of spontaneous hypertension in rats. In: Genest J, Koiw E, Kuchel O, editors. Hypertension: physiopathology and treatment. New York: McGraw-Hill, 1977;507–29.
12. Korner PI, Oliver JR, Casley DJ. Effect of dietary salt on hemodynamic of established renal hypertension in the rabbit. Implications for the autoregulation theory of hypertension. Hypertension 1980;2:794–801.
13. Broughton A, Korner PI. Basal and maximal inotropic state in renal hypertensive dogs with cardiac hypertrophy. Am J Physiol 1983;245:H33–41.
14. Pfeffer MA, Frohlich ED. Hemodynamic and myocardial function in young and old normotensive and spontaneously hypertensive rats. Circ Res 1972;32 (Suppl I):28–38.
15. Sen S, Tarazi RC, Khairallah PA, Bumpus FM. Cardiac hypertrophy in spontaneously hypertensive rats. Circ Res 1974;35:775–81.
16. Adams MA, Bobik A, Korner PI. Differential development of vascular and cardiac hypertrophy in genetic hypertension. Relationship to sympathetic function. Hypertension 1989;14:191–202.
17. Carlier P, Radelet M, Montrieux C, Greimers R, Rorive GL. Réponse proliférative de la paroi artérielle dans l'HTA: hyperplasie vs polyploïdie. Arch Mal Coeur Vaisseaux 1985;78:1710–5.

18. Pickering GW. High blood pressure. 2nd ed. London: J. & A. Churchill, 1968.
19. Levine RA, Gillam LD, Weyman AE. Echocardiography in cardiac research. In: Fozzard HA, Jennings RB, Haber H, Katz AM, editors. The heart and cardiovascular system: scientific. New York: Raven Press, 1986;369–452.
20. Abi-Samra F, Fouad FM, Tarazi RC. Determinants of left ventricular hypertrophy and function in hypertensive patients. An echocardiographic study. Am J Med 1983;75(3A):26–33.
21. Hammond IW, Devereux RB, Alderman MH, et al. The prevalence and correlates of echocardiographic left ventricular hypertrophy among employed patients with uncomplicated hypertension. J Am Coll Cardiol 1986;7:639–50.
22. Devereux RB, Casale PN, Hammond IW, et al. Echocardiographic detection of pressure overload left ventricular hypertrophy: effect of criteria and patient population. J Clin Hypertens 1987;3:66–78.
23. Laufer E, Jennings GL, Korner PI, Dewar E. Prevalence of cardiac structural and functional abnormalities in untreated primary hypertension. I published erratum appears in Hypertension 1989 May 13(5):498J. Hypertension 1989;13:151–62.
24. Fisher RA. Statistical methods for research workers. 9th ed. Edinburgh: Oliver & Boyd 1946;285–98.
25. Korner PI. Cardiac structure and function in animal models and in human hypertension. In: Safar ME, Fouad-Tarazi FM, editors. The Heart in Hypertension: a tribute to Robert Tarazi (1925–1986). Dordrecht: Kluwer Academic Publishers, 1989;145–68.
26. Bevan RD, Eggena P, Hume WR, van Marthens E, Bevan JA. Transient and persistent changes in rabbit blood vessels associated with maintained elevation in arterial pressure. Hypertension 1980;2:63–72.
27. Owens GK, Rabinovitch PS, Schwartz SM. Smooth muscle cell hypertrophy vs hyperplasia in hypertension. Proc Natl Acad Sci USA 1981;78:7759–63.
28. Carlier PG, Rorive GL, Barbason H. Kinetics of proliferation of rat aortic smooth muscle cells in Goldblatt one-kidney, one-clip hypertension. Clin Sci 1983;65:351–7.
29. Carlier PG, Rorive GL. Pathogenesis and reversibility of aortic changes in experimental hypertension. J Cardiovasc Pharmacol 1985;7 (Suppl 2):S46–51.
30. Wolinsky H. Effects of hypertension and its reversal on the thoracic aorta of male and female rats. Morphological and chemical studies. Circ Res 1971;28:622–37.
31. Foidart JM, Rorive GL, Nusgens BV, Lapiere CM. The relationship between blood pressure and aortic collagen metabolism in renal hypertensive rats. Clin Sci Mol Med (Suppl) 1978;4:27s–9s.
32. Foidart JM, Rorive GL, Carlier PG, Nusgens B, Lapiere CH, Lambotte R. Hypertension expérimentale: modifications précoces du métabolisme du collagène. Rev Med Liege 1983;38:537–49.
33. Rorive GL, Carlier PG, Foidart JM. The structural responses of the vascular wall in experimental hypertension. In: Zanchetti A, Tarazi RC, editors. Pathophysiology of hypertension. Amsterdam: Elsevier, 1986;428–53.
34. Wolinsky H. Long-term effects of hypertension on the rat aortic wall and their relation to concurrent aging changes. Morphological and chemical studies. Circ Res 1971;30:301–9.
35. Nakada T, Lovenberg W. Lysine incorporation in vessels of spontaneously hypertensive rats: effect of adrenergic drugs. Eur J Pharmacol 1978;48:87–96.
36. Weiss L, Lundgren Y. Chronic antihypertensive drug treatment in young spontaneously hypertensive rats: effects on arterial blood pressure, cardiovascular reactivity and vascular design. Cardiovasc Res 1978;12:744–51.
37. Owens GK. Differential effects of antihypertensive drug therapy on vascular smooth muscle cell hypertrophy, hyperploidy, and hyperplasia in the spontaneously hypertensive rat. Circ Res 1985;56:525–36.
38. Carlier PG. Contribution expérimentale à la prévention des altérations de structure cardiovasculaires associées à l'hypertension artérielle [dissertation]. Liège: Université de Liège 1987.

39. Ehrhart LA, Ferrario CM. Collagen metabolism and reversal of aortic medial hypertrophy in spontaneously hypertensive rats treated with methyldopa. Hypertension 1983;3:479–84.

40. Sen S, Bumpus FM. Collagen synthesis in development and reversal of cardiac hypertrophy in spontaneously hypertensive rats. Am J Cardiol 1979;44:954–8.

41. Ruskoaho HJ, Savolainen ER. Effects of long-term verapamil treatment on blood pressure, cardiac hypertrophy and collagen metabolism in spontaneously hypertensive rats. Cardiovasc Res 1985;19:355–62.

42. Udenfriend S, Cardinale G, Spector S. Hypertension-induced fibrosis and its reversal by antihypertensive drugs. In: Laragh JH, Buhler FR, Seldin DW, editors. Frontiers in hypertension research. Springer, 1981;404–11.

43. Carlier PG, Warling X, Rorive GL. Prevention of the cardiovascular structural changes in the spontaneously hypertensive rat. J Hypertens 1984;2:429–36.

44. Oshima T, Matsushita Y, Miyamoto M, Koike H. Effects on long-term blockade of angiotension converting enzyme with captopril on blood pressure and aortic prolyl hydroxylase activity in spontaneously hypertensive rats. Eur J Pharmacol 1983;91:283–6.

45. Carlier PG, Smelten NS, Rorive GL. Reversion of cardiac, arteriolar, and arterial changes following antihypertensive treatment. In: Safar ME, Fouad-Tarazi FM, editors. The heart in hypertension: a tribute to Robert Tarazi (1925–1986). Dordrecht: Kluwer Academic Publishers 1989;395–410.

46. Hamrell BB, Low RB. The relationship of mechanical V_{max} to myosin ATPase activity in rabbit and marmot ventricular muscle. Pflugers Arch 1978;337:119–24.

47. Lompre AM, Mercadier JJ, Wisnewsky C, et al. Species-dependent and age–dependent changes in the relative amounts of cardiac myosin isozymes in mammals. Dev Biol 1981;84:286–90.

48. Mercadier JJ, Lompre AM, Wisnewsky C, et al. Myosin isozyme changes in several models of rat cardiac hypertrophy. Circ Res 1981;49:525–32.

49. Gorza L, Pauletto P, Pessina AC, Sartore S, Schiaffino S. Isomyosin distribution in normal and pressure overloaded rat ventricular myocardium. An immunohistochemical study. Circ Res 1981;49:1003–9.

50. Hoh YF, Yeoh GP, Thomas MA, Higginbottom L. Structural differences in the heavy chains of rat ventricular myosin isozymes. FEBS Lett 1979;97:330–4.

51. Sinha AM, Umeda PK, Kavinsky CJ, et al. Molecular cloning of mRNA sequence for cardiac alpha- and beta-form myosin heavy chains: expression in ventricles of normal, hypothyroid and thyrotoxic rabbits. Proc Natl Acad Sci USA 1982;79:5847–51.

52. Mahdavi V, Chambers AP, Nadal-Ginard B. Cardiac alpha- and beta- myosin heavy chain genes are organized in tandem. Proc Natl Acad Sci USA, 1984;81:2626–30.

53. Sen S, Young DR. Role of sodium in modulation of myocardial hypertrophy in renal hypertensive rats. Hypertension 1986;8:918–24.

54. Dussaule JC, Michel JB, Auzan C, Schwartz K, Corvol P, Menard J. Effect of antihypertensive treatment on the left ventricular isomyosin profile in one-clip, two-kidney hypertensive rats. J. Pharmacol Exp Ther 1986;236:512–8.

55. Sen S. Regression of cardiac hypertrophy: experimental animal model. In: Safar ME, Fouad-Tarazi FM, editors. The heart in hypertension: a tribute to Robert Tarazi (1925–1986). Dordrecht: Kluwer Academic Publishers, 1989;301–20.

56. Sen S. Alteration in myocardial collagen phenotypes in spontaneously hypertensive rats (abstract). J Moll Cell Cardiol 1982;14 (Suppl I):60.

57. Weber KT, Janicki JS, Pick R, et al. Collagen in the hypertrophied, pressure-overloaded myocardium. Circulation 1987;75(1 pt 2):I40–7.

58. Sen S, Tarazi RC, Bumpus FM. Cardiac hypertrophy and antihypertensive therapy. Cardiovasc Res 1977;11:427–33.

59. Motz W, Strauer B. Regression of structural cardiovascular changes by antihypertensive therapy. Hypertension 1984;6:III133–9.

60. Tarazi RC, Fouad FM. Reversal of cardiac hypertrophy in humans. Hypertension 1984;6:III140–6.

61. Fletcher PJ. Baroreceptor heart rate reflex in rabbits after reversal of renal hypertension. Am J Physiol 1984;246:H261-6.
62. Casale PN, Devereux RB, Alonso DR, Campo E, Kligfield P. Improved sex-specific criteria of left ventricular hypertrophy for clinical and computer interpretation of electrocardiograms: Validation with autopsy findings. Circulation 1987;75:565-72.
63. Reichek N, Devereux RB. Left ventricular hypertrophy: relationship of anatomic, echocardiographic and electrocardiographic findings. Circulation 1981;63:1391-8.
64. Frohlich ED. Left ventricular hypertrophy as a risk factor. Cardiol Clin 1986;4:137-44.
65. Kannel WB, Dannenberg AL, Levy D. Population implications of electrocardiographic left ventricular hypertrophy. Am J Cardiol 1987;60:85I-93I.
66. Kannel WB, Doyle JT, McNamara PM, Quickenton P, Gordon T. Precursors of sudden coronary death: Factors related to the incidence of sudden death. Circulation 1975;51:606-13.
67. Messerli FH, Ventura HO, Elizardi DJ, Dunn FG, Frohlich ED. Hypertension and sudden death. Increased ventricular ectopic activity in left ventricular hypertrophy. Am J Med 1984;77:18-22.
68. McLenachan JM, Henderson E, Morris KI, Dargie HJ. Ventricular arrhythmias in patients with hypertensive left ventricular hypertrophy. N Engl J Med 1987;317:787-92.
69. Devereux RB, Reichek N. Echocardiographic determination of left ventricular mass in man. Anatomic validation of the method. Circulation 1977;55:613-8.
70. Eichstädt H, Bubenheimer P, Ferber B, Riesterer H. Welche Bedeutung hat die Echokardiographie zur Beurteilung der linksventrikulären Hypertrophie? Verh Dtsch Ges Kreislaufforsch 1977;43:400-1.
71. Eichstädt H, Felix R, Langer M, Schmutzler H. Left ventricular hypertrophy regression under therapy with the ACE-inhibitor Ramipril – a study with magnetic resonance imaging (abstract). Chest 1986;89(6 Suppl):496.
72. Eichstädt H, Felix R, Langer M, Schmutzler H. Hypertrophy regression under therapy with the ACE-inhibitor Ramipril – a study with magnetic resonance imaging (abstract). Abstracts of the Xth World Congress of Cardiology; 1986 Sept. 14-19; Washington. Abstr. Nr. 3939.
73. Eichstädt HW, Felix R, Langer M, et al. Use of nuclear magnetic resonance imaging to show regression of hypertrophy with ramipril treatment. Am J Cardiol 1987;59:98D-103D.
74. Eichstädt H, Langer M, Skarupke W, Felix R, Schmutzler H. Hypertrophy regression in hypertensive hearts during long-term treatment with Nitrendipine – measurements with MR-tomography (abstract). 12th Scientific Meeting of the International Society of Hypertension. 1988, May 22-26, Kyoto, Abstractbook No. 1277.
75. Eichstädt H, Richter W, Baeder M, et al. Demonstration of hypertrophy-regression with magnetic resonance tomography under the new adrenergic inhibitor Moxonidine. Cardiovasc Drugs Ther 1989;3:583-9.
76. Eichstädt H, Mertens D, Del N, Rupp C. Magnetic resonance measurements for quantification of left ventricular hypertrophy regression under the treatment with Lisinopril. J Mol Cell Cardiol 1990 (abstract); 22 (Suppl 5):S14.
77. Strauer BE. The heart in hypertension. Berlin: Springer 1981.
78. Eichstädt H, Kraemer R, Dougherty FC, Schneider R, Felix R, Schmutzler H. Hypertrophieregression unter chronischer Betablockade. Nachweis durch quantitative Schichtszintigraphie. Z Kardiol 1983;72:69-74.
79. Büll U, Strauer BE, Hast B, Niendorf HP. Die 201-Thallium-Szintimetrie des Herzens als neues Verfahren zur funktionellen Differenzierung der koronaren Herzkrankheit. ROFO 1979;124:434-43.
80. Büll U, Strauer BE. Assessment of left ventricular muscle mass with 201-thallium myocardial imaging. In: Strauer BE, editor. The heart in hypertension. Berlin, Springer, 1981;345-56.
81. Wollam GL, Hall WD, Porter VD, et al. Time course of regression of left ventricular hypertrophy in treated hypertensive patients. Am J Med 1983;75(3A):100-10.

82. Kazda S, Garthoff B, Thomas G. Antihypertensive effect of calcium antagonists in rat differs from that of vasolidators. Clin Sci 1982;63 (Suppl 8):363s-5s.

83. Smith VE, White WB, Meeran MK, Karimeddini MK. Improved left ventricular filling accompanies reduced left ventricular mass during therapy of essential hypertension. J Am Coll Cardiol 1986;8:1449-54.

84. Sen S, Tarazi RC, Bumpus FM. Effect of converting enzyme inhibitor (SQ14,225) on myocardial hypertrophy in spontaneously hypertensive rats. Hypertension 1980;2:169-72.

85. Nakashima Y, Fouad FM, Tarazi RC. Regression of left ventricular hypertrophy from systemic hypertension by enalapril. Am J. Cardiol 1984;53:1044-9.

86. Frohlich ED, Tarazi RC. Is arterial pressure the sole factor responsible for hypertensive cardiac hypertrophy? Am J Cardiol 1979;44:959-63.

87. Pfeffer MA, Pfeffer JM, Weiss AK, Frohlich ED. Development of SHR hypertension and cardiac hypertrophy during prolonged beta blockade. Am J Physiol 1977;232:H639-44.

88. Lindpaintner K, Sen S. Role of beta 1–adrenoreceptors in hypertensive cardiac hypertrophy. J Hypertens 1987;5:663-9.

89. Franz IW, Wiemel D, Behr DW, Ketelhut R. Ruckbildung der Myokardhypertrophie Hochdruckkranker unter chronischer beta-rezeptorenblockade. Dtsch Med Wochenschr 1986;111:530-4.

90. Dunn FG, Ventura HO, Messerli FH, Kobrin I, Frohlich D. Time course of regression of left ventricular hypertrophy in hypertensive patients treated with atenolol. Circulation 1987;76:254-8.

91. Rowlands DB, Glover DR, Stallard TJ, Littler WA. Control of blood pressure and reduction of echocardiographically assessed left ventricular mass with once-daily timolol. Br J Clin Pharmacol 1982;14:89-95.

92. Ishise S, Pegram BL, Frohlich ED. Disparate effects of methyldopa and clonidine on cardiac mass and haemodynamics in rats. Clin Sci 1980;59 (Suppl 6):449S-52S.

93. Pegram BL, Ishise S, Frohlich ED. Effect of methyldopa, clonidine, and hydralazine on cardiac mass and haemodynamics in Wistar Kyoto and spontaneously hypertensive rats. Cardiovasc Res 1982;16:40-6.

94. Feisal K, Eckstein JW, Horsley AW, Keasling HH. Effects of chlorothiazide on forearm vascular responses to norepinephrine. J Appl Physiol 1961;16:549-52.

95. Gifford RW. Management of hypertensive patients with cardiac problems. In: Safar ME, Fouad-Tarazi FM, editors: The heart in hypertension: a tribute to Robert Tarazi (1925–1986). Dordrecht: Kluwer Academic Publishers 1989:221-30.

96. Farmer RG, Gifford RW Jr, Hines EA Jr. Effect of medical treatment on severe hypertension. A follow-up study of 161 patients with group 3 and group 4 hypertension. Arch Intern Med 1963;112:118-28.

97. Dorph S, Leth A, Degnbol B, From A. Visceral changes in severe hypertension and their response to drug treatment. Acta Med Scand 1970;187:411-7.

98. Five-year findings of the Hypertension Detection and Follow-up Program. Prevention and reversal of left ventricular hypertrophy with antihypertensive drug therapy. Hypertension Detection and Follow-up Program Cooperative Group. Hypertension 1985;7:105-12.

99. Freis ED. Electrocardiographic changes in the course of antihypertensive treatment. Am J Med 1983;75(3A):111-5.

100. Bolli P, Burkart F, Vesanen K, Baker JL, Pinto M, Buhler FR. Electrocardiographic changes during antihypertensive therapy in the International Prospective Primary Prevention Study in Hypertension. Hypertension 1987;9(6 pt 2):III69-74.

101. The effect of treatment on mortality in 'mild' hypertension: results of the hypertension detection and follow-up program. N Engl J Med 1982;307:976-80.

24. Magnetic resonance imaging in cardiology: Attractive for clinical cardiologists?

RODERIC I. PETTIGREW*

Summary

The large body of present data generated by cardiac magnetic resonance imaging (MRI) presents a data presentation and analysis challenge. More unified, integrated presentations of the three-dimensional anatomy, function, perfusion, regional and global response to stress, and contrast enhancement will likely be achieved using high-capacity/high-speed computers and specialized software display programs. These should offer near-life-like visualizations of the functioning heart in three dimensions. They should also permit the physician to interact with and manipulate the display so that the beating heart can be rotated and electronically dissected to offer any view or perspective imaginable. Existing and developing technology seems to indicate that dynamic three-dimensional cardiac MRI will soon be a cost-effective tool for evaluating almost all major types of cardiovascular disease and addressing many of the major needs in diagnostic cardiology. As such, it should become increasingly more attractive to clinical cardiologists.

1. Introduction

The diagnostic needs in routine clinical cardiology are broad. In general, these include: 1) defining cardiac structure, 2) evaluating biventricular function and valvular dysfunction, 3) evaluating the myocardium post-infarction to establish residual viable tissue vs scar, 4) detection and characterization of paracardiac or intracardiac masses or infiltrative disease, 5) detection of pericardial disease, 6) assessing great vessel anatomy and quantifying blood flow, and 7) noninvasive detection and evaluation of the physiologic significance of coronary artery disease - which is perhaps the greatest need.

Although several effective diagnostic methodologies currently exist, answering this broad spectrum of clinical questions often requires that the clinical cardiologist employ several tests in his/her practice. This is required since no routine existing examination is comprehensive enough to meet all of these needs. Of the available diagnostic tools which are suitable for evaluating the heart, MRI offers the most comprehensive current capabilities

*This work was supported in part by a grant from the Robert Wood Johnson Foundation.

Johan H.C. Reiber & Ernst E. van der Wall (eds.), Cardiovascular Nuclear Medicine and MRI, 369–395.
© 1992 Kluwer Academic Publishers.

Table 1. Cardiovascular Applications of MRI

Disorder	MRI Information
Congenital heart disease	3–dimensional structure Biventricular function, pre- and post operative Shunt identification Valve areas Severity of valvular insufficiency
Aortic aneurysm, dissection, coarctation	Cross-sectional area Site of dissection/intimal flap Thrombus identification Location of important branches Flow quantification
Ischemic heart disease	Site and extent of infarction and sequelae Viable myocardium vs scar Ventricular aneurysms, thrombi Segmental wall motion and systolic thickening Global function and indexes, eg, RVEF, LVEF, CO
Cardiac masses	Lesions, site, and extent Resectability Functional consequence Limited tissue characterization
Cardiomyopathies	Myocardial function/dysfunction Hypertrophic site and distribution Myopathic vs reactive hypertrophy Ventricular mass
Valvular heart disease	Visualization of regurgitant jets Regurgitant fractions/volumes Valve area Chamber volumes
Pericardial disease	Thickened pericardium Intrapericardial adhesions Effusion volume Transudative vs exudative Functional consequence

From, Pettigrew RI, Dynamic Magnetic Resonance Imaging in Acquired Heart Disease. Sem in Ultrasound, CT, and MR 12:61–91, 1991, with permission

and shows considerable promise for being applicable to all major cardiovascular diseases in the intermediate future [1,2]. It is this comprehensive feature of MRI, in addition to its clarity and relative definitiveness that make it potentially attractive for clinical cardiologists (Tables 1 and 2).

State-of-the-art cine MRI images the heart in a series of dynamic tomographic slices encompassing the entire thoracic cardiovascular structures, thus permitting both global and regional evaluation over 3 dimensions (3–D). When performed in this way, it is comprehensive and time-effective in

Table 2. Comparison of resting noninvasive imaging modalities

Feature	Modality*			
	ECHO	1st Pass	GBP	MRI
3–Dimensional structure	+ +	0	+	+ + + +
Wall tissue character	+	0	0	+ +
3–D Wall motion	+ + +	+	+ + +	+ + + +
3–D Wall thickening	+ + +	0	0	+ + + +
Functional indexes	+ +	+ +	+ +	+ + +
Valvular disease	+ + + +	0	0	+ + +
Blood flow/ regurg	+ + + +	0	0	+ + + +
Body habitus-independence	+ +	+ + + +	+ + + +	+ + + +
Lack of non-viz area	+	0	+ + +	+ + + +
Noninvasiness	+ + + +	+ + +	+ + +	+ + + +

*ECHO = two-dimensional color echocardiography; 1st Pass = first pass angiocardiography; FBP = gated equilbrium blood pool imaging. 0, of no utility; + , little utility; + +, fair utility; + + +, good utility, + + + +, excellent utility.

Adapted from Pettigrew RI, Magnetic Resonance Imaging of the Heart and Great Vessels, in *The Heart*, 7th ed., J. Willis Hurst ed., McGraw Hill, 1990, with permission.

that it can provide in a single examination (typically about 1 hr) the following: 1) precise depictions of normal and pathologic structure over 3D, 2) some information on the character of cardiac masses and pericardial effusion (e.g. solid vs cystic, fat vs tumor, transudate vs exudate) and extensive functional information including 3) myocardial mass, 4) both right and left ventricular enddiastolic and endsystolic volumes from which ejection fractions, stroke volumes, cardiac output, single-valve regurgitant and shunt fractions can be calculated, 5) evaluation of valvular insufficiency by direct jet visualization, 6) vascular time-flow velocity curves from which either right or left ventricular forward output, regurgitant volumes, and pulmonic to systemic flow ratios can be calculated, and 7) enddiastolic wall thickness and systolic wall thickening to identify scar and establish myocardial viability [1–3].

Recent innovations which are on the horizon as future routine techniques include: 1) ultra-fast methods which could image the entire heart in seconds and assess regional myocardial perfusion when used in conjunction with paramagnetic or high susceptibility contrast agents, 2) pharmacologic stress to detect ischemia and identify stunned myocardium, and 3) 3–D display techniques to aid in depicting cardiac and great vessel anatomy, particularly in pre-operative and post-operative congenital heart disease.

In this chapter, the current applications of cardiac MRI which make it potentially attractive for clinical cardiologists are reviewed. Ongoing advances which promise a greater MRI role in the detection and management of coronary artery disease, and which should considerably enhance its attractiveness as a routine clinical tool, are also briefly described.

2. Current clinical applications

2.1. *Cardiac structure and ventricular function*

MRI is now well established as a superlative technique for defining cardiac and vascular anatomy over 3-D [1-4]. Images may be obtained with either the spin-echo sequence which is characterized by 'dark blood' and high soft tissue contrast, or by the fast gradient-echo sequence, characterized by 'bright blood'. While cine studies may be obtained with both techniques, the faster speed of the gradient-echo sequence makes it more practical for this application. This allows both cardiac structure and function to be evaluated simultaneously [1,2].

The dimensions of all chambers of the heart and the great vessels can be measured to within approximately 2 mm at any desired phase of the cardiac cycle. Both right ventricular and left ventricular volumes can be measured directly by planimetry of the endocardium in each slice, and subsequent summation of the volumes contained within all of the slices spanning the ventricular cavities (Fig. 1) [1,2,5-7]. Consequently, these volumes are directly measured without significant geometry assumptions, in contrast to the ventricular volumes obtained by either contrast ventriculography or first-pass radionuclide techniques. The ventricular stroke volume, ejection fraction, and cardiac output are calculated from these measurements of enddiastolic and endsystolic volumes (Fig. 2). In the presence of a single valvular lesion or an isolated shunt, the regurgitant or shunt volume can be calculated by subtracting the measured stroke volumes for the two ventricles [6].

Measurements of systolic wall thickening are readily obtained for any segment of myocardium by direct measurement of the enddiastolic and endsystolic thickness (Fig. 3). This provides an excellent index of myocardial contractility [8]. This particular parameter has also been shown to correlate with myocardial perfusion. In addition, systolic wall thickening is a more specific indicator of myocardial function than is radial shortening or wall motion, which may occur passively in a segment due to the active contraction of the adjacent segments [1,2].

Qualitative assessment of myocardial function can also be easily obtained by simple visual inspection of the cine displays. This allows a visual identification of regions that are relatively hypokinetic, akinetic or dyskinetic, in a fashion similar to the interpretation of contrast or radionuclide ventriculograms [9].

Recently, an even more sophisticated method for evaluating regional myocardial function has been introduced in which the myocardium is noninvasively 'tagged' with dark stripes. These stripes are created by planes of saturated magnetization which are thus non-signal producing and which intersect the imaged slice in either a radial or grid-like pattern [10-12]. These tagging stripes or grids can be produced within the myocardium at enddiastole so that the functional behavior of a specifically tagged segment can

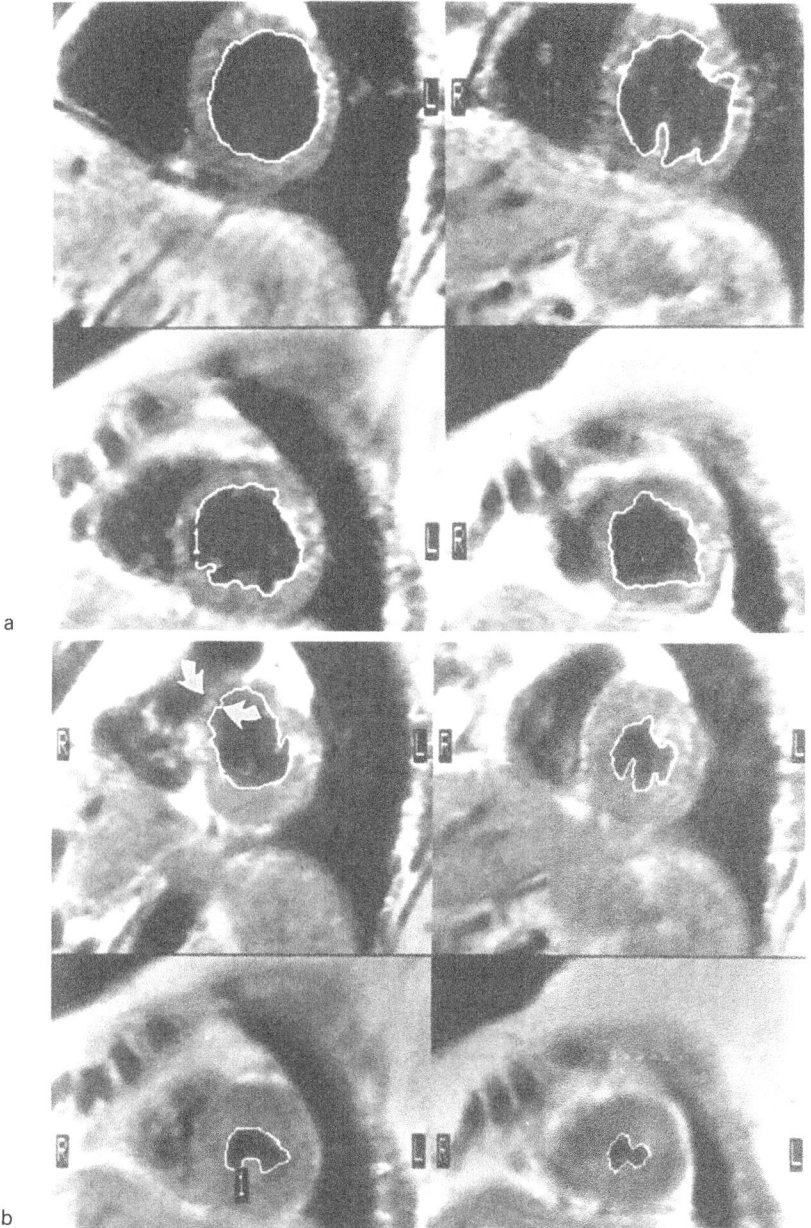

Figure 1. (a) The central four of six successive short-axis sections that span the ventricles from base (upper left) progressing towards apex (bottom right). Each section is at enddiastole. Planimetry and summation for the ventricular volume of each section yield direct determination of enddiastolic volume. (Reprinted with permission [70]) (b) The ventricular measurement process shown in Fig. 12 is repeated with endsystolic images to obtain endsystolic volume. Note that no geometric assumptions about ventricular shape are made. Also note that the membranous septum (curved arrows) has descended into the basal plane at upper left. (Reprinted with permission [9])

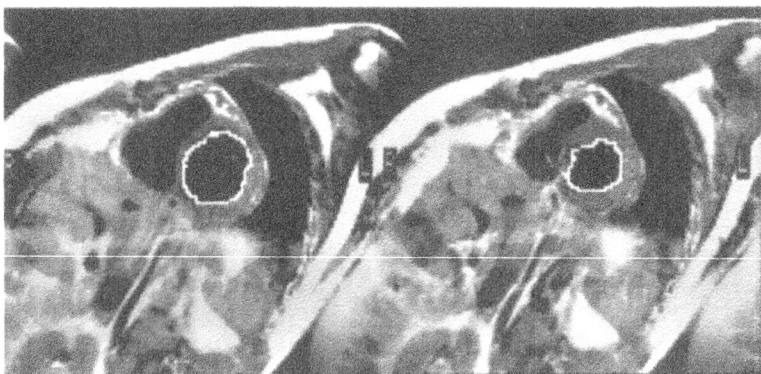

Figure 2. Console display of functional data obtained from a complete set of planimetered tomographic images at enddiastole and endsystole. Ejection fraction (EF), enddiastolic volume (EDV), endsystolic volume (ESV), stroke volume (SV), and cardiac output (CO) are given. EF = 47 %; EDV = 149 ml; ESV = 79 ml; SV = 70 ml; CO = 5.7 l/min; ED phase No. 1: 9 msec; ES phase 4: 261 msec. (Reprinted with permission [9])

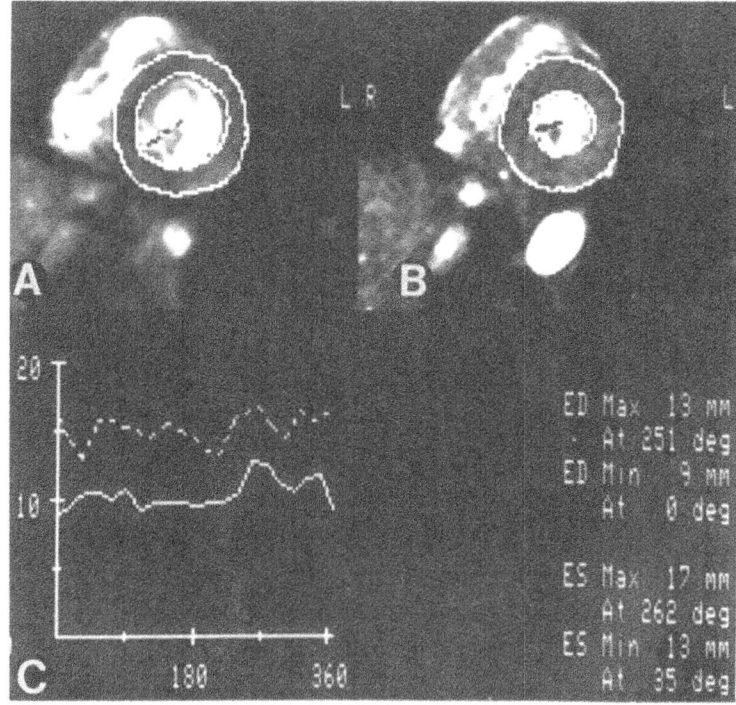

Figure 3. (A) Typical paired normal enddiastolic and (B) endsystolic gradient-echo images from which (C) systolic wall thickening is circumferentially measured and displayed. Zero degrees is at the inferoseptal site of the right ventricular insertion, with a clock-wise progression. (Reprinted with permission [9])

ED   ES

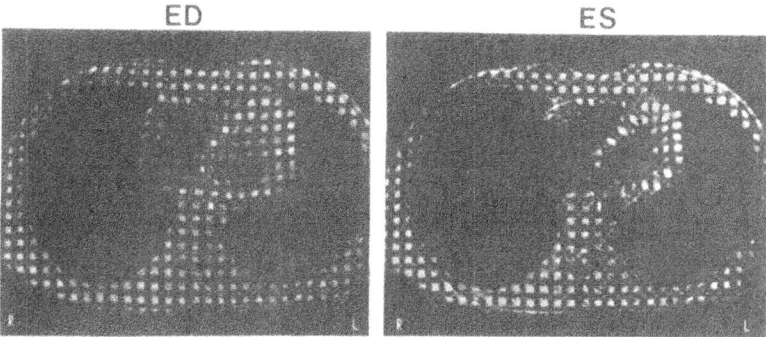

Figure 4. Myocardial tagging of a transaxial section using the spatial modulation of magnetization technique is shown at enddiastole (ED) and endsystole (ES). Note the regional and transmural differences in systolic deformation of the initially tagged squares or tiles [71].

be observed throughout the remainder of the cardiac cycle. Because regions across the transmural thickness of the myocardium can be tagged in this fashion, this technique allows for the evaluation of intrawall dynamics as well as simply observing transmural wall thickening. Consequently, subendocardial vs subepicardial mechanics can be assessed (Fig. 4).

Clinically, myocardial tagging has potential utility in 1) objectively assessing wall motion abnormalities, 2) assessing regional myocardial stress and strain, 3) distinguishing thrombus (no grid deformation) from slow flow (grid deformation), and 4) observing the effects of drug therapy on regional function of the myocadium by observing variances in the mechanical deformation of the tagged segments [10–13].

Validation of both the qualitative and quantitative assessments of ventricular function obtained by conventional cine techniques have been performed by several investigators [1,2,5–9,14,15]. Studies comparing qualitative analysis of wall motion by MRI vs that assessed by both nuclear and contrast ventriculography have shown excellent agreement [1,8,9]. The quantitative measurements of ejection fraction have also correlated closely in many studies ($r \approx 0.9$) [2,5–9]. The measurements of ventricular volumes have also correlated closely with reference measurements in several studies, as have the measurements of myocardial mass ($r > 0.9$) [16–18].

2.2. *Valvular function*

Regurgitant jets created by insufficient valves may be directly visualized as flame shaped regions of slow signal intensity or signal void within the receiving chamber of otherwise normal bright blood signal (Fig. 5). This signal loss, associated with the disturbed flow pattern characteristic of a regurgitant jet, is due to a loss of coherence between the individual spins contained within the imaging voxel. Since the blood within cardiac chambers is normally

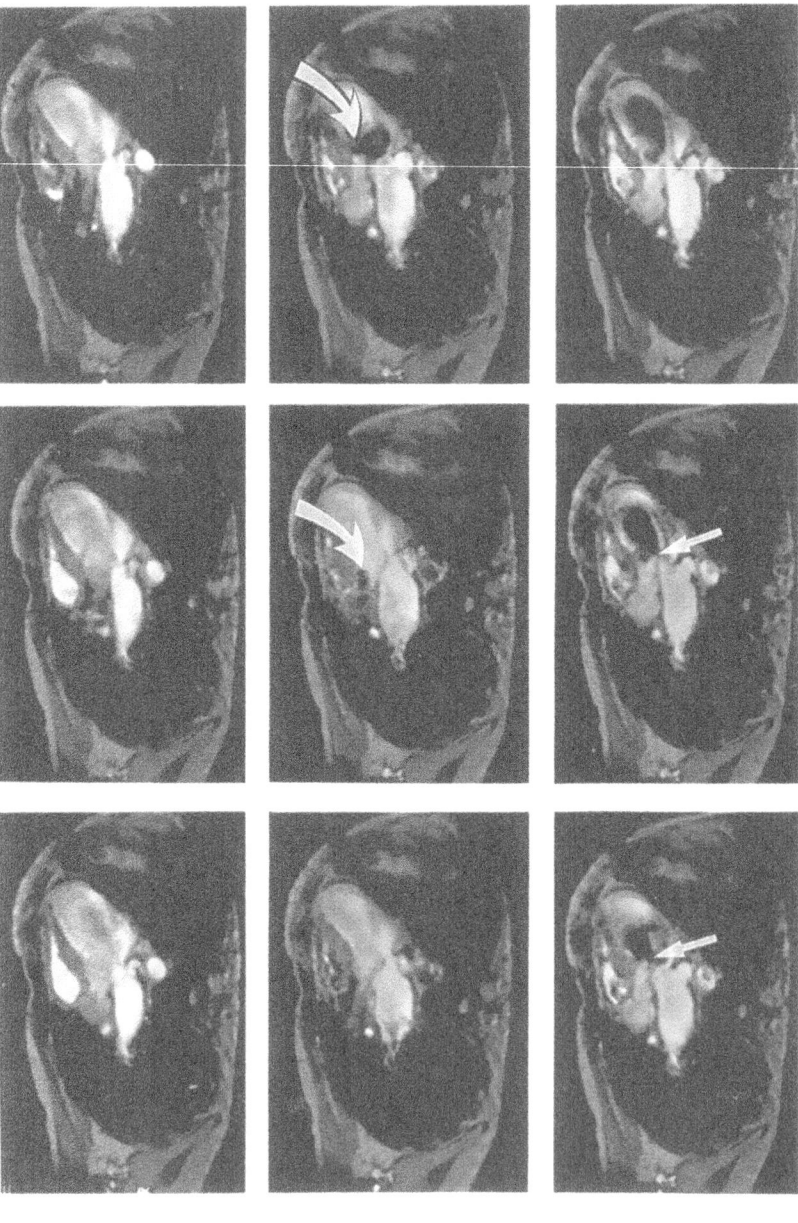

Figure 5. Aortic regurgitation and mitral stenosis. Mitral stenosis produces a dark, flame-shaped jet of signal void (arrows) across the mitral valve during diastole (phases 7–9). Moderate aortic regurgitation (curved arrows) is also present in phases 5–9. The two jets become confluent in the latter three phases [71].

bright when imaged with the fast gradient-echo sequence, the signal loss provides an excellent contrast mechanism [19–21]. Because the regurgitant jet is directly visualized, the severity of regurgitation can be evaluated and graded in a fashion analogous to that used in conventional echocardiography. For example, a grading of mild regurgitant is commonly assigned for jets that are less than 1/3 the size of the receiving chamber, moderate regurgitation for jets greater than 1/3 the size of the receiving chamber, and severe regurgitation for jets greater than 2/3 the size of the receiving chamber. Alternatively, a 1+ to 4+ scale may be used where the receiving chamber is divided into quadrants extending from the valve to the opposing chamber wall. A 1+ regurgitation is that which extends to within the first quadrant, while 2+, 3+, 4+ grades are given to regurgitant jets that extend to within the second, third, and fourth quadrants respectively.

Comparative studies of cine MRI color flow Doppler echocardiography have shown excellent agreement between these modalities in assessing valvular insufficiency, although with either technique multiple technical factors may influence the apparent size of the regurgitating jet [22–30]. Thus, caution should be utilized when comparing studies where these are variances in the MR parameters, particularly matrix size and echo time (TE).

More recently, with the advent of very short gradient-echo times of approximately 4 msec, the imaging of jets through stenotic valves has become possible. This permits some degree of flow quantification by using the technique of phase-velocity mapping [31–38]. This may routinely allow the estimation of pressure gradients across stenotic regions by using a modification of the Bernoulli equation, as is currently done with Doppler echocardiography.

2.2.1. *Phase-velocity mapping for flow qualification*

In addition to the qualitative visualization of intracardiac and intravascular flow, blood velocity (cm/sec) and flow rates (ml/min) can be measured.

Blood velocity can be quantified by utilizing the observation that as spins move along an imaging gradient (G) with a velocity (V) they acquire a spin phase shift f, which is proportional to the velocity with which the spins move. This phase shift is given by the relationship: $0 = V \cdot G \cdot t^2$, where t equals the time during which the spins move along the gradient. This shift in the phase angle of the spins, relative to that of stationary spins, is a parameter contained within the detected NMR signal and can be readily computed [31–34]. Since the gradient strength G, and the time of its application t, are known, the velocity of the spins can be computed from the above equation. Phase, or velocity images, can be generated where the signal intensity within the image is proportional to the spin phase and thus the spin velocity. This phase data is extracted from the same NMR signal which is used to generate the conventional modulus image, where the image signal intensity is simply related to the magnitude of the NMR signal. In phase images, however, a gray scale is used where zero velocity is typically represented by medium gray. The positive phase shifts of 0–180° are displayed as proportional increasing shades of gray to white, while negative phase shifts of 0 to −180° are displayed as proportional darker shades from medium gray to black. This allows display of flow in two opposite directions while retaining the linear intensity mapping characteristic of gray scale displays (Fig. 6).

2.3. *Ischemic heart disease*

Currently, there are two major areas of clinical application of MRI in the management of ischemic heart disease. These are 1) the assessment of post-infarction prognosis, and 2) the identification of viable myocardium vs scar, particularly in the setting of remote infarction.

2.3.1. *Myocardial infarction and prognosis*

Remotely infarcted regions of the myocardium (greater than several weeks) are typically readily identified on MR images as 1) segments with diastolic wall thinning, 2) decreased segmental systolic wall thickening and motion, and 3) on occasion, decreased myocardial signal intensity on spin-echo images [1,2,8,9,39].

Segmental diastolic wall thinning is seen as a discrete area that is significantly thinner than the adjacent segments (Fig. 7). The normal left ventricular wall thickness at enddiastole is approximately 10 ± 2 mm, which increases by approximately 30–70 % at endsystole [2,8]. Decreased wall thickening during systole, in conjunction with segmental thinning at enddiastole is consistent with remote infarction and scar (Fig. 8). It should be noted, however, that post-inflammatory sarcoidosis can also produce this type of finding.

The signal intensity of remotely infarcted regions may also be decreased on T2–weighted spin-echo images. This T2 signal reduction is due to a decrease in the water content of scar tissue as compared with normal myocardium.

Acute myocardial infarction (less than approximately 2–3 weeks of age) can be typically identified as regions which demonstrate decreased systolic wall thickening and motion, as well as locally increased signal intensity on T2 weighted spin-echo images [2,40–42]. This increase in signal intensity is due to the intracellular edema which accompanies acute infarction (Fig. 9A). Since the severity of the edema may vary from patient to patient and with the stage of the infarction, the bright signal intensity findings on MR images may be somewhat variable [42].

Perhaps the most reliable indicator of acute infarction is a segmental decrease in systolic thickening [2,8,42] (Fig. 10). Since the fibrosis and scar typically develop approximately 2–3 weeks post-infarction, the enddiastolic wall thickness for acute infarction will usually appear normal, although on occasion some degree of early segmental thinning also may be seen. When

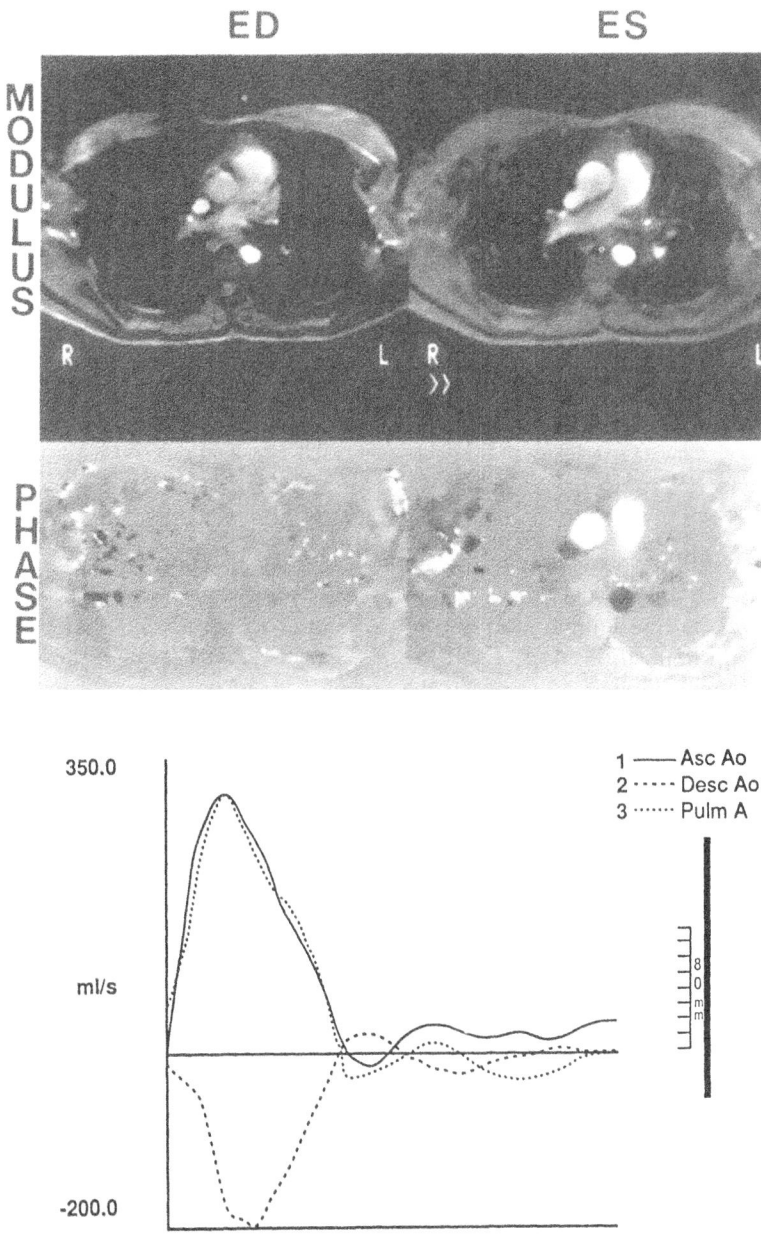

Figure 6. (a) Modulus and phase images at enddiastole (ED) and endsystole (ES) of a normal transsexual section at the level of the main pulmonary artery.

(b) Flow-time curves obtained after quantification of the aortic and pulmonic flow velocities at 16 points through the cardiac cycle. Measurement of cross-sectional vascular areas was used to compute flow in mL/sec from directly measured velocities in cm/sec. — ascending aorta, – – – descending aorta, · · · · pulmonary artery [71].

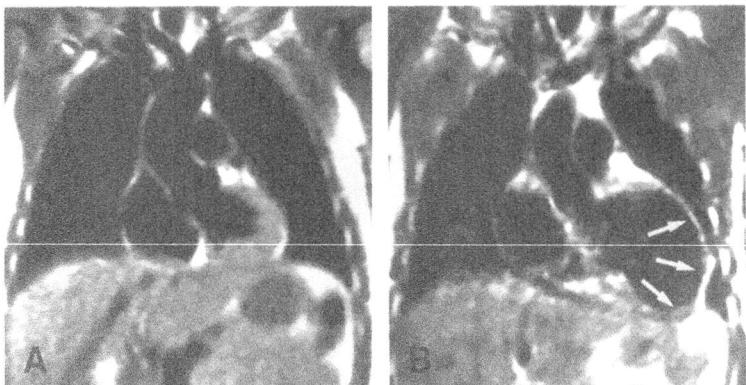

Figure 7. Coronal sections showing (A) normal left ventricular wall thickness and (B) marked anteroapical thinning exemplary of a remote transmural infarction (arrows). (Adapted with permission [72])

imaged with the gradient-echo technique, one may also observe the infarcted region as an area of decreased signal intensity [43]. This signal alteration, as suggested by one animal study, may be related to hemorrhage with subsequent iron deposition [44].

This agent appears to improve the conspicuity of the infarcted region by increasing the contrast between the normal and infarcted myocardium and the image contrast-to-noise ratio [45–47]. Enhancement of the acutely infarcted region may be achieved by using Gd-DTPA (Fig. 11). Future agents which are more cardiac specific may improve the detection of acute infarction regions further as has been suggested by a study using an iron oxide based agent [48]. The potential to delineate non-transmural vs transmural acute infarction by direct visualization of the infarction within the wall thickness is possible and has been demonstrated [48]. Additional studies with these and other agents are needed to define the ultimate clinical role. However, it appears highly likely that a perfusion that infarct enhancement agent will become a part of the diagnostic technique used in the MR assessment of the heart.

In post-infarction patients, MRI can be quite useful not only in identifying the site and size of an infarction but also in measuring the ejection fraction and the endsystolic volumes, as the most significant determinant of survival. The measurement of endsystolic volumes should prove quite beneficial in this regard, since recent studies have demonstrated the importance of this parameter in the management of post-infarction patients. In a series of infarct patients who were followed for approximately 7 years, White et al. [49] have reported that the endsystolic volume is the most significant determinant of survival. Additional studies have also indicated that therapy with angiotensin-converting enzyme inhibitors to shrink dilated ventricles with endsystolic volumes >96 ml, appears to prolong survival [49,50].

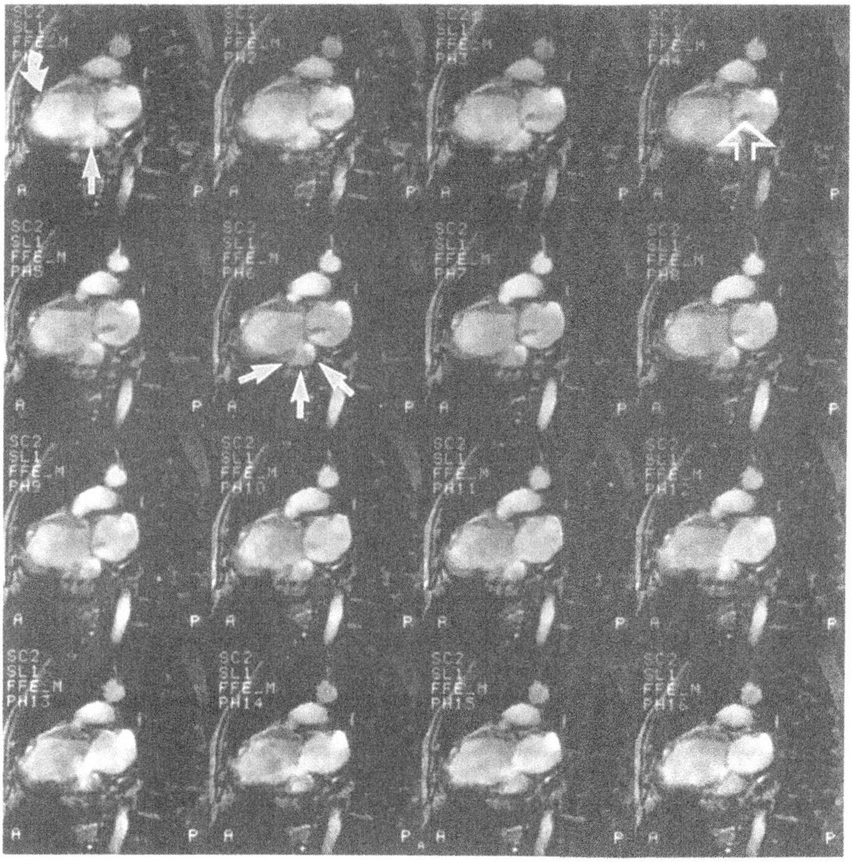

Figure 8. Sequential vertical long-axis images of a patient with poor global contraction, remote anterior infarction (curved arrow) and an inferobasal aneurysm (arrows). Also note mild mitral regurgitation (open arrowhead) [71].

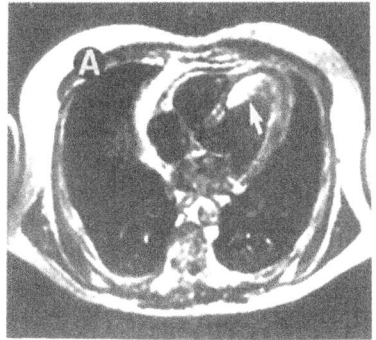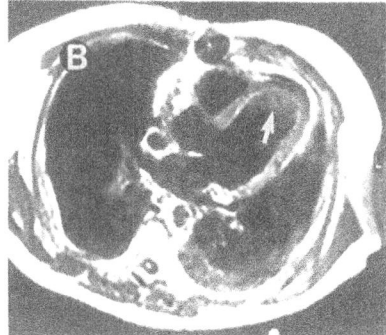

Figure 9. Acute infarction. (A) This image shows an acute infarction with distinctly increased signal intensity (arrows) on a second echo image (TE = 60 msec). (B) The same patient imaged 6 weeks later shows apical thrombus (arrow). (Reprinted with permission [72])

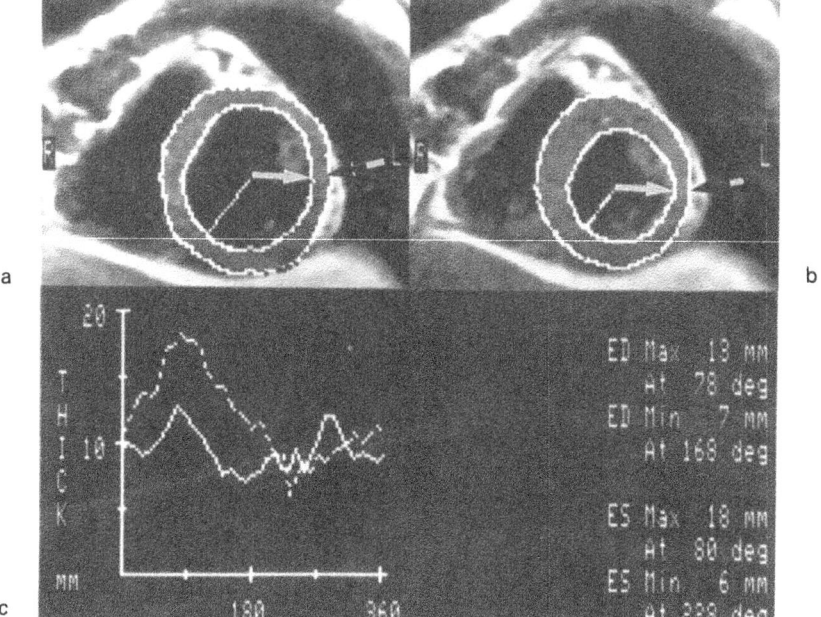

Figure 10. Acute non-Q wave infarction. Enddiastolic (a) and endsystolic (b) images of same short-axis section, with the endocardial and epicardial margins outlined. Circumferential plots of enddiastolic and endsystolic thickness are shown (c) with 0° at the inferoseptal segment, and progressing clockwise. Note the normal enddiastolic thickness but absence of systolic thickening of lateral/inferolateral segment (arrows) 1 week postinfarction treated with thrombolytic therapy. (Reprinted with permission [9])

2.3.2. *Viable myocardium vs scar*

In post-infarction patients for whom the question of residual viable myocardium arises, cine MRI can be quite useful in distinguishing viable myocardium from scar. The presence of viable myocardium is established when active systolic thickening is observed. Scar, on the other hand, is identified as a region having the combination of segmental diastolic thinning with absent systolic thickening. In cases of non-transmural infarction, the viable subepicardial layer may demonstrate some degree of thickening while the transmural thickness at enddiastole will be somewhat reduced. Our experience today, indicates that for this type of characterization of the myocardium, dynamic MRI may be more definitive than conventional tomographic thallium-201 studies which are on occasion plagued by artifactual 'perfusion' defects due to soft tissue attenuation, asymmetric ventricular hypertrophy, or atypical cardiac axises resulting in atypical attenuation patterns [51].

The primary limitation of MRI in ischemic heart disease at the current time, is its inability to routinely assess myocardial functions under stress.

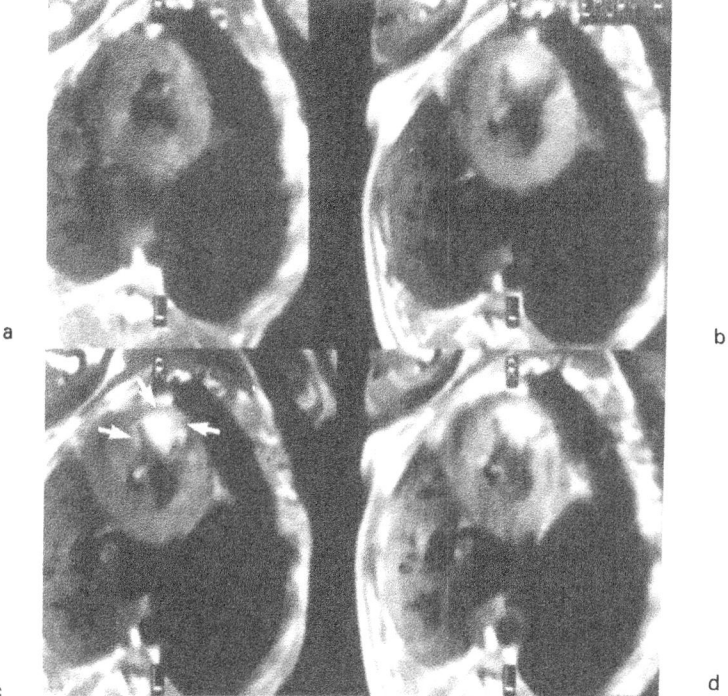

Figure 11. Transverse spin-echo (TE = 30 msec, TR = R-R) section of a dog's heart before intervention (a). Following LAD ligation (b) there are equivocal apical intensity changes that enhance (arrows) after GD-DTPA (c). In the final image (d), obtained 15 min after Gd-DPTA, clearance of the agent reduced previous enhancement [71].

Ongoing studies to develop and evaluate pharmacologic stress methodologies indicate that this current limitation will likely be resolved in the future.

2.4. *Cardiomyopathies*

All of the major types of cardiomyopathies are readily assessed by cine MRI. This includes the hypertrophic, congestive, and restrictive forms [1,2,52,53]. In hypertrophic cardiomyopathy, the precise site, and extent of hypertrophy, and site of outflow tract obstruction can be visualized and accurately evaluated. The ventricular mass can also be determined [16–18]. The volume of the planimetered left ventricular myocardium can be converted to mass by simple multiplication by the specific mass of tissue, which is approximately 1.05 g/ml. In addition, the presence or absence of partial obstruction of the left ventricular outflow tract can be determined from simple inspection of the functional sections in which the outflow tract is imaged (Fig. 12).

In congestive cardiomyopathy, ventricular dilatation and poor global sys-

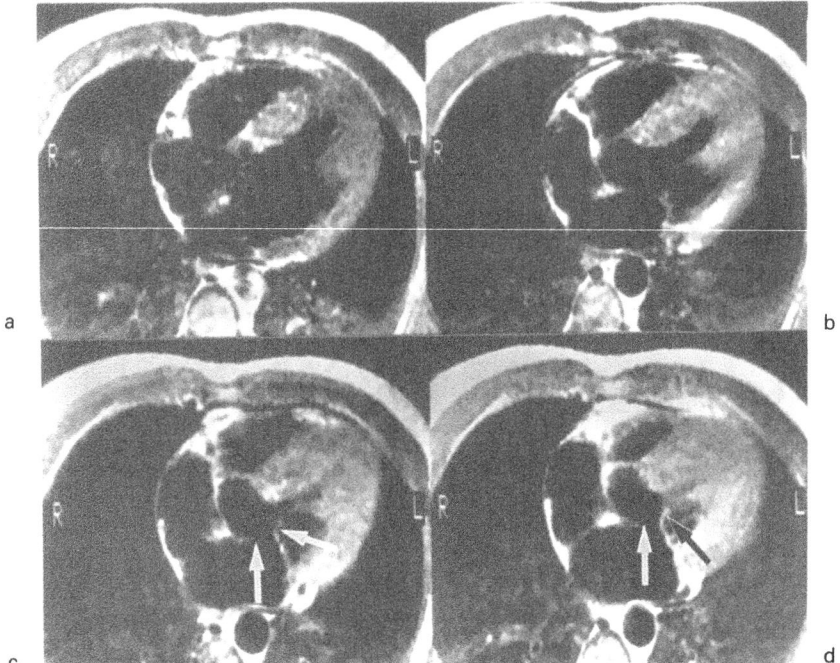

Figure 12. Four of six multiphase images of a transaxial ection of a patient with left ventricular hypertrophy. The first four phases (left to right, top to bottom) show systolic anterior motion (SAM) of the mitral valve (arrows) with partial obstruction of the left ventricular outflow tract [71].

tolic function can be evaluated both qualitatively and quantitatively. In particular, ventricular volumes and ejection fractions can be quantified and followed as indices of responsiveness to medical therapy.

Restrictive cardiomyopathies may have normal systolic function, but should have small enddiastolic volumes consequent to the restricted diastolic filling. In addition, diastolic relaxation (i.e. diastolic function) may be abnormal. Although there has been some early investigation of the right ventricle, at present this parameter has not been fully explored or well characterized by cardiac MRI, and remains an area for additional investigation [52].

2.5. *Cardiac and paracardiac masses*

Three basic types of clinically useful information about cardiac masses can be obtained by MRI. These are: 1) the precise location, size, and site of attachment of a mass, which impacts on its surgical resectability, 2) limited characterization of the nature of the mass (i.e. cystic vs solid, fat vs tumor, etc.), and 3) the impact of the mass on cardiac function or vascular patency.

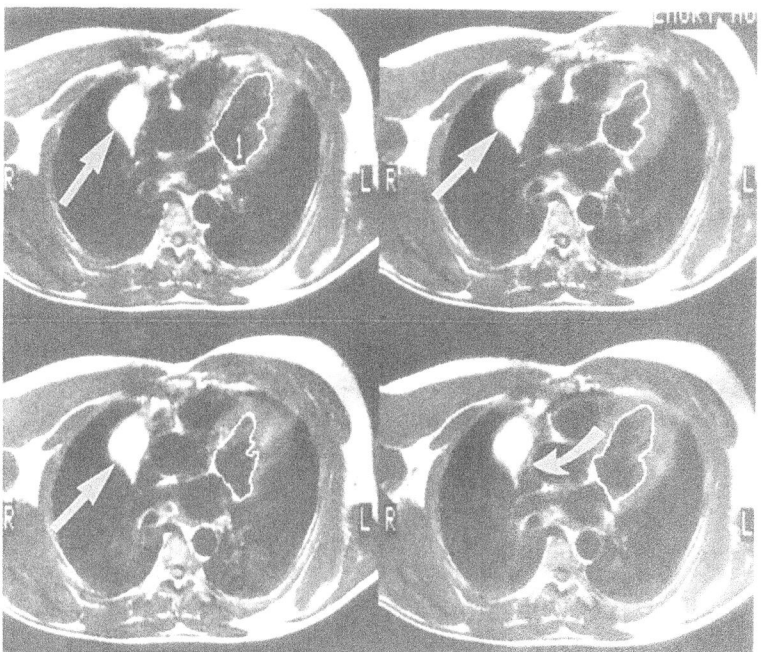

Figure 13. Single horizontal long-axis spin-echo section shown at four successive phases (left to right, top to bottom) of the cardiac cycle. Typically, images at 12 successive points throughout the first ≈ 500 msec of the cardiac cycle are obtained for cine display and quantitative assessment of function by planimetry of ventricular cavity (as shown). Evaluation of structure and tissue character is also possible with this sequence. Note the large, high signal intensity mass (arrows) adjacent to the pericardium. Attachment to the cardiac wall can be excluded by review of the dynamic study; note that in the latter two phases the left atrial wall (curved arrow) has separated from the mass found to be a cyst upon surgical removal. (Reprinted with permission [9])

In some instances, the lesion signal intensity relative to that of the myocardium indicates whether or not it has a prolonged T2, and its overall appearance may well suggest the nature of the lesion. For example, pericardial cysts are typically very bright, probably due to a short T1 consequent to the increased protein in cystic fluid (Fig. 13). Lipomas generally have a signal intensity equivalent to that of subcutaneous fat, where lymphomas on T2–weighted spin-echo images are slightly brighter than the myocardium due to a prolonged T2. Myxomas are typically isointense or slightly brighter than the myocardium (Fig. 14). Calcified tumors of any type generate little to no signal, and thus, are dark on both spin-echo and gradient-echo imaging. Calcified intracavitary tumors may not be seen on spin-echo imaging, but should be seen as a typical filling defect on gradient-echo images [54–55].

Intracavitary thrombus may also be imaged by MRI (Fig. 9B). Depending on the age of the thrombus, it may be slightly less intense than the myocardium or isointense on the first echo image. This intensity, however, should not fluctuate with changes in slice orientation or with the phase of the cardiac

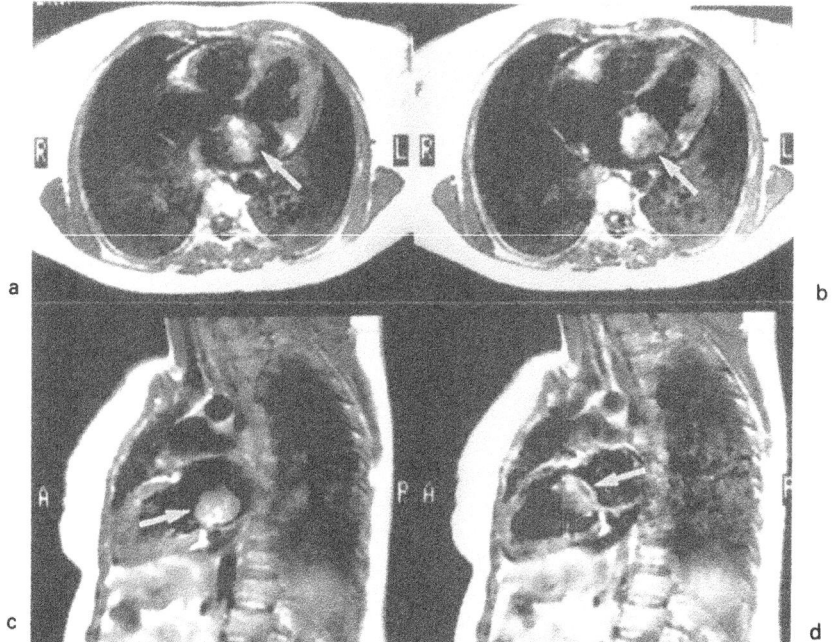

Figure 14. Left atrial myxoma (arrows) seen in transverse images at two systolic phases (a,b) and in vertical long axis images during systole (c) and diastole (d). During diastole, the myxoma prolapses across the mitral valve plane into the LV and partially out of the image plane, thus appearing smaller [71]).

cycle. Variation in signal intensity with either of these changes indicates that the increased signal intensity is more likely due to slow flow rather than thrombus. Typically, thrombus has a slightly increased signal intensity on the first echo image and a slightly dark appearance on the second echo image. This is unlike slow-moving blood, which may appear similar on the first echo image but should get considerably brighter on the second echo image due to even-echo rephasing [56]. Finally, when a section is viewed dynamically, it becomes immediately apparent whether or not an area of increased signal intensity seen in spin-echo images represents flow or thrombus. When imaged with a gradient-echo sequence, thrombus is seen as a constant filling defect throughout the cardiac cycle [34].

2.6. *Pericardial disease*

The utility of MRI in clearly visualizing the abnormal pericardium has been well described. MRI may identify and characterize pericardial effusions, pericardial cysts, and exudative processes, such as uremic or inflammatory pericarditis [3,57,58]. Normally the pericardium is a thin dark line, approximately 2 mm in thickness, and is best seen along the anterior margin of the right heart border. The dark appearance of the pericardium and pericardial space in normal individuals is due to the thin fibrous composition of the pericardial layers in conjunction with the rapid motion of the pericardial fluid which causes considerable intravoxel spin dephasing is likely, resulting in absent signal [19]. Similarly, transudative effusions have been noted to have signal intensity less than that of myocardium. Exudative effusions have signal intensity equivalent to or greater than that of myocardium [58]. This difference is probably due to a short T1 of the exudative fluid in which the protein content is high. The relatively increased signal of exudative effusions has been reported specifically in uremic peracarditis where the inflamed pericardium and intrapericardial adhesions may be visualized [3,58]. In constrictive pericarditis, the pericardium may appear as a thickened area of variable but likely increased signal intensity (relative to myocardium). In addition, the functional consequence of the pericardial abnormality may be assessed by both qualitative inspection and quantitative analysis of the cine MR images (Fig. 15).

2.7. *Vascular disease*

MRI is particularly well-suited to the evaluation of vascular disease [1–3, 59–61]. This is due to the high contrast between flowing blood and the vascular walls seen with both the spin-echo or 'dark blood' technique, and the gradient-echo or 'bright blood' technique. Because of the flow void associated with the spin-echo technique, this sequence is excellent for defining vascular anatomy and distinguishing the vascular tree from surrounding structures. Cine MRI studies with the gradient-echo technique are excellent for establishing the presence or absence of flow within vessels. Phase images reconstructed from the cine gradient-echo acquisitions also permit quantitative evaluation of intravascular flow. In aortic dissection, direct visualization of the intimal flap and the true and false lumina can be made (Fig. 16). In addition, the location of important branches, and the presence of flow in the false lumen usually can be established without the need for an intravascular contrast agent. The ability to image in any plane permits the acquisition of images in the plane of the vascular abnormality, facilitating optimal depiction of the true and false lumina [2,3].

In pulmonary hypertension, characteristic enlargement of the pulmonary artery can be assessed and the pulmonary artery can be measured. In addition, increased signal intensity within the enlarged pulmonary artery during the systolic phases on spin-echo images correlates with severe pulmonary artery hypertension with pressures greater than 90 mm Hg [3]. This increased signal intensity is indicative of abnormally slow flow comparable to, or less than that typically present at enddiastole.

Using phase velocity mapping in aortic dissection, the total flow per

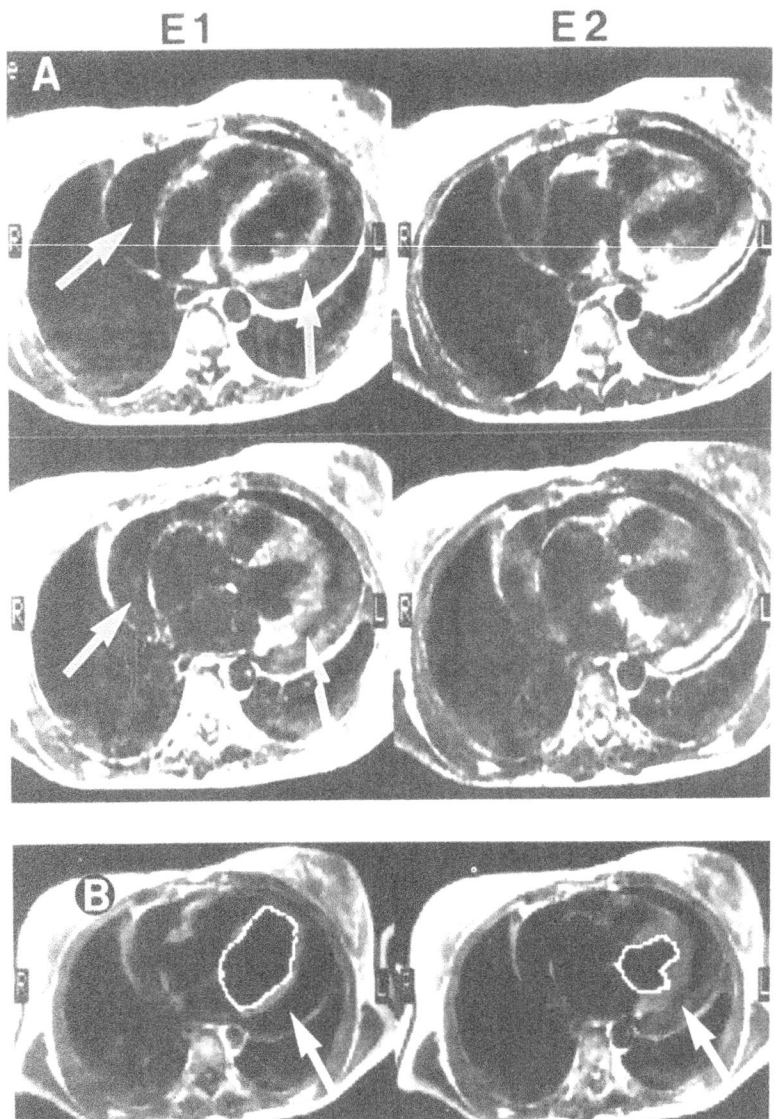

Figure 15. (A) Large transudative pericardial effusion in a patient with scleroderma. A large pericardial space (arrows) in two slices (above and below) is noted on the first echo image, TE = 30 msec (E1) and second echo image, TE = 60 msec (E2). Note that despite the size of the effusion (≈ 400 ml), signal intensity is decreased relative to normal myocardium on the first echo. Second echo brightness is due to even echo rephasing of slow flow. (Reprinted with permission [70]). (B) Same patient with a single section through the large transudative pericardial effusion (arrows) seen at enddiastole (upper right). Planimetry of all sections spanning the ventricular cavity permits measurement of the enddiastolic volume (EDV) and endsystolic volume (ESV) from which the stroke volume (SV), cardiac output (CO) and ejection fraction (EF) are calculated. Effusion volume was also planimetered and found to be ≈400 ml. Despite the size of the effusion, global ventricular function is still normal, as shown quantitatively. EF = 60 %; EDV = 105 ml; ESV = 42 ml; SV = 63 ml; CO = 4.9 l/min; ED phase No. 1: 9 msec; ES phase No. 4: 274 msec. (Reprinted with permission [9])

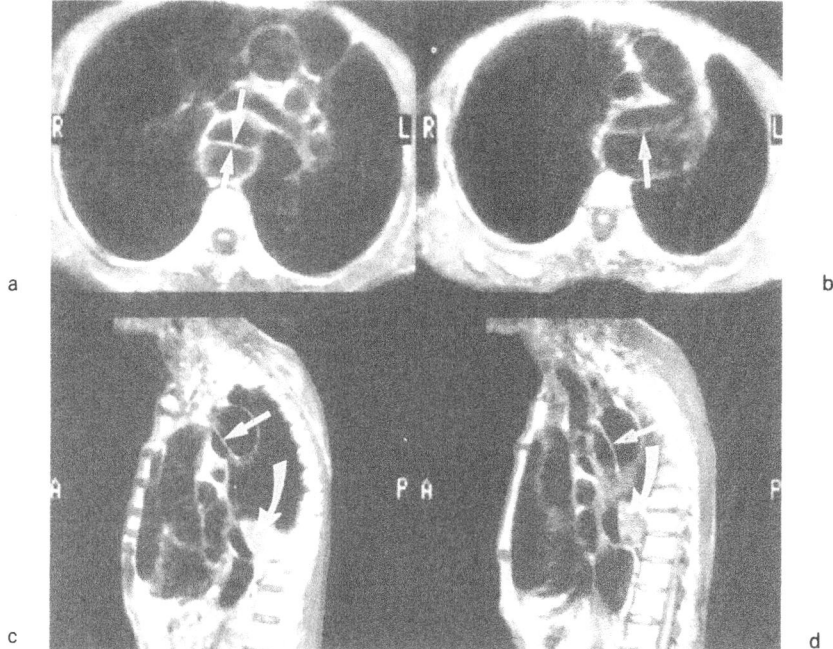

Figure 16. Aortic dissection, type II, is established by demonstrating an intimal flap (arrows) in the descending aorta in transverse sections just below (a) and through (b) the aortic arch. Two sagittal sections (c,d) show the flap and increased signal in the false lumen due to slow flow (curved arrow) [71].

cardiac cycle in the true lumen and in the false lumen can be accurately determined. Velocities also can be measured in regions of stenoses and, in the future, these measurements may be routinely converted to estimated pressure gradients as is currently done with Doppler echocardiography.

3. Future developments

The major current diagnostic limitations of cardiac MRI are the inability to detect coronary artery disease and evaluate myocardial dynamics (ventricular function) under stress. Several developments that are in progress indicate that these diagnostic goals will be realized. These specific developments include: 1) very high speed scanning techniques that generate an MRI image in as little as 300 msec using conventional hardware, or in 40 msec to real-time using modified hardware (Figs. 17,18), 2) MRI contrast agents that can be used to image relative myocardial perfusion and may even mark residual viable myocardium post-infarction, 3) pharmacologic stress methodologies to assess the response of regional myocardial function to stress and thereby detect coronary artery disease as well as distinguish stunned myocardium

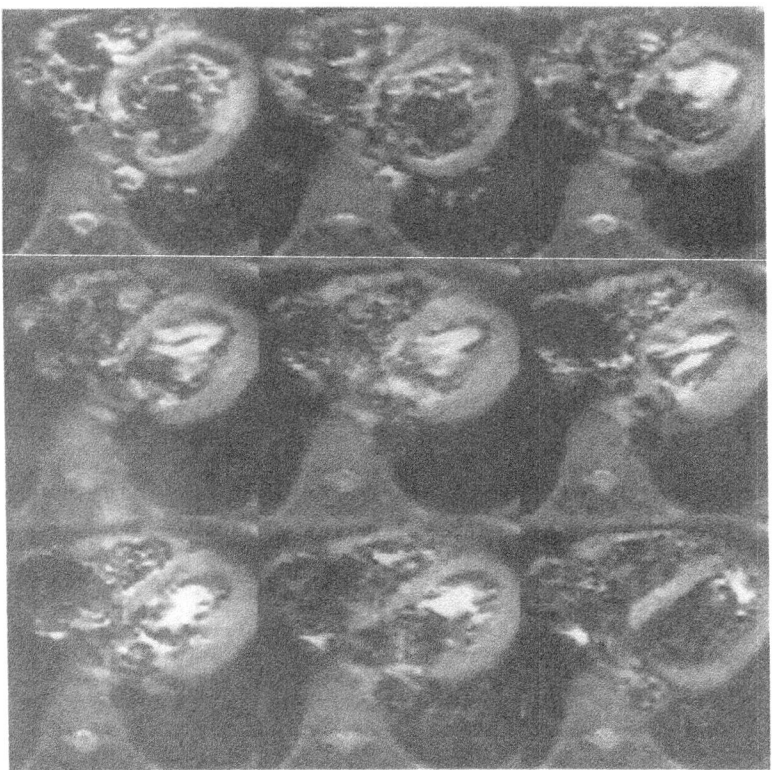

Figure 17. Ultrafast spin-echo cine MRI. By incrementing the delay from the R-wave trigger over 16 successive cycles, a series of instant 56 msec images are acquired at 16 points in the cardiac cycle. To minimize T1-related signal loss, one image was acquired every other heart-beat. TE = 26 msec, matrix = 128 × 128. Images at nine of the points are shown. (Courtesy of R. Rzedzian, Ph.D., Advanced NMR, Inc)

from acute infarction, and 4) displays of the dynamic MR images in a 3–D perspective, permitting the diagnostician to interactively review the images in 3–D [48,62–69]. MR coronary angiography remains a distinct theoretical possibility, but requires further technological advances.

Differential myocardial perfusion due to coronary occlusion has been imaged using ultra-high speed to real-time imaging in patients in combination with magnetic perfusion agents and dipyridamole. Other investigators have used catecholamine stress (dobutamine and isoproterenol) with conventional cine MRI to detect stress-induced ischemic dysfunction of the myocardial regions [66–67]. With real-time MRI, examinations under physical stress (e.g. supine bicycle) might also be possible.

We have also observed in animals that stunned myocardium can be identified with catecholamine stress cine MRI by demonstrating a stress-induced improvement in resting hypofunction [67].

Ischemic but viable myocardium vs infarcted myocardium might also be readily imaged and differentiated with a superparamagnetic contrast agent.

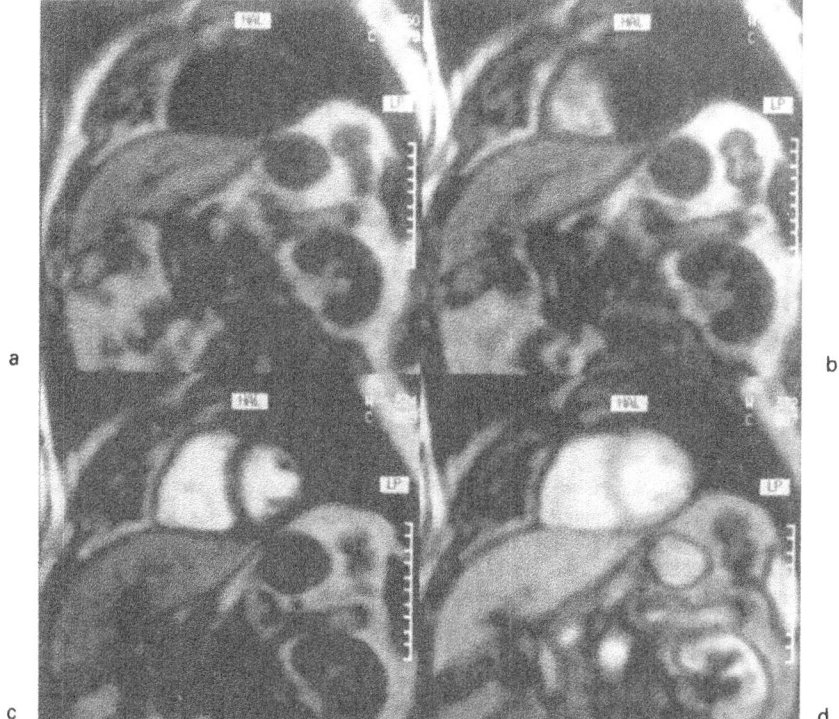

Figure 18. First-pass cardiac perfusion. Ultrafast (340 msec) sequential turboFLASH short-axis images of the heart obtained following a bolus injection of Gd-DTPA. Contrast agent is seen to enter the right ventricle (b), then the left ventricle (c), and myocardium (d). (Courtesy of Daniel Finelli, University Hospitals of Cleveland, Ohio, and Siemens Medical Systems)

This differentiation may be comparable to positron emission tomography imaging with combined ammonia perfusion and glucose metabolism imaging [48]. This type of contrast agent (iron oxide) apparently decreases the signal of both normal and ischemic but viable myocardium, thereby causing the adjacent acutely infarcted segments to be highlighted as very bright regions [48]. When used in conjunction with cine imaging, one could identify the ischemic or jeopardized regions as dysfunctional dark zones. While the MRI contrast agent that may be ultimately used routinely in patients has yet to be developed, these studies indicate the feasibility and tremendous clinical potential for such an agent.

4. Conclusion

The large body of data generated by cardiac MRI presents a data presentation and analysis challenge. More unified, integrated presentations of the 3–D anatomy, function, perfusion, regional and global response to stress, and contrast enhancement will likely be achieved using high-capacity/high-speed computers and specialized software display programs. These should offer near-life-like visualizations of the functioning heart in three dimensions. They should also permit the physician to interact with and manipulate the display so that the beating heart can be rotated and electronically dissected to offer any view or perspective imaginable [69].

In summary, existing and developing technology seems to indicate that dynamic 3–D cardiac MRI will soon be a cost-effective tool for evaluating almost all major types of cardiovascular disease and addressing many of the major needs in diagnostic cardiology. As such, it should become increasingly more attractive to clinical cardiologists.

References

1. Higgins CB, Holt W, Pflugfelder P, Sechtem U. Functional evaluation of the heart with magnetic resonance imaging. Magn Reson Med 1988;6:121–39.
2. Pettigrew RI. Dynamic cardiac MR imaging. Techniques and applications. Radiol Clin North Am 1989;27:1183–203.
3. Higgins CB. Overview of MR of the heart. Am J Roentgenol 1986;146:907–18.
4. Herfkens RJ, Higgins CB, Hricak H, et al. Nuclear magnetic resonance imaging of the cardiovascular system: normal and pathologic findings. Radiology 1983;147:749–59.
5. Utz JA, Herfkens RJ, Heinsimer JA, et al. Cine MR determination of left ventricular ejection fraction. Am J Roentgenol 1987;148:839–43.
6. Sechtem U, Pflugfelder PW, Gould RG, Cassidy MM, Higgins CB. Measurement of right and left ventricular volumes in healthy individuals with cine MR imaging. Radiology 1987;163:697–702.
7. Rehr RB, Malloy CR, Filipchuk NG, Peshock RM. Left ventricular volumes measured by MR imaging. Radiology 1985;156:717–9.
8. Pflugfelder PW, Sechtem UP, White RD, Higgins CB. Quantification of regional myocardial function by rapid cine MR imaging. Am J Roentgenol 1988;150:523–9.
9. Pettigrew RI, Eisner RL, Ziffer J, et al. Dynamic cardiac MRI using dual spin echoes. Dynamic Cardiovasc Imaging 1988;1:214–9.
10. Zerhouni EA, Parish DM, Rogers WJ, Yang A, Shapiro EP. Human heart: tagging with MR imaging – a method for noninvasive assessment of myocardial motion. Radiology 1988;169:59–63.
11. Axel L, Dougherty L. MR imaging of motion with spatial modulation of magnetization. Radiology 1989;171:841–5.
12. Axel L, Dougherty L. Heart wall motion: improved method of spatial modulation of magnetization for MR imaging. Radiology 1989;172:349–50.
13. Palmon L, Reichek N, Yeon S, et al. Circumferential myocardial segment shortening in concentric left ventricular hypertrophy due to hypertension. In: Ninth annual scientific meeting and exhibition; August 18–24,1990; New York. Berkeley: Society of Magnetic Resonance in Medicine, 1990:271.
14. Cranney GB, Lotan CS, Dean L, Baxley W, Bouchard A, Pohost GM. Left ventricular volume measurement using cardiac axis nuclear magnetic resonance imaging. Validation by calibrated ventricular angiography. Circulation 1990;82:154–63.
15. Stratemeier EJ, Thompson R, Brady TJ, et al. Ejection fraction determination by MR imaging: comparison with left ventricular angiography. Radiology 1986;158:775–7.
16. Caputo GR, Tscholakoff D, Sechtem U, Higgins CB. Measurement of canine left ventricular mass by using MR imaging. Am J Roentgenol 1987;148:33–8.

17. Katz J, Milliken MC, Stray-Gundersen J, et al. Estimation of human myocardial mass with MR imaging. Radiology 1988;169:495–8.
18. Maddahi J, Crues J, Berman DS, et al. Noninvasive quantification of left ventricular myocardial mass by gated proton nuclear magnetic resonance imaging. J Am Coll Cardiol 1987;10:682–92.
19. von Schulthess GK, Higgins CB. Blood flow imaging with MR: spin-phase phenomena. Radiology 1985;157:687–95.
20. Evans AJ, Blinder RA, Herfkens RJ, et al. Effects of turbulence on signal intensity in gradient echo images. Invest Radiol 1988;23:512–8.
21. Evans AJ, Hedlund LW, Herfkens RJ. A cardiac phantom and pulsatile flow pump for magnetic resonance imaging studies. Invest Radiol 1988;23:579–83.
22. Holmvang G, Edelman R, Pearlman, Marshall JE, Brady TJ, Kantor HL. Study of valvular regurgitation by cine-NMR: comparison to color Doppler flow maps (abstract). Circulation;76 Suppl 4:IV30.
23. Pflugfelder PW, Landzberg JS, Cassidy MM, et al. Comparison of cine MR imaging with Doppler echocardiology for the evaluation of aortic regurgitation. Am J Roentgenol 1989;152:729–35.
24. Nishimura T, Yamada N, Itoh A, Miyatake K. Cine MR imaging in mitral regurgitation: comparison with color Doppler flow imaging. Am J Roentgenol 1989;153:721–4.
25. Sechtem U, Pflugfelder PW, Cassidy MC, Holt W, Wolfe L, Higgins CB. Ventricular septal defect: visualization of shunt flow and determination of shunt size by cine MR imaging. Am J Roentgenol 1987;149:689–92.
26. Pettigrew RI, Churchwell A, Dannels W, et al. Fast-multiphase magnetic resonance imaging to detect mitral regurgitation in mitral valve prolapse (MVP): correlation with two-dimensional Doppler echocardiography (2–DDE) (abstract). Circulation; 74 Suppl 2:II318.
27. Shiebler M, Axel L, Reichek N, et al. Correlation of cine MR imaging with two-dimensional pulsed Doppler echocardiography in valvular insufficiency. J Comput Assist Tomogr 1987;11:627–32.
28. Utz JA, Herfkens RJ, Heinsimer JA, Shimakawa A, Glover G, Pelc N. Valvular regurgitation: dynamic MR imaging. Radiology 1988;168:91–4.
29. Aurigemma G, Reichek N, Schiebler M, Axel L. Evaluation of mitral regurgitation by cine magnetic resonance imaging. Am J Cardiol 1990;66:621–5.
30. Sechtem U, Pflugfelder PW, Cassidy MM, et al. Mitral or aortic regurgitation: quantification of regurgitant volumes with cine MR imaging. Radiology 1988;167:425–30.
31. Moran PR. A flow velocity zeugmatographic interlace for NMR imaging in humans. Magn Reson Imag 1982;1:197–203.
32. van Dijk P. Direct cardiac NMR imaging of heart wall and blood flow velocity. J Comput Assist Tomogr 1984;8:429–36.
33. Nayler GL, Firmin DN, Longmore DB. Blood flow imaging by cine magnetic resonance. J Comput Assist Tomogr 1986;10:715–22.
34. Pettigrew RI, Dannels W. Use of standard gradients with compound oblique angulation for optimal quantitative MR flow imaging in oblique vessels. Am J Roentgenol 1987;148:405–9.
35. Pettigrew RI, Dannels W, Galloway JR, et al. Quantitative phase-flow MR imaging in dogs by using standard sequences: comparison with in vivo flow-meter measurements. Am J Roentgenol 1987;148:411–4.
36. Meier D, Maier S, Bosiger P. Quantitative flow measurements on phantoms and on blood vessels with MR. Magn Reson Med 1988;8:25–34.
37. Firmin DN, Nayler GI, Klipstein RH, Underwood SR, Rees RS, Longmore DB. In vivo validation of MR velocity imaging. J Comput Assist Tomogr 1987;11:751–6.
38. Firmin DN, Nayler GL, Kolner PJ, Longmore DB. The application of phase shifts in NMR for flow measurement. Magn Reson Med 1990;14:230–41.
39. McNamara MT, Higgins CB. Magnetic resonance imaging of chronic myocardial infarcts in man. Am J Roentgenol 1984;146:315–20.

40. Wesbey G, Higgins CB, Lanzer P, Botvinick E, Lipton MJ. Imaging and characterization of acute myocardial infarction in vivo by gated nuclear magnetic resonance. Circulation 1984; 69:125–30.

41. McNamara MT, Higgins CB, Schechtmann N, et al. Detection and characterization of acute myocardial infarction in man with use of gated magnetic resonance. Circulation 1985;71:717–24.

42. Peshock RM, Filipchuk NG, Mallor CR, et al. Magnetic resonance imaging of patients with recent myocardial infarction: comparison with normal volunteers (abstract). J Am Coll Cardiol 1985;5:435.

43. Meese RB, Herkens RJ, Negro-Vilan R, Spritzer C, Bashore TM. Rapid dynamic magnetic resonance images of the heart in evaluation of acute myocardial infarction. Circulation 1987;76 Suppl 4:IV31.

44. Lotan C, Miller SK, Reeves R, Elgarish GA, Pohost GM. High-field MR imaging: evidence of the presence of hemorrhagic regions in infarcted canine myocardium (abstract). Radiology 1988;169 Suppl P:37.

45. McNamara MT, Tscholakoff D, Revel D, et al. Differentiation of reversible and irreversible myocardial injury by MR imaging with and without gadolinium-DTPA. Radiology 1986;158:756–9.

46. de Roos A, Doornbos J, van der Wall EE, van Voorthuisen AE. MR imaging of acute myocardial infarction: value of Gd-DTPA. Am J Roentgenol 1988;150:531–4.

47. Nishimura T, Kobayashi H, Ohara Y, et al. Serial assessment of myocardial infarction by using gated MR imaging and Gd-DTPA. Am J Roentgenol 1989;153:715–20.

48. Pettigrew RI, Brownell AL, Holmvang G, et al. Iron oxide MRI of myocardial tissue blood delivery post acute infarction: comparison with quantitative PET (abstract). Circulation 1989;80 Suppl 2:II231.

49. White HD, Norris RM, Brown MA, Brandt PN, Whitlock RM, Wild LJ. Left ventricular end-systolic volume as the major determinant of survival after recovery from myocardial infarction. Circulation 1987;76:44–51.

50. Pfeffer JM, Pfeffer MA. Angiotensin converting enzyme inhibition and ventricular remodeling in heart failure. Am J Med 1988;84(3A):37–44.

51. Ziffer J, Pettigrew RI. Dynamic cardiac MRI to assess viable vs scarred myocardium: comparison with SPECT T1–201 (abstract). Magn Reson Imaging 1988;6 Suppl 1:98.

52. Markiewicz W, Sechtem U, Higgins CB. Evaluation of the right ventricle by magnetic resonance imaging. Am Heart J 1987;113:8–15.

53. Maron BJ, Dwyer AJ, Knop R, Bonow RO, Doppman JL. Efficacy of nuclear magnetic resonance in the diagnosis and the identification of distribution of left ventricular hypertrophy in hypertrophic cardiomyopathy. J Am Coll Cardiol 1985;5:434.

54. Lund JT, Ehman RL, Julsrud PR, Sinak LJ, Tajik AJ. Cardiac masses: assessment by MR imaging. Am J Roentgenol 1989;152:469–73.

55. Rienmuller R, Lloret JL, Tiling R, et al. MR imaging of pediatric cardiac tumors previously diagnosed by echocardiography. J Comput Assist Tomogr 1989;13:621–6.

56. Waluch V, Bradley WG. NMR even echo rephasing in slow laminar flow. J Comput Assist Tomogr 1984;8:594–8.

57. Soulen RL, Stark DD, Higgins CB. Magnetic resonance imaging of constrictive pericardial disease. Am J Cardiol 1985;55:480–4.

58. Mulvagh SL, Hohnston DL, Vick GW, et al. Augmentation of the echocardiographic diagnosis of pericardial effusion by NMR imaging and spectroscopy. Am J Cardiol. In press.

59. Amparo EG, Higgins CB, Hoddick W, et al. Magnetic resonance imaging of aortic disease: preliminary results. Am J Roentgenol 1984;143:1203–9.

60. Amparo EG, Higgins CB, Hricak H, Sollitto R. Aortic dissection: magnetic resonance imaging. Radiology 1985;155:399–406.

61. Dinsmore RE, Liberthson RR, Wismer GL, et al. Magnetic resonance imaging of thoracic aortic aneurysms: comparison with other imaging methods. Am J Roentgenol 1986;146:309–14.

62. Atkinson DJ, Burstein D, Edelman RR. First-pass cardiac perfusion: evaluation with ultrafast MR imaging. Radiology 1990;174:757–62.
63. Mansfield P. Real-time echo-planar imaging by NMR. Br Med Bull 1984;40:187–90.
64. Chapman B, Turner R, Ordidge RJ, et al. Real-time movie imaging from a single cardiac cycle by NMR. Magn Reson Med 1987;5:246–54.
65. Rzedzian RR, Pykett IL. Instant images of the human heart using new, whole-body MR imaging system. Am J Roentgenol 1987;149:245–50.
66. Kantor HL, Rzedzian RR, Pykett IL, Berliner E, Brady TJ, Baxton R. Transient effects of gadolinium-DTPA and dysprosium-DTPA intravenous infusion on myocardial NMR image intensity using high speed NMR imaging. In: Seventh annual meeting and exhibition; August 20–26, 1988; San Francisco. Berkeley: Society of Magnetic Resonance in Medicine, 1988:246.
67. Pennell DJ, Underwood R, Manzara CC, et al. Detection of reversible myocardial ischemia with MR imaging during dobutamine infusion (abstract). Radiology 1990;177 Suppl P:101.
68. Pettigrew RI, Martin S, Eisner R, et al. Quantitative catecholamine stress MR imaging to evaluate ischemic heart disease (abstract). Radiology 1990;177 Suppl P:278.
69. Brummer ME, Pettigrew, RI, Pearlman J. Multi-perspective 4–D display of dynamic cardiac MR images. In: Ninth annual scientific meeting and exhibition; August 18–24, 1990; New York. Berkeley: Society of Magnetic Resonance in Medicine, 1990:460.
70. Pettigrew RI. Cardiovascular magnetic resonance imaging in acquired disease. In: Sandler M (ed): Correlative Imaging. Baltimore, MD, Williams & Wilkins, 1989.
71. Pettigrew RI. Dynamic magnetic resonance imaging in acquired heart disease. Sem in Ultrasound, CT, MR 1991; 12:61–91.
72. Casarella WJ, Ball T, Bernardino ME et al. Magnetic resonance imaging: Current clinical applications, Part 2. Emory Univ J Med 1987;1:200.

Index

Developments in Cardiovascular Medicine

1. Ch.T. Lancée (ed.): *Echocardiology.* 1979   ISBN 90-247-2209-8
2. J. Baan, A.C. Arntzenius and E.L. Yellin (eds.): *Cardiac Dynamics.* 1980
                                                     ISBN 90-247-2212-8
3. H.J.Th. Thalen and C.C. Meere (eds.): *Fundamentals of Cardiac Pacing.* 1979
                                                     ISBN 90-247-2245-4
4. H.E. Kulbertus and H.J.J. Wellens (eds.): *Sudden Death.* 1980   ISBN 90-247-2290-X
5. L.S. Dreifus and A.N. Brest (eds.): *Clinical Applications of Cardiovascular Drugs.*
    1980   ISBN 90-247-2295-0
6. M.P. Spencer and J.M. Reid: *Cerebrovascular Evaluation with Doppler Ultrasound.*
    With contributions by E.C. Brockenbrough, R.S. Reneman, G.I. Thomas and D.L.
    Davis. 1981   ISBN 90-247-2384-1
7. D.P. Zipes, J.C. Bailey and V. Elharrar (eds.): *The Slow Inward Current and Cardiac
    Arrhythmias.* 1980   ISBN 90-247-2380-9
8. H. Kesteloot and J.V. Joossens (eds.): *Epidemiology of Arterial Blood Pressure.* 1980
                                                     ISBN 90-247-2386-8
9. F.J.Th. Wackers (ed.): *Thallium-201 and Technetium-99m-Pyrophosphate. Myocar-
    dial Imaging in the Coronary Care Unit.* 1980   ISBN 90-247-2396-5
10. A. Maseri, C. Marchesi, S. Chierchia and M.G. Trivella (eds.): *Coronary Care Units.*
    Proceedings of a European Seminar, held in Pisa, Italy (1978). 1981
                                                     ISBN 90-247-2456-2
11. J. Morganroth, E.N. Moore, L.S. Dreifus and E.L. Michelson (eds.): *The Evaluation of
    New Antiarrhythmic Drugs.* Proceedings of the First Symposium on New Drugs and
    Devices, held in Philadelphia, Pa., U.S.A. (1980). 1981   ISBN 90-247-2474-0
12. P. Alboni: *Intraventricular Conduction Disturbances.* 1981   ISBN 90-247-2483-X
13. H. Rijsterborgh (ed.): *Echocardiology.* 1981   ISBN 90-247-2491-0
14. G.S. Wagner (ed.): *Myocardial Infarction.* Measurement and Intervention. 1982
                                                     ISBN 90-247-2513-5
15. R.S. Meltzer and J. Roelandt (eds.): *Contrast Echocardiography.* 1982
                                                     ISBN 90-247-2531-3
16. A. Amery, R. Fagard, P. Lijnen and J. Staessen (eds.): *Hypertensive Cardiovascular
    Disease.* Pathophysiology and Treatment. 1982   IBSN 90-247-2534-8
17. L.N. Bouman and H.J. Jongsma (eds.): *Cardiac Rate and Rhythm.* Physiological,
    Morphological and Developmental Aspects. 1982   ISBN 90-247-2626-3
18. J. Morganroth and E.N. Moore (eds.): *The Evaluation of Beta Blocker and Calcium
    Antagonist Drugs.* Proceedings of the 2nd Symposium on New Drugs and Devices,
    held in Philadelphia, Pa., U.S.A. (1981). 1982   ISBN 90-247-2642-5
19. M.B. Rosenbaum and M.V. Elizari (eds.): *Frontiers of Cardiac Electrophysiology.*
    1983   ISBN 90-247-2663-8
20. J. Roelandt and P.G. Hugenholtz (eds.): *Long-term Ambulatory Electrocardiography.*
    1982   ISBN 90-247-2664-6
21. A.A.J. Adgey (ed.): *Acute Phase of Ischemic Heart Disease and Myocardial
    Infarction.* 1982   ISBN 90-247-2675-1
22. P. Hanrath, W. Bleifeld and J. Souquet (eds.): *Cardiovascular Diagnosis by
    Ultrasound.* Transesophageal, Computerized, Contrast, Doppler Echocardiography.
    1982   ISBN 90-247-2692-1

Developments in Cardiovascular Medicine

Developments in Cardiovascular Medicine

Developments in Cardiovascular Medicine

Developments in Cardiovascular Medicine

78. M.M. Scheinman (ed.): *Catheter Ablation of Cardiac Arrhythmias*. Basic Bioelectrical Effects and Clinical Indications. 1988   ISBN 0-89838-967-4
79. J.A.E. Spaan, A.V.G. Bruschke and A.C. Gittenberger-De Groot (eds.): *Coronary Circulation*. From Basic Mechanisms to Clinical Implications. 1987
    ISBN 0-89838-978-X
80. C. Visser, G. Kan and R.S. Meltzer (eds.): *Echocardiography in Coronary Artery Disease*. 1988   ISBN 0-89838-979-8
81. A. Bayés de Luna, A. Betriu and G. Permanyer (eds.): *Therapeutics in Cardiology*. 1988   ISBN 0-89838-981-X
82. D.M. Mirvis (ed.): *Body Surface Electrocardiographic Mapping*. 1988
    ISBN 0-89838-983-6
83. M.A. Konstam and J.M. Isner (eds.): *The Right Ventricle*. 1988   ISBN 0-89838-987-9
84. C.T. Kappagoda and P.V. Greenwood (eds.): *Long-term Management of Patients after Myocardial Infarction*. 1988   ISBN 0-89838-352-8
85. W.H. Gaasch and H.J. Levine (eds.): *Chronic Aortic Regurgitation*. 1988
    ISBN 0-89838-364-1
86. P.K. Singal (ed.): *Oxygen Radicals in the Pathophysiology of Heart Disease*. 1988
    ISBN 0-89838-375-7
87. J.H.C. Reiber and P.W. Serruys (eds.): *New Developments in Quantitative Coronary Arteriography*. 1988   ISBN 0-89838-377-3
88. J. Morganroth and E.N. Moore (eds.): *Silent Myocardial Ischemia*. Proceedings of the 8th Annual Symposium on New Drugs and Devices (1987). 1988
    ISBN 0-89838-380-3
89. H.E.D.J. ter Keurs and M.I.M. Noble (eds.): *Starling's Law of the Heart Revisited*. 1988   ISBN 0-89838-382-X
90. N. Sperelakis (ed.): *Physiology and Pathophysiology of the Heart*. (Rev. ed.) 1988
    ISBN 0-89838-388-9
91. J.W. de Jong (ed.): *Myocardial Energy Metabolism*. 1988   ISBN 0-89838-394-3
92. V. Hombach, H.H. Hilger and H.L. Kennedy (eds.): *Electrocardiography and Cardiac Drug Therapy*. Proceedings of an International Symposium, held in Cologne, F.R.G. (1987). 1988   ISBN 0-89838-395-1
93. H. Iwata, J.B. Lombardini and T. Segawa (eds.): *Taurine and the Heart*. 1988
    ISBN 0-89838-396-X
94. M.R. Rosen and Y. Palti (eds.): *Lethal Arrhythmias Resulting from Myocardial Ischemia and Infarction*. Proceedings of the 2nd Rappaport Symposium, held in Haifa, Israel (1988). 1988   ISBN 0-89838-401-X
95. M. Iwase and I. Sotobata: *Clinical Echocardiography*. With a Foreword by M.P. Spencer. 1989   ISBN 0-7923-0004-1
96. I. Cikes (ed.): *Echocardiography in Cardiac Interventions*. 1989
    ISBN 0-7923-0088-2
97. E. Rapaport (ed.): *Early Interventions in Acute Myocardial Infarction*. 1989
    ISBN 0-7923-0175-7
98. M.E. Safar and F. Fouad-Tarazi (eds.): *The Heart in Hypertension*. A Tribute to Robert C. Tarazi (1925-1986). 1989   ISBN 0-7923-0197-8
99. S. Meerbaum and R. Meltzer (eds.): *Myocardial Contrast Two-dimensional Echocardiography*. 1989   ISBN 0-7923-0205-2

Developments in Cardiovascular Medicine

Developments in Cardiovascular Medicine

Previous volumes are still available

KLUWER ACADEMIC PUBLISHERS – DORDRECHT / BOSTON / LONDON